Migraine

Migraine

Russell Lane

Charing Cross Hospital
Imperial College
London, U.K.

Paul Davies

Radcliffe Infirmary
University of Oxford
Oxford, U.K.

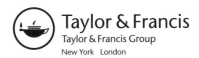

Taylor & Francis
Taylor & Francis Group
New York   London

Taylor & Francis is an imprint of the
Taylor & Francis Group, an informa business

The *migraine fire* (conceptual illustration located on the spine). The migraine mechanism underlying the primary headaches is envisaged to involve activation of brainstem neural networks extending from the hypothalamus to the area postrema. (The image was generated by probabilistic tractography, mapping connections between a locus in the lateral hypothalamus used as a target for the abolition of intractable cluster headache using deep brain stimulation, and other parts of the pain network. Particularly strong connections (paler colors) were found with the reticular formation. Courtesy of The Centre for Functional MRI of the Brain, University of Oxford, England.)

Published in 2006 by
Taylor & Francis Group
270 Madison Avenue
New York, NY 10016

International Standard Book Number-10: 0-8247-2957-9 (Hardcover)
International Standard Book Number-13: 978-0-8247-2957-8 (Hardcover)

Library of Congress Cataloging-in-Publication Data

Lane, Russell J. M., 1949-
    Migraine / by Russell Lane, Paul Davies.
        p. ; cm. -- (Neurological disease and therapy ; v. 84)
    Includes bibliographical references and index.
    Contents: A brief history of migraine -- The migraine mechanism -- Aura -- Complications -- Variants -- Conceptualizing primary headache -- Management of migraine.
    ISBN-13: 978-0-8247-2957-8 (Hardcover : alk. paper)
    ISBN-10: 0-8247-2957-9 (Hardcover : alk. paper)
    1. Migraine. I. Davies, Paul, 1955- II. Title. III. Series. [DNLM: 1. Migraine Disorders. 2. Headache Disorders, Primary. 3. Migraine with Aura. W1 NE33LD v.84 2006 / WL 344 L266m 2006]

RC392.L33 2006
616.8'4912--dc22   2006043860

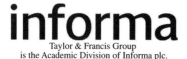
Taylor & Francis Group
is the Academic Division of Informa plc.

Visit the Taylor & Francis Web site at
http://www.taylorandfrancis.com

Dedication

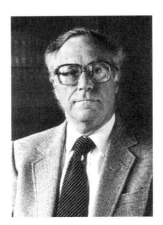

Frank Clifford Rose
Past Secretary General, World Federation of Neurology
Past President World Headache Society

We are pleased to dedicate this book to a special friend and colleague, Dr. Frank Clifford Rose. We both owe him a great deal in terms of our careers, and it was Frank who kindled and nurtured our interest in headache. Frank spent most of his career as Consultant Neurologist to the Charing Cross Hospital in London, and we worked in his department in the late 1980s and early 1990s. This was a time when there were relatively few neurologists in the United Kingdom, and hardly any had an interest in headache. Frank was already a pioneer in British neurology and had a particular interest in conditions that were rather unfashionable or neglected, such as motor neurone disease and stroke, in addition to headache. For example, he instituted an emergency domiciliary stroke service in the early 1980s, a concept that may perhaps resurface one day if safe protocols for acute thrombolysis in the community are developed.

He had a talent for getting things done and for involving and inspiring people. He would often suggest a solution to a problem that might be unconventional, but was nearly always effective. Perhaps our witness to his challenge to establishment views has been part of the inspiration for our work. The seed to some extent was sown twenty years ago and has grown steadily. *Migraine* represents the culmination of our experience and thinking about headache to date.

It is difficult to do justice to Frank's achievements. His entry under "Who's Who" is a full A4 page of small print! He has a huge number of publications to his credit, including some 70 books on various neurological conditions. The following is but a brief précis, concentrating on the headache side of Frank's work.

Frank was born on August 29, 1926 and was educated at King's College and Westminster Hospital Medical School. He worked at the National Hospital, Queen Square, and was Consultant Neurologist to the Medical Ophthalmology Unit at St. Thomas' Hospital between 1963 and 1985. He then became Physician in Charge at Charing Cross Hospital, where he formed the Department of Neurology, and over time, he developed the Academic Unit of Neurosciences, which was officially opened by Princess Anne in November 1986. This was to evolve into the present Department of Clinical Neurosciences of the Hammersmith Hospitals NHS Trust, affiliated to Imperial College and one of the largest departments of neurology in the United Kingdom. It was in the Academic Unit that he established the Princess Margaret Migraine Clinic, which has been the starting point for a number of neurologists from the United Kingdom and across the world, who went on to specialize in headache.

Some of his achievements in headache include the Harold Wolff Award of the American Association for the Study of Headache (1981 and 1984); the Distinguished Clinician Award (1986); Senior Editor of the American Association for the Study of Headache; and Co-editor of Headache Quarterly; and Trustee and Chairman (1988–1996) of the Migraine Trust in the United Kingdom. Frank also helped in the formation of the International Headache Society and the European Headache Federation. Some of his other neurological achievements also cannot go unmentioned. In 1989, he became Secretary-Treasurer General of the World Federation of Neurology (WFN) and Editor of the WFN newsletter *World Neurology*; he was President of the Section of Neurology of the Royal Society of Medicine, edited *Historical Aspects of the Neurosciences*; and the Founding Editor-in Chief of the *Journal of the History of the Neurosciences*, receiving its Lifetime Contribution Award in 2002.

How did he do it all? We don't really know, but if you arrived early in the department, you always new Frank had been there for at least two hours! He had probably been jogging beforehand as well. It was fantastic to train in a department with such a dynamic driving force. It was inspiring, but it wasn't all work. Frank is also an extraordinary *bon viveur* and raconteur, an expert on wine and champagne, and his regular Friday lunches, at which we as juniors were invariably his guests, are among our fondest recollections.

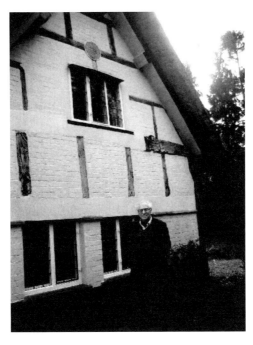

FCR outside the birthplace of the "Father of Neurology,"
Thomas Willis, in great Bedwyn, Wiltshire, England,
March 2006

Foreword

Migraine is recognized by the World Health Organization as a major cause of disability, but it is widely under-diagnosed, misdiagnosed, and poorly managed. Interest in migraine and other primary headache syndromes has grown considerably over the last twenty years. There are many books available that cover the current thinking on the diagnosis and classification of headache, our rapidly advancing understanding of migraine pathophysiology, and the latest developments in migraine treatment and headache management. So, why is this book necessary and what does it add to our knowledge base?

The authors state that it is a "concept book" that introduces new ideas about primary headache. They put forward three basic and at times controversial hypotheses: that all primary headache is migraine; that all human brains are potentially susceptible to the migraine mechanism and its many manifestations; and that the neural basis of primary headache syndromes is spreading depression, a process that can be generated in both the cerebral cortex and brainstem. The evidence for these concepts is a large database of headache case histories that the authors have accumulated over many years of practice, examined in the light of our current understanding of headache pathogenesis.

A key factor in the analysis is that a number of these cases illustrate the principle of primary headache "transformation," wherein one headache syndrome changes to another during a patient's lifetime; a feature Edward Liveing first recognized in the late 19th Century. Other cases illustrate the principle of what the authors call "overlaps" and "intermediate forms," in which patients' symptoms do not strictly conform to the primary headache syndromes as classified by the International Headache Society, but have either features of two or more primary headache types or lie somewhere in between. On this basis, the authors propose that primary headaches are probably not clear-cut, discrete entities but lie within a continuum, bounded by dimensions of headache severity, duration and frequency, and the occurrence of trigeminal autonomic symptoms.

This book is comprehensive and authoritative. It starts with a detailed review of the history of migraine and the evolution of our ideas on pathogenesis over the centuries and, in particular, how the current "neural" basis of migraine gradually supplanted the popular "vascular" theory. In the next chapter, the authors explore the migraine mechanism, summarize the latest research findings on migraine pathophysiology, and try to provide some understanding of what is a very complex but extremely common human condition. Chapter 3 uses many case histories to describe the florid, vivid, and variable nature of migraine auras that may be encountered, and how migraine probably accounts for a substantial proportion of otherwise inexplicable neurological symptoms. Chapter 4 looks at the complications of migraine, such as stroke in young people and epilepsy, and Chapter 5, concerning what the authors consider to be "Migraine Variants," looks at the relationship between "typical" migraine and other primary headache syndromes. Chapter 6 brings this all together and synthesizes the book's main premise: that all primary headaches are fundamentally manifestations of migraine.

No headache book is complete without a careful look at headache management, and the final chapter covers ideas on therapy and some of the common myths surrounding headache causation. It reflects on how we arrived at where we are, and looks to the increasingly exciting future of migraine treatment. The case database covers the treatment of most of the headache syndromes that one is likely to encounter in clinical practice.

In an era of ever-increasing reliance on technology and tests, this book is a welcome return to one of the fundamental tenets of medical science—that listening to patients can teach us how things really are. The authors' views are certainly challenging and provocative, and they will no doubt be the basis for much future debate—which is as it should be.

Stephen Silberstein
Professor of Neurology
Thomas Jefferson University
Jefferson Headache Center
Philadelphia, Pennsylvania, U.S.A.

Preface

Headache is the commonest of all human maladies. For most of us, it is an infrequent and relatively minor inconvenience but for a substantial minority, recurrent or persistent headache is a serious disability and handicap, with significant consequences for the wider community in terms of time lost from work and treatment costs, in addition to the suffering of affected individuals.

This, however, is not just another book about headache, although inevitably this aspect is covered in depth. Rather, we have focussed on the "migraine mechanism," its clinical manifestations, and the occasional serious consequences that it can cause. Our observations and conclusions are based on the case histories of over 250 headache patients seen in a general neurology outpatient clinic between 1990 and 2004. Based on these observations and the extensive scientific literature on migraine, we propose two main hypotheses.

First, we believe that migraine is a fundamental property of the normal human brain; we are all potential migraineurs. Migraine is not a disease but a pathophysiological process. Anyone can experience the symptoms of migraine if their genetically determined threshold for initiation of the migraine mechanism is breached. Indeed, we would predict that almost all of us will sooner or later experience some manifestation of this process, although many may not realize the origin of the symptoms. In particular, the symptoms may not include headache. Thus, while migraine attacks are thought to afflict 'only' 15% to 20% of the population, and most people will deny they "suffer from migraine," we suspect that symptoms of migrainous origin are frequently ignored or attributed to other causes. For example, one of the authors had his first migraine aura while conducting an outpatient clinic in Liverpool about twenty years ago. He felt increasingly strange and "distant" over a number of minutes and then became aware of a bright, shimmering, partly-colored, snake-like hallucination that migrated to the left for about thirty minutes before disappearing. There was a little nausea but no headache. The cause was immediately recognized but might well have caused consternation to someone unfamiliar with such symptoms. He had a further identical attack about eight years later at a medical conference and took the opportunity to confirm that the newly developed medication sumatriptan had no effect on the aura. He has since had one or two minor headaches with some migrainous qualities, but if asked, "Do you suffer from migraine?" the author would respond, "No." No doubt many readers will have had similar experiences. It is interesting to note that the "prevalance" of migraine is substantially higher among physicians than the general population and higher still among neurologists and headache specialists.

The migraine mechanism can produce a wide range of neurological symptoms in addition to the classical visual, somasthetic, and dysphasic auras. These can be as non-descript as vague episodic visual blurring or shimmering, which might be attributed to the effects of bright lights or the "wrong glasses"; funny turns, faints, and episodes of amnesia, often erroneously ascribed to "blood pressure" or "transient ischemia"; recurrent attacks of vertigo without evidence of underlying vestibular dysfunction; and episodic non-specific headaches or head pains, which may be attributed to "sinus" or "arthritis in the neck." We suspect that many unnecessary visits to opticians, dentists, and ear, nose, and throat surgeons are made because the many manifestations of the migraine mechanism are not widely appreciated.

Our second contention is that *all* primary headaches are caused by the same fundamental migraine mechanism. While we are firm supporters of the attempts by the International Headache Society to provide detailed definitions of individual forms of primary headache, it must be realized that many patients do not conform to these stereotypes. "*Overlap*" cases are very common, and we have seen many examples of patients with typical migraine who subsequently develop features of other primary headache disorders. We have also seen examples of aura in cluster headache, and features of trigeminal autonomic dysfunction, and Horner's syndrome, in otherwise typical migraine. While most patients certainly experience stereotyped headache attacks conforming to a particular primary headache syndrome, *transformation* to another form is not uncommon, and there is probably no clinical symptom that is exclusive to any particular headache syndrome. We think it is unlikely that an individual who experiences different forms of primary headache actually has several different disorders; rather, the symptoms result from the same basic process, which varies in output characteristics at different times.

All recurrent, episodic, and stereotyped primary headaches probably begin with neural activation in the brain, although whether this occurs first in the cortex or brainstem remains unclear and it is likely that the cortex and brainstem activations occur independantly. If the process starts in the cortex, the patient may experience an aura. The neural activation leads to a complex sequence of events involving principally the trigeminocervical complex and its outflow pain pathways, resulting in a headache or head pain, with characteristics depending on the specific pathways involved and the extent of autonomic activation via the trigeminal-autonomic reflex. Presumably the neural activation sometimes fails to excite the pain pathways, resulting in aura symptoms without headache (acephalalgic migraine). This is hardly a new idea but rather a modern restatement of Edward Liveing's 19th century thesis of "nerve-storms." The process underlying aura is almost certainly cortical spreading depression. From observations on migrainous ventigo, increasingly recognized as a common manifestion of the migraine mechanism, we speculate that brainstem neural activation demonstrated during migraine attacks is also caused by spreading depression.

The book starts with a review of the historical development of our understanding of the migraine mechanism, and then explores the current views of migraine pathogenesis, based largely on recent revelations from neuroimaging. Chapter 3 deals with auras, the clinical manifestations of the migraine mechanism, including what we refer to as "atypical auras," which include a number of common neurological symptoms not usually considered to be of migrainous origin. Chapter 4 deals with the neurological complications of the migraine mechanism. Current evidence suggests that no matter how severe the symptoms, the migraine mechanism normally does not damage the brain. Conversely, however, migraine attacks can sometimes lead to blackouts, amnesic attacks, and stroke, and the reasons for this are considered.

The chapter on "Variants" deals with the relationship between migraine and other primary headache disorders. We begin with a review of the history of headache classification, and then give illustrative examples of typical cases of migraine variants and other primary headache syndromes. In each instance, however, we also give examples of "overlap" cases in which symptoms of one or more additional primary headache disorders have occurred in association with, or instead of, the habitual headache syndrome to another and also provide illustrative cases of "transformation" of one primary headache syndrome in individual patients. We then consider the difficult clinical problem of "symptomatic migraine," in which the migraine mechanism is provoked by systemic diseases or structural lesions in the brain. The final chapters include an overview of our findings and conclusions and our current strategies for managing headache.

Our hypotheses are simple. All primary headaches are "migraine" and the migraine mechanism is responsible for many other recurrent and stereotypical neurological symptoms. Secondly, everyone has migraine—we are all susceptible. Finally, we suggest that the migraine mechanism is fundamentally, spreading depression. We appreciate that some of our views are likely to prove controversial, perhaps even heretical, but we trust they are at least thought provoking. Criticism will no doubt encourage debate and further experiment.

ACKNOWLEDGMENTS

We wish to thank a number of our colleagues who have provided cases to help illustrate the ideas set out in this book:

Dr. Sunil Wimalaratna	Swindon and Oxford	Cases 13 and 238
Dr. Nick Silver	Liverpool	Cases 27 and 28
Dr. Wojtek Rakowicz	London	Case 123
Drs. Michael Johnson and Pankaj Sharma	London	Case 239
Dr. Alidz Pambakian	London	Case 240
Dr. Paul Hughes	Haywards Heath	Case 258
Dr. Nikos Evangelou	Nottingham	Case 259

We also had useful discussions with Drs. David Kernick, Shazia Afridi, and Anish Bahra.

We have been admirably supported (and sometimes cajoled) by our editors and producers at Informa Healthcare (Joseph Stubenrauch and Susan B. Lee) and The Egerton Group Ltd. (Jan Goldsworthy and Joanne Jay). Finally, writing a major text inevitably imposes restrictions on all other aspects of life, and we therefore especially wish to thank and acknowledge the support, tolerance, and patience of our partners Mary McSweeney and Diane Lane.

Russell Lane
r.lane@imperial.ac.uk

Paul Davies
paul.davies@ngh.nhs.uk

Contents

Landmarks in Migraine

3000 B.C.	Mesopotamia	First descriptions of possible migrainous symptoms
2000 B.C.	Ancient Egypt	First written descriptions of headache treatments
400 B.C.	Hippocrates	First description of migraine with visual aura
A.D. 81	Arateus	"Heterocrania" distinguished from "cephalalgia" and "cephalea"
A.D. 150	Galen	Hemicrania
A.D. 1000	Avicenna	Recognition of primary headaches
A.D. 1597		First citation of hemicrania in Oxford English Dictionary
A.D. 1618	Le Pois	First description of hemisensory aura
A.D. 1672	Willis	Anatomical and pathological basis of head pain
A.D. 1723	Vater	First description of hemianopic migrainous scotoma
A.D. 1778	Fothergill	Description of "fortification" spectrum
A.D. 1868	Woakes	Ergot stops migraine headache
A.D. 1870	Airy	Teichopsia
A.D. 1873	Latham	Vascular theory of migraine
A.D. 1873	Liveing	Theory of "nerve-storms"
A.D. 1883	Eulenberg	Ergotinin effective in migraine attacks
A.D. 1916	Stoll	Ergotamine synthesized
A.D. 1925	Rothlin	Ergotamine found to be effective in terminating migraine attacks
A.D. 1938	Graham and Wolff	Ergotamine relieves headache by constricting branches of the dilated external carotid artery during migraine attacks

(Continued)

xvii

A.D. 1941	Lashley	Mapping of progression of migrainous scotoma
A.D. 1944	Leão	Spreading depression
A.D. 1945	Horton	Dihydroergotamine (DHE) effective for migraine headache
A.D. 1948	Page	5-HT identified in human blood
A.D. 1949	Rapport	Isolation of 5HT
A.D. 1957	Gaddum and Picarelli	5-HT D and M receptors
A.D. 1958	Milner	Spreading depression causes migraine aura
A.D. 1961	Sicuteri	Increased urinary 5-HIAA excretion in migraine attacks links migraine to 5-HT metabolism
A.D. 1962	Ad Hoc Committee	First classification of headache
A.D. 1965	Curran	Blood serotonin falls in acute migraine attacks
A.D. 1966	Rabin	Propranolol found to be effective prophylactic treatment
A.D. 1967	Anthony	Fall in serotonin is specific to acute migraine attacks
A.D. 1978	Hannington	Migraine is proposed to be a primary platelet disorder
A.D. 1979	Peroutka and Snyder	Basis laid for the modern classification of 5-HT receptors
A.D. 1979	Moskowitz	Trigeminovascular system
A.D. 1981		International Headache Society founded
A.D. 1980s	Olesen	Regional cerebral blood flow studies—vascular changes in migraine are secondary
A.D. 1988		International Headache Society first classification of headache (ICH1)
A.D. 1991	Humphrey	Introduction of sumatriptan, the first 5-HT$_1$ receptor agonist
A.D. 1993	Goadsby and Edvinsson	CCRP release into jugular venous blood during migraine attacks blocked by sumatriptan
A.D. 1993	Olesen	Nitric oxide and glyceryl trinitrate model of migraine
A.D. 1993	Joutel	First migraine gene identified
A.D. 1995	Weiller	Brainstem activation imaged during migraine headache
A.D. 2000	Burstein	Basis of allodynia
A.D. 2001	Sanchez del Rio	Spreading depression underlying visual aura illustrated by functional MRI

(Continued)

A.D. 2002	Strong	First direct recording of cortical spreading depression in man
A.D. 2004		IHC2 published
A.D. 2005	Janssen-Cilag	Largest ever controlled clinical trials confirm efficacy of the anticonvulsant topiramate, as migraine prophylactic

A Brief History of Migraine

Life is short, the art is long, opportunity fleeting, experience fallacious,
judgement difficult.
—Hippocrates

"MIGRAINE"—THE ETYMOLOGY OF A CLINICAL SYNDROME

Migraine has fascinated physicians and scientists throughout the ages. The
early literature abounds with the personal observations and insights of some
of the most distinguished figures of the times. Although headache is the most
prominent feature, the syndrome encompasses many other neurological
phenomena that are encountered frequently in clinical practice. Yet it has
no "pathological signature." Even today, it is defined and recognized
entirely by clinical history.

Mesopotamia and Egypt

Did our ancient forebears suffer from migraine? We believe that migraine is
a function of the normal human brain, and because it is a very common and
sometimes disabling disorder, we would expect to find some reference to
migrainous symptoms in the earliest medical writings.

Headache has been recognized as an important and sometimes omi-
nous symptom of disease for thousands of years. Trepanation or trephination
(Fig. 1), which dates from at least 6000 B.C., is thought to have been used to
release the demons and evil spirits that were believed to cause convulsions
(1,2), but it might also have been performed to "relieve" headache. Its practice continues even today in some cultures (3). The earliest records from
the ancient civilizations of Mesopotamia (Sumeria, Babylonia, and Assyria,

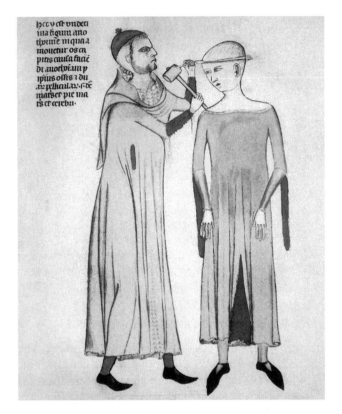

ब्रूट vcl vnद
ula figuu ano
द्गणुnie म quua a
mouctur os m
prus caufa facie
ठि auodviun p
lpuis ostis 1 ठu
.x:px1aulax:.f∙ठc
ंम्नासcr pic uua
ts cr ctrcbu∙

Figure 1 Headache relief? Trepanation. Plate XI from the *Anothomia Designata per Figuras* (1345) by Guido de Vigevano, physician to Emperor Henri VII and Queen Jeanne de Bourgogne. *Source*: Reproduced by permission from the front cover of *Journal of Neurology, Neurosurgery and Psychiatry* 2004, Volume 75, Issue 4.

Fig. 2) include references to headache, and Sumerian poetic literature written about 3000 B.C. speaks of the "sick-headed" (4). Writings from Babylon later in that millennium describe headaches "flashing like lightning." It has been argued that such descriptions probably referred to head symptoms caused by serious diseases (5), but we believe that migraine would still have been the commonest cause of "sick headache" and visual disturbance even in those times.

Much of our knowledge of the medicine of ancient Egypt is embodied in the *papyri*. There were about forty-two of these, written in hieratic, the cursive analogue of hieroglyphics, of which seven dealing with medical issues still exist. The Edwin Smith papyrus contains the first reference to the brain, in which its sulci and gyri are compared to the corrugations on metal slag (6). Priests and teachers at this time were already aware that injury to

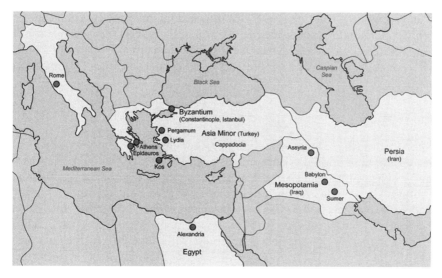

Figure 2 (*See color insert*) The Ancient World of Eurasia, the Cradle of Medicine. The countries of the Mediterranean and Middle East in the fifth century, showing areas and cities that played an important part in the migraine story.

one side of the brain affected the control of the opposite side of the body, so unilateral headache had particular significance. In the Papyrus Leiden, the god Horus, a sufferer of unilateral headache, beseeches the goddesses Isis and Nyphthys for a substitute head (5). Migraine patients sometimes express similar sentiments during an attack!

Concepts of the causes and treatment of illness in the ancient world were based almost entirely on religion and magic. The Papyrus Ebers, written in about 1552 B.C. but based on much older writings from around 4000 B.C., includes remedies for various ills, among which were treatments for head pains. Many of these involved the application of "healing" materials to the head. In one such treatment, recommended for King Usaphais in 2700 B.C., a clay crocodile holding grain in its mouth was firmly bound to the sufferer's head by a linen strip bearing the names of the gods (7). Remedies of this type may have been based on the observation that pressure on the painful area of the head during a migraine attack can sometimes give some relief.

Greece, Alexandria, and Rome

Greek and Roman physicians were also well aware of the significance of headache as a feature of disease. Zeus, the Father of the Gods, suffered from severe headache that was relieved when Hephaestus opened his head with an axe, giving birth to Athena (5). Inscriptions on stone tablets found in the temple at Epidauros, dedicated to Aesculapius, include the case history of Agaestratos, who suffered headache that was cured after he slept in a temple (6), possibly a reference to the fact that sleep sometimes terminates a migraine attack.

Hippocrates

Hippocrates (Fig. 3) was without doubt the most important and influential medical figure of this era. Born in Kos circa 460 B.C., he was a prolific writer and teacher with some sixty major texts written in his name over the next century. He was the first physician to base diagnosis on careful observation and verifiable facts rather than mysticism and speculation. In his *Aphorisms*, he decreed that headaches were not visitations of the gods, and while credit for the first description of migraine with aura (MA) is debated (5),

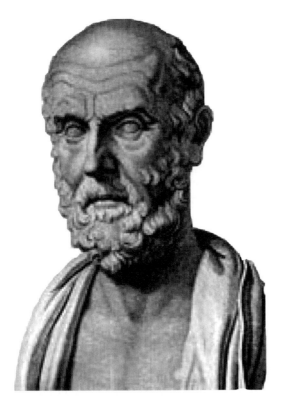

Figure 3 Hippocrates (*circa* 460–370 B.C.). First description of migraine with visual aura.

Hippocrates described a patient with severe unilateral headache associated with visual disturbance (8,9).

> He seemed to see something shining before him like a light, usually in part of the right eye; at the end of a moment a violent pain supervened in the right temple, then in all the head and neck, ... vomiting, when it became possible, was able to divert the pain and render it more moderate.

Arateus and "Heterocrania"

Arateus (Fig. 4) is credited as the first to distinguish cases of what we would recognize as migraine from other types of headache (5,8–12). He was born in Cappadocia, now a Turkish province, and later moved to Rome. In about 81 A.D., he described *cephalalgia* (severe but infrequent short-lasting headaches), *cephalea* (protracted but relatively mild headaches—presumably

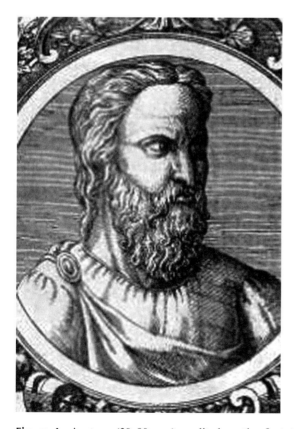

Figure 4 Arateus (30–90 A.D.) credited as the first to distinguish what we now recognize as migraine from other forms of headache.

our chronic daily headache), and *heterocrania*, which we would now recognize as migraine. He characterized this as:

> An illness by no means mild, even though it intermits, and although it appears to be slight . . . In certain cases the whole head is pained, and the pain is sometimes on the right, and sometimes on the left, or the forehead, or the fontanelle, and such attacks shift their place during the same day . . . It sets in acutely, it occasions unseemly and dreadful symptoms . . . nausea, vomiting of bilious matters; collapse of the patient . . . there is much torpor, heaviness of the head, anxiety; and life becomes a burden . . . For they flee the light; the darkness soothes their disease; nor can they bear readily to look upon or hear anything agreeable . . .

He therefore recognized that this form of headache was commonly but not invariably unilateral, and he appreciated that it was usually associated with nausea, vomiting, and photo and phonophobia. These defining symptoms remain the basis of the clinical diagnosis of migraine today. Like Hippocrates, he also recognized that such headaches could be heralded by a visual disturbance.

> Flashes of purple or black colours before the sight, or all mixed together, so as to exhibit the appearance of a rainbow expanded in the heavens.

Arateus' teachings and conceptual frameworks formed the basis for many neurology texts up until the 19th century, and the fundamentals of his headache classification are still discernable in the first modern classification produced by the International Headache Society in 1988. A late contemporary of Arateus, Soranus of Ephesus (90–118 A.D.) of the Alexandrian school, also referred to pounding unilateral headache with vomiting in one of the chapters of his book on chronic diseases, but in combination with vertigo (6). We will see in Chapter 3 that the association between migraine and vertigo is of considerable significance.

Galen and "Hemicrania"

The great library in Alexandria established by Ptolemy, a vast repository of the accumulated wisdom of the time, was destroyed in 391 A.D., but much of our knowledge of the medicine of Alexandria survived in the writings of Claudius Galen. Galen (129–199 A.D., Fig. 5) was born in Pergamum in what is now Turkey and was appointed surgeon to the gladiators in 157 A.D. He worked in both Alexandria and Rome (6). His teachings and writings were based on the *humoral theory*, originally propounded by Empedocles (circa 490–430 B.C.) and later taught by Hippocrates. Humoral theory contended that illnesses arose from an imbalance among the four essential body "humors": sanguis (blood), pituita (cerebral secretion, or "phlegm"), chole (bile), and melanchole (black bile). Galen did not systematize disease on this basis, but the humoral theory was later developed extensively in the Middle Ages and the early Renaissance. The theory had the advantage that physical and emotional aspects of illness could be viewed holistically

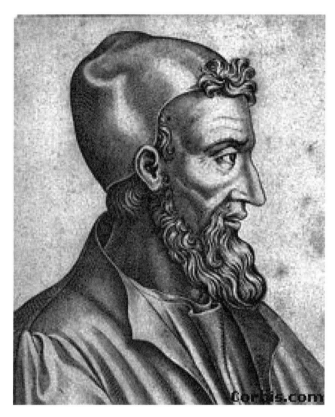

Figure 5 Claudius Galen (*circa* 129–199 A.D.). The gladiators' physician referred to migraine as "hemicrania."

without recourse to an understanding of the anatomy or pathology—an idea that finds sympathy even today among exponents of "alternative medicine"! Such views sat uneasily with later anatomical knowledge, but the Galenic theory was by then so ingrained that it remained the basis of medical practice until the 15th century. Among Galen's vast output of medical works were five tomes on neurological matters (6). Galen referred to unilateral headache attacks as "hemicrania" (hem–ee–crania, Greek for "half skull").

> A painful disorder affecting approximately one half of the head, either the right or left side, and which extends along the length of the longitudinal suture...

Hemicrania, he suggested, resulted from excessive "choler" irritating intracranial structures on one side of the head, the opposite side being shielded by the falx cerebri. Galenic theory considered the throbbing quality of the headache to be caused by arterial pulsation, while pain from nerves and tendons caused "tension-type" headache (*tonodes* in Greek) (5).

Byzantium and Persia

Following the fall of Rome, physicians such as Oribasius and Aëtios in Byzantium (successively Constantinople and then Istanbul), the eastern part of the old Roman Empire, kept the ideas of Galen alive through the compilation of medical encyclopedia (6). In the sixth century, Alexander of Tralleis (in Lydia, now in Turkey) wrote a twelve-volume textbook of medicine, and concentrated particularly on the nervous system. He provided a detailed account of headaches based on the writings of Arateus and Galen and from his own practice (5,6). He was of the view that hemicrania was caused by toxins connected with abdominal disorders. By the 10th century, the focus of medical and scientific development had moved still further east. Arabic medicine built and expanded on the earlier concepts, and Abu Ibn Sina, better known by his Hebrew name Avicenna (980–1037 A.D.), was particularly influential. Born in Afshaneh near Bukhara in what is now Uzbekistan, Avicenna was a gifted child and later a scientific polymath. His immense work *Qanun fi al-Tibb* (Canon of Medicine) surveyed all that was then known of medicine from ancient and Islamic sources and it remained a standard text in medical schools until the Renaissance. He recognized that headaches were not always associated with brain injury or disease and also that some headaches could be triggered by light, sound, and odors, indicating increased sensitivity to such inputs—an important factor in the modern interpretation of the migraine mechanism (5,6).

Evolution of "Migraine"

Galen's "hemicrania" was translated into Low Latin as *hemigranea*. Successive transliterations and abbreviations (*"emigranea," "migranea," "migrana,"* and others) evolved by the 16th century into *megrim* in England (sick headache, blind headache, and bilious headache). The *Shorter Oxford English Dictionary* cites the first appearance of "hemicrania" with reference to headache in English texts as 1597 (11), but the term was already used to refer to "vertigo"(1595) and a "whim or fancy" (1593). It was also used around this time to denote "low spirits" or "vapors," and feelings of dysequilibrium, and was later used to refer to "staggers" in horses (1693). In France, "migrana" was called *"migraine,"* and in Germany, *"migräne."* "Migraine" is therefore a French word, and from an historical perspective, it should be pronounced "mee-graine" and not "my-grain" (11).

EARLY DESCRIPTIONS OF AURAS

The term "aura" has been used for some two thousand years to describe the hallucinations that sometimes precede certain epileptic seizures. Sir William Gowers attributed the term to Pelops, a contemporary of Aretaeus who had taught Galen (11). Pelops noted that some epileptic attacks began with a feeling like a "cold vapor" in a hand or foot, which would ascend to the head—what we would now describe as a hemisensory aura. It was believed in those times that blood vessels contained air, and Pelops reasoned that this sensation might be due to the passage of a "spirituous vapor" through the vessels. "*Aura*" is the Greek word for "breeze." Hippocrates' and Arateus' descriptions of visual aura have already been noted, but use of the term "aura" to describe similar phenomena preceding migraine headache did not come into common usage until much later.

It is now recognized that neurological manifestations of migraine can encompass very many other symptoms, including sensory hallucinations, disorders of cognitive function, altered perception of time and space, and forms of delirium and impaired consciousness. Medieval medical literature attributed such experiences to various recognized mechanisms, from hemicrania, epilepsy and apoplexy, to hysteria, psychosis, toxicity, and onanism (surprisingly, the latter attribution may in fact have some factual basis—see p. 131, 221).

Mood changes during migraine aura can rarely include sensations of awe, rapture, and wonderment (11), and it is conceivable that certain experiences, described as "visions" or "trances" in religious literature and conceived to be evidence of divine revelation, might have had a basis in migraine. For example, "visions" typically include images with a brilliant, radiant luminosity (Fig. 6). Is it possible, for example, that the blinding light experienced by Saul on the road to Damascus was caused by a migrainous visual aura?

The visions of the Abbess Hildegard of Bingen (1098–1179) have also been attributed to migraine (11,12).

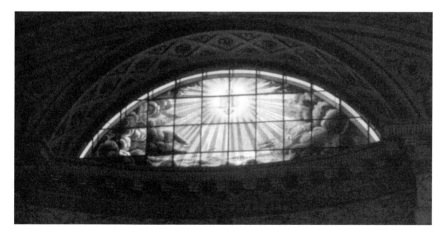

Figure 6 (*See color insert*) In hoc signo or International Headache Society? Stained glass window in the Chapel of All Saints, Wardour, Wiltshire in England.

I saw a great star, most splendid and beautiful, and with it an exceeding
multitude of falling sparks with which the star followed southward . . . and
suddenly they were all annihilated, being turned into black coals . . . and cast
into the abyss so that I could see them no more.

However, Singer (13), in an extensive review of Hildegard's descriptions, suggested that she was possibly experiencing hallucinations produced
(ironically) by ergot. Furthermore, her illustrations, interpreted as possibly
showing teichopsic aura, generally have a square wave boundary rather than
the zigzag or serrated edge typical of fortification spectra (see below).
Demonstrating typical female intuition, the Abbess is said to have decreed
that the pain of hemicrania was unilateral because it was of such severity that
it would be impossible to bear if it was bilateral!

The visual hallucinations associated with migraine can be dramatic,
and most references in the ancient literature relate to this form of aura.
But in 1618, the French physician Charles le Pois (1563–1633) became the
first person to report hemisensory aura in migraine (5). He described a
12-year-old girl who suffered episodes of severe left temporal headache preceded by left-sided numbness, stiffness, and formication, starting in the little
finger and ascending up the arm ("aurae cujusdam instar ascendentis"—as
an ascending breeze). He referred to her symptoms as *hemicraniae insultus*.
He was also the first to record *premonitory* symptoms in migraine. His
own attacks were preceded by "febricula" or "little fever," and also by thirst
(see Chapter 3, p. 48). Johann Jakob Wepfer (1620–1695), who together
with Le Pois and Thomas Willis is credited with the foundation of clinical
neurology, also made important contributions to the understanding of
migraine, including the first description of migrainous infarction (see
Chapter 4, p. 141) and basilar-type migraine (see Chapter 5, p. 209).
Wepfer's posthumous description of visual aura (1727) was published just
after Vater's report of hemianopic migrainous scotoma in 1723 (5).

"Ophthalmic Migraine"

Visual aura became the focus of particular attention in the late 17th century
and early 18th century, when a number of eminent French and English
scientists and astronomers began to publish their personal experiences of
migraine attacks. These observations not only helped clarify the characteristics of visual aura, but also led to the elucidation of a fundamental piece
of neuroanatomy—the hemidecussation of the optic nerves (14). John
Fothergill (1712 1780), in a paper to the Select Society of Licentiates in
December 1778, gave a description of his personal experience of a particular
visual aura characterized by an obscuration with a "zigzag border," describing the spectral appearance as being *"surrounded by luminous angles, like
those of a fortification"* (15). His account of "sick headache" is considered
a seminal contribution. He particularly emphasized dietary factors as triggers

> The head-ach proceeds from the stomach; not the reverse, as has been the opinion of many who suffer by it.

He is also celebrated for providing the first comprehensive description of the condition later called trigeminal neuralgia by his great-nephew Samuel Fothergill, although John Locke, a pupil of Willis and later his successor as Professor of Natural Philosophy in Oxford, had first described the condition.

Sir David Brewster (1781–1868), another child prodigy and polymath, who had invented the kaleidoscope in 1816 and later a giant lens that led to the development of lenses for lighthouses (his ancestor William Elder Brewster led the pilgrims on the Mayflower in 1610), concluded that the appearance of visual aura was due to the retinal blood vessels, but he had ignored the fact that the pattern of the retinal vessels did not correspond in homonymous fields (14). Up to this time, none had questioned the view of Descartes, that the optic nerves and tracts from the two eyes were separate. But in 1824, William H. Wollaston (1766–1828), celebrated chemist, physicist, physiologist, and inventor of the camera lucida, presented a paper in which he brilliantly deduced the correct anatomy from accounts of his own hemianopic auras (16).

Sir John F.W. Herschel (1792–1871), the Astronomer Royal of the day, reported his own similar experience of this type of visual hallucination in 1866, again referring to the aura as "fortification" (17). He seems to have been unaware that his symptoms were a manifestation of migraine; they were evidently not associated with headache. However, he made two important observations: that the hallucination migrated, and that it persisted with the eyes closed. He also surmised that the straight-lined angular forms, with some colored elements, were generated subconsciously and could not be accounted for by disturbance of the retina or optic nerves.

Sir George Biddell Airy, another Astronomer Royal, took to describing and illustrating his colored auras (which also occurred without headache), but his illustrations were relatively crude. However, in 1870, his son Dr. Hubert Airy published a most important paper entitled "On a distinct form of transient hemiopsia," in which he provided a beautiful illustration of his own visual aura (Fig. 7) (18). It was Airy who popularized the term "teichopsia" (Greek for "town wall vision") to refer to this distinctive zig-zag-edged scotoma, which he recognized was distinct from the hemianopic auras described by Wollaston. He was apparently unaware of Fothergill's observation. Airy's illustration was reproduced in 1873 in a monograph on hemicrania by Latham (19) and also in Edward Liveing's magnum opus published in the same year entitled *On Megrim, Sick Headache and Some Allied Disorders* (20). This work is considered by many to be the best descriptive text on the subject ever written. Indeed, the contribution of Liveing to our understanding of the clinical manifestations of migraine cannot

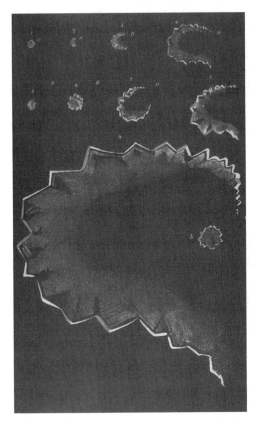

Figure 7 (*See color insert*) Dr. Hubert Airy's "sinistral teichopsia." His drawing shows a teichopsia starting in the left paracentral area and expanding into the left hemifield, eventually obscuring most of the left field of vision. A second aura then begins in its wake.

be overstated. His accounts were the first to include aura types other than visual, and to clearly make the connection between these experiences and hemicranial headaches. In particular, he realized that the auras and neurological complications of "megrim" were legion. We will return to his contributions later in this chapter.

The manifestations of migraine with visual aura were thought so compelling and distinct that physicians in Paris began to refer to it as "ophthalmic migraine," a new entity completely distinct from migraine without aura (MO). However, this notion was scotched in an 1887 book by Thomas (21), who pointed out that migraine with visual aura could also occur in patients who had migraine but who did not usually have aura, and that optic nerve dysfunction could not account for some of the symptoms considered to be features of the condition, such as eyelid edema and conjunctival injection. He accepted that these features were actually manifestations of the trigeminovascular reflex, whose existence had been proposed in 1855 by Hasse, and again in 1878 by Galezowski (5), as we will discuss in Chapter 2.

EARLY CONCEPTS OF CAUSALITY: THE 1ST TO THE 16TH CENTURY A.D.

As noted, Hippocrates was clearly familiar with the manifestations of what we now term migraine, and he believed that attacks could be triggered by exertion or sexual intercourse (11). Although not a physician, Cornelius Celsus (25 B.C.–50 A.D.), a friend of the Roman Emperors Tiberius and Caligula, wrote what is generally accepted as the best account of Roman medicine, *De Re Medicina*, a medical encyclopedia for the Roman gentry (5,6,8), in which he stated his belief that migraine headache was contracted by

> Drinking wine, or crudity, or cold, or heat of a fire, or the sun. And all of these pains are sometimes accompanied by a fever, and sometimes not; sometimes they afflict the whole head, at other times a part of it.

Galen believed in the Hippocratic view that migraine was caused by a disturbance of the parts of the body believed to be responsible for the dispatch of vapors or liquids that could harm the brain

> It is caused by the ascent of vapours, either excessive in amount, or too hot, or too cold . . .

He believed that vomiting during the attack would redress the balance of humors by eliminating "choler" (bilious humor) (11).

According to Adams (22), the 7th century Greek physician Paulus Aeginata (Paul of Aegina) wrote that the factors that provoked migraine included

> Noises, a brilliant light, drinking of wine and strong smelling things which fill the head. Some as if the whole head were struck, and some as if one half, in which case the complaint is called hemicrania.

Treatments of the day emphasized the use of low-fat diets (much in vogue now for other reasons), emetics, and purgatives, the latter also favored by Alexander Trallianus (11)

> If therefore headache frequently arises on account of a superfluity of bilious humor, the cure of it must be affected by means of remedies which purge and draw away the bilious humor.

An alternative theory, which evolved contemporaneously with the humoral concept, considered that migraine originated peripherally in one or more of the viscera, the affects then being propagated by some mysterious subconscious means, termed "sympathy" by the Greeks and "consensus" by the Romans (11). Little further advance on the understanding of the condition appears to have been made until the 17th century, although the Arabic literature includes lengthy descriptions of the syndrome. Surgical techniques, including trephination, scalp incision, cautery, and bloodletting, were variously recommended for treatment, in addition to medical remedies.

THE 17TH CENTURY: THE INFLUENCE OF THOMAS WILLIS

Thomas Willis (1621–1675) (Fig. 8) was Professor of Natural Philosophy at Oxford University. He is often described as the "Father of Neurology" and indeed first coined the term "neurology"—the "doctrine of the nerves"—in his seminal work *Cerebri Anatome* (1664). In 1672, Willis published *De Anima Brutorum* (Concerning the Souls of Brutes) (23). This work described "the nature, parts, powers and affections of the soul and the pathological states affecting the brain and nervous system" and was the first study

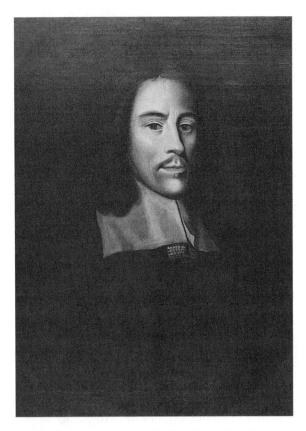

Figure 8 Thomas Willis (1621–1675). The "Father of Neurology" made many important observations concerning primary headache. Painting by J. Wollaston, displayed in the Lower Reading Room of the Bodleian Library, University of Oxford. *Source*: By permission of the Royal Society of Medicine, London, England.

of the comparative and functional anatomy of the nervous system. Willis' work was republished in several later volumes, including his 1684 *Practise of Physick* (Fig. 9). Among many important observations in this work, he described the anatomy of the cerebral blood vessels and also provided the first description of myasthenia gravis in a woman who periodically lost her voice, becoming "mute as a fish." In a section entitled *De Cephalalgia*, he wrote on headache. It is interesting to see how arguably the most eminent physician, anatomist, and physiologist of the latter part of the 17th century viewed its origins.

Willis had been schooled in the traditional humoral theory, but his studies provided considerable new advances and insights. The following are extracts from his work in modern English. Of headache, he commented that

> The causes are manifold and very diverse and they can hardly be methodologically recited. Hence it is that the cure is often instituted empirically.

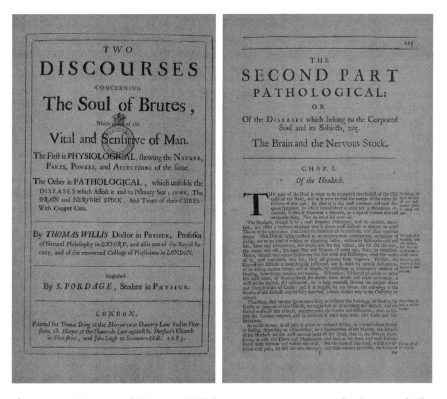

Figure 9 Title page of Thomas Willis' *De Anima Brutorum. The Brain and The Nervous Stock*, and the title page of *The Second Part (Pathological)* beginning with "*Of the Headach.*" From Willis' *Practise of Physick,* London, 1684. *Source*: By permission of the Royal Society of Medicine, London, England.

Willis went on to discuss the possible anatomical basis for headache, noting that the brain parenchyma is essentially insensate.

> What things belong to its pathology? The most nervous part of the head that is the nerves themselves and also the membranes which are sensible both within and without the skull. Of these parts, the first are the meninges and their various processes, the coats of the nerves, the pericranium or skin over the skull, the muscles and lastly the skin itself. As to the brain and cerebellum and their medullary dependencies, we affirm that these bodies are free from pain since they lack sensory fibres . . .

He then considered the reasons for the variable severity of headache, in particular the role of the very pain-sensitive meninges.

> As to the differences of the headache, the common distinction is, that the pain of the head is either without the skull, or within its cavity: the former is a more rare and a more gentle disease, because the parts above the skull are not so sensible as the interior meninges; nor are they watered with so plentiful a flow of blood that by sudden and vehement incursion, they may be easily distended, or inflamed above measure. Secondly, the other kind of headache, to wit, within the skull, is more frequent, and much more cruel, because the membranes, clothing the brain, are very sensible, and the blood is poured upon them by a manifold passage, and by many greater arteries.

He reasoned that the focal nature of "meagrim" might reflect the variable distribution of blood to the meninges

> Further, because the blood or its serum, sometimes passing through all the arteries at once, both the carotids and the vertebrals, and sometimes apart, through these or those, on the one side or the opposite, bring hurt to the meninges, hence the pain is caused that is interior; which is either universal, infesting the whole head, or its greater part; or particular, which is limited to some private region; and sometimes produces a meagrim on the side, sometimes in the forepart; and sometimes in the hinder part of the head.

Willis believed that headache resulted from the affects of one or more "excrementous humours" on the pain-sensitive structures. Accumulation of blood, serum, "chyme" (or "nutritious juice"), and nervous liquor (cerebrospinal fluid) could mediate headache, singly or in concert, resulting in "painful corrugations or wrinkings" of the nerve fibers. Some of his observations were probably based on cases of meningitis and subarachnoid hemorrhage, which he extrapolated to the understanding of what we now classify as primary headaches.

> Pain in the head can be either accidental, or occasional and habitual. The former can happen to most men after the drinking of wine, surfeit, lying in the sun or exercise and result from the blood being incited and boiling up immoderately, extending the membranes it passes through. Yea, the serum and

vapors copiously sent forth from it then growing hot and rushing on the membranes pull and provoke the nervous fibres.

Willis then described a number of cases from his practice to illustrate these principles. These included a patient with probable parasagittal meningioma, who died from coning with evident local cerebral edema ("dropsy of the brain"), and cases of meningitis and subarachnoid hemorrhage. He noted, for example, that some headaches tended to occur chiefly in the morning, as with raised intracranial pressure due to hydrocephalus.

He also recorded details of several cases of headache that he recognized as being benign despite the severity of the symptoms. For example, in the case of Anne, Countess of Conway (Fig. 10), whom William Harvey had also attended because of frequent and protracted headache attacks dating from the age of 12, Willis wrote

> But although this distemper, most grievously afflicting this noble lady, above 20 years (when I saw her) having pitched its tents near the confines of the brain, had so long besieged its regal tower, yet it had not taken it: for the sick lady, being free of vertigo, swimming in the head, convulsive

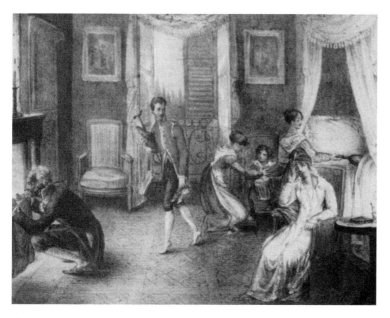

Figure 10 (*See color insert*) The Countess of Conway, a patient of both William Harvey and Thomas Willis. "A lady of most beautiful form, and a great wit, for that she was skilled in the liberal arts and in all forms of literature." She suffered from disabling attacks of migraine and underwent many treatments without success, including "opening of the jugular veins" rather than trepanation, in France.

distempers and any soporiferous symptoms, found the chief faculties of her soul sound enough.

Willis was well aware of hereditary influences in migraine and also recorded cases following injury and emotional upset. He observed that episodes could sometimes be preceded by hunger and terminated by vomiting.

A beautiful young woman with a slender habitus was subject to hereditary headache. On the day before a spontaneous headache, she would grow very hungry in the evening and would eat a most plentiful supper, even greedily. Following this, a headache would almost certainly follow the next morning. This was present as soon as she awaked and affected the whole of her forehead. She was also troubled with vomiting (sometimes acid, sometimes bile). Thus, vomiting will sometimes succeed a headache; yet pain of the head would rarely follow vomiting.

He also noted that polyuria may follow attacks.

Sometimes the watery humour suffering of flux offends the head. Hence, in those that have the headache as in convulsive diseases, there is often a clear and copious urine.

In addition to the humoral theory, Willis also favored the "sympathy" concept and embodied it in his theory of *"idiopathy,"* the tendency to periodic and explosive neurological reactions such as hemicrania, which could be triggered by a variety of internal and external factors and transmitted throughout the body by "sympathetic" nerves, whose existence at that time could only be inferred. However, in one important case, a patient with a left-sided headache was found at necropsy to have occlusion of the right internal carotid artery. Willis suggested that the headache had been due to compensatory dilatation of the vessels of the left carotid tree, an observation that echoes the vascular theory later to be propounded by Latham (see below). It also supported the importance of the anastomotic vessels at the base of the brain, which he had described earlier, with ultimately eponymous distinction (24).

THE 18TH AND 19TH CENTURIES: VASCULAR AND NEURAL HYPOTHESES

In 1758, John Fordyce published *De Hemicrania*, based largely on documentation of his own migraine attacks. He experienced prodromal depression, and was among the first to attribute attacks to dietary factors such as eating chocolate (8). The Scot, Robert Whytt (1714–1766), a student of Boerhaave of Leiden, wrote extensively on the incompatibility of the "Galenic Corpus" with the growing understanding of neurophysiology, and in particular the lack of evidence to support the concept of "nervous fluid" as the means by which nerves affected muscular function (5). In 1764, he wrote a book on nervous diseases in which, with remarkable insight, he proposed that "altered sensitivity of the nerves" could cause vascular reactions in response to

> Sudden changes of weather, errors of diet, fatigue of body, strong passions, suppression of ordinary evacuations...

He believed that in migraine, the blood vessels were either in continuous spasm or acting in a pulsatile fashion, causing pain (5). Again, this theory has elements of the later vascular hypothesis of migraine. He also observed the relationship between migraine attacks and menstruation.

In 1790, Simon-Andre Tissot of Lausanne (1728–1797) published an enormous treatise entitled *Traite des nerfs met leurs maladies*, the most comprehensive account of neurological disorders to that date. He gave an extensive account of migraine in Volume 13. He noted the importance of emotional factors in precipitating migraine, and suggested that the gastric symptoms of attacks might occasionally *initiate* the headache, consistent with the sympathy concept (5,8,11).

> A focus of irritation is formed little by little in the stomach, and that when it has reached a certain point the irritation is sufficient to give rise to acute pains in all the ramifications of the supraorbital nerve.

He also recognized hemianopia and hemiplegia as migraine manifestations. However, Tissot is more famously remembered for convincing the medical world of the harmful affects of masturbation. (As above, was he right? See Chapters 3 and 5.) The medical scientists of the 18th century made no distinction between the physical and emotional components of nervous dysfunction, but the rapid advances in physiology and medicine during the 19th century were to provide significant advances in our understanding of such disorders. Conditions began to be described as "organic," determined by defined pathological changes; and "functional," caused by disturbed physiology—and not as the term is used today, incorrectly, to denote ostensible "psychogenic" origins. Many celebrated physicians of the time wrote vividly on their personal experiences of migraine, but dwelt largely on the physical constituents of attacks, rather than emotional elements.

The Vascular Theory

Several observations dating from the mid-19th century began to emphasize the importance of changes in the extracranial blood vessels in the pathogenesis of migraine headache. Two schools of thought emerged. Parry in 1825 noted that compression of the carotid artery in the neck could abort migraine headache temporarily (25), and the theory that such headache was caused by vasodilatation resulting from sympathetic deficit was supported by Brown-Sequard and Claude Bernard (5). Conversely, Emil Du Bois-Réymond (1818–1896), the discoverer of the nerve action potential, noted, when describing changes in his own superficial temporal artery during migraine attacks (8), that the headache was "increased by motion to a high degree of violence" and "responds to each beat of the temporal artery." He found that the artery on the affected side was "like a hard cord" while that on the unaffected side was normal. He also noted that during his migraine attacks, he appeared very pale. He referred to this as "white migraine" and attributed it to sympathetic excitation on the affected side, via the "regio cilio-spinalis," resulting in painful vasoconstriction of cerebral arteries (angiospastic migraine). He reasoned that oscillations of blood pressure in the visual apparatus and brain would account for the neurological symptoms (5,8). In this regard, his views were similar to those of Robert Whytt.

However, shortly afterwards, Möllendorf described "red migraine" (or "angioparalytic migraine"), describing cases with prominent facial flushing (5). The beneficial effects of the rye fungus, ergot, on migraine headache, first reported by the British otorhinolaryngologist Edward Woakes in 1868 (26), supported the view that migraine headache resulted from vasodilatation; ergot was known to cause intense vasoconstriction, the basis of ergotism or "St. Anthony's fire." Eulenberg and his successors subsequently reconciled the contradictory views of Du Bois-Réymond and Möllendorf by correctly suggesting that these different manifestations of migraine attacks reflected the relative activations of the sympathetic and parasympathetic nervous systems. Eulenberg later reported the successful use of a subcutaneous ergot preparation (*ergotinin*) in the treatment of migraine attacks (27). We will return to this story in Chapter 7, p. 281.

Sir Samuel Wilks, in 1872 (11), also attached significance to the superficial vascular changes that occur during attacks, that he believed

> Alter the current of blood through the head; thus, while the face is pale, the larger vessels are throbbing, the head is hot, and the remedies which instinct suggests are cold and pressure to the part.

Latham (19) subsequently extended these observations in his vascular theory of migraine, explaining that aura and subsequent headache resulted from

> Contraction of the blood vessels of the brain, and so diminished supply of blood, produced by the excitation of the sympathetic; and that the exhaustion of the sympathetic following on this excitement causes the dilatation of the vessels and the headache.

The idea that migraine aura was the result of cerebral vasoconstriction and headache was due to vasodilatation, remained accepted orthodoxy for the next three centuries. Further reports of the benefits of ergot in migraine followed during the 1880s (28). Gowers and other prominent physicians of the time recommended ergot preparations such as ergotinin for the treatment of "red migraine," while the vasodilator nitroglycerine was favored for "white migraine." One wonders how successful this treatment could have been in light of recent evidence that glyceryl trinitrate is in fact a potent migraine trigger, now being used to study migraine pathogenesis (see Chapter 2, p. 68)! Gowers also advocated prophylactic treatment with a potion based on bromide and nitroglycerine in alcohol ("Gowers' mixture"—see Chapter 7) (29). We would presume that the beneficial effects of Gowers' mixture as a prophylactic were largely dependent on the bromide content, because bromides are anticonvulsant, and as we will see, migraine shares some pathogenetic characteristics with epilepsy.

Nerve-Storms

Edward Liveing (Fig. 11) published his treatise *"On Megrim"* in 1873, although a brief summary had appeared in the British Medical Journal the previous year (30). He proposed a radically different view of migraine

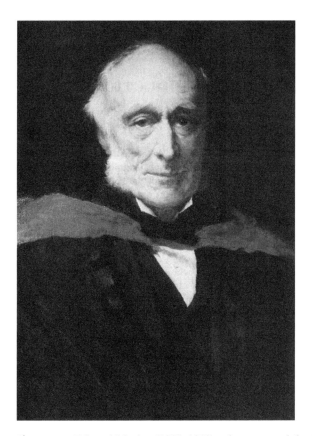

Figure 11 Edward Liveing (1832–1919), who proposed the theory of "nerve-storms." Painting by Walter William Ouless (1910). *Source*: Copyright The Royal College of Physicians of London.

pathogenesis. His hypothesis was based on evidence collected over a number of years, but he had been reluctant to publish because his ideas flew in the face of the prevalent orthodoxy. Liveing conducted a meticulous analysis of personal cases and previously published descriptions, amounting to 67 cases in all, recording the nature of migraine headache in terms of site, frequency, duration, periodicity and interval, and the co-occurrence of symptoms such as nausea, vomiting, affection of sight, vertigo, affection of speech, emotional and intellectual disorders, and sensory disorders, together with observations on factors possibly related to causation, such as hereditary predisposition. He also referred to what he termed "metamorphosis" or "transformation"—the tendency for this paroxysmal syndrome to be replaced or transformed periodically into other "functional" paroxysmal syndromes, such as epilepsy, gastrointestinal disorders, vasovagal syncope, and even asthma. He arranged his cases in a hierarchy of complexity: "simple" cases in which the paroxysm was represented by a single feature such as violent headache, usually unilateral but sometimes bilateral; or an attack of nausea, vomiting, and prostration, like seasickness; or perhaps hemianopia: and *complex* cases in which several symptoms such as sensory abnormalities, aphasia, confusion, or memory disturbance would develop sequentially. He confirmed that such symptoms usually preceded the headache phase and that vomiting was often the last event in the sequence. He noted that the syndrome affected females more than males, that there was a strong familial predisposition, and that migraine attacks exhibited some regularity of occurrence, although a severe attack might result in a more prolonged remission. Attacks seemed to be provoked at vulnerable periods by "various forms of peripheral irritation … excitement … ovarian irritation, eyestrain, strong odors," and in particular, "mental emotion and excessive brain work."

Although these clinical observations are perhaps the most important part of his work, Liveing's book also included a lengthy consideration of the many theories of causation prevalent at the time. These included the doctrine of biliousness, based on the humoral theory, the theory of "sympathy," noted above, and a detailed analysis of the "determination of blood to the head," including cerebral congestion (plethora) and the vascular theories of Du Bois-Reymond, Mollendorf, and Latham. Liveing was sceptical of Du Bois-Reymond's view that migraine originated not in the brain or nerves of the brain, but in the "regio cilio-spinalis," having been unable to confirm any abnormality in the retinal vasculature by ophthalmoscopy while observing a patient during an attack of "ophthalmic migraine," and being unable to confirm changes in the temporal arteries in another patient, during a "well-marked hemicranial paroxysm."

Liveing believed that migraine originated in the "sensory tract and ganglia of sensory nerves from the optic thalamus above to the nucleus of the vagus below." He considered migraine to be an exemplar of the "neurosal disorders" or neuroses, functional disorders that included asthma, epilepsy, angina, tic doloreux, "temporary insanity," and others. He accepted that the headache of migraine might be mediated by arterial dilatation, but he rejected this as an explanation for the aura and other neurological manifestations, because the symptoms could sometimes be bilateral and crossed anatomical vascular territories, and were often highly pleomorphic in individual cases. Instead, he proposed the theory of "nerve-storms."

> A form of centrencephalic seizure, the activity of which is projected rostrally upon the cerebral hemispheres, and peripherally via the ramifications of the autonomic nervous system.

He proposed that migraine and similar "neuroses" were the consequence of the tendency of the nervous system to periodically resolve the accumulation of "nerve-force" in paroxysmal or sometimes truly "explosive" symptoms. Liveing concluded

> No hypothesis seemed to me so well adapted to explain the phenomena as that of a nerve-storm traversing more or less of the sensory tract from the optic thalami to the ganglia of the vagus, or else radiating from the same tract from a focus in the neighbourhood of the quadrigeminal bodies.

In this regard, his views were more in keeping with our current understanding of migraine pathogenesis than those of his peers.

Hughlings Jackson (Fig. 12), the founding father of epileptology, was of the view that migraine was a form of sensory epilepsy. He noted that (8)

> Dr. Latham thinks the paroxysm in migraine to be due to arterial constriction in the region of the posterior cerebral artery; Dr. Liveing that there is a "nerve storm" traversing the optic thalamus and other centres. I think the sensory symptoms of the paroxysm are due to a "discharging lesion" of convulsions evolved out of the optic thalamus, i.e., of "sensory middle centres" analogous to the "motor middle centres." I believe the headache to be post-paroxysmal.

Jackson's view was therefore essentially in keeping with Liveing's: migraine was a primary neurogenic disorder, with vascular changes being secondary. Sir William Gowers' (Fig. 13) influential two-volume work *Manual of Diseases of the Nervous System*, published in 1886, included a chapter on "Migraine; paroxysmal headache," which provided an overview of the manifestations and pathogenesis of migraine, and included a discussion of the "vascular" and "neural" theories (8,9). Gowers viewed migraine as one of a number of disorders, which included "vagal attacks" (syncope), vasomotor attacks, vertigo, and sleep disorders that inhabited the "borderland of epilepsy." Like Liveing and Jackson, he considered neural factors to be primary, but he believed the cortex rather than the thalamus to be the origin of the dysfunction. He could conceive the headache to be of vascular origin,

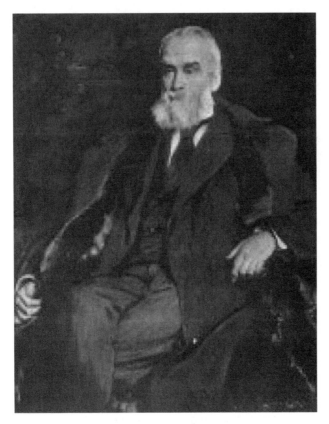

Figure 12   John Hughlings Jackson (1834–1911). The "Father of Epileptology" supported Liveing's concept that migraine was fundamentally a neurogenic disorder.

although he described the notion as "obscure," and like Liveing, he dismissed a vascular mechanism for aura on the basis that

> To explain (migraine) on the vasomotor hypothesis, we must assume first, an initial spasm of the arteries in a small portion of the brain; secondly, that the contraction always begins in the same place; and thirdly that it can give rise to a definite, uniform and very peculiar disturbance of function. There is no evidence of the truth of any of these assumptions.

Thus, by the end of the 19th century, the battle lines were drawn between the advocates of two principal theories of causation—the vascular and the neural. In many respects, this debate continues today. However, the observers of yesteryear based their reasoning on clinical deductions alone. There was no experimental evidence. There had been no experiments.

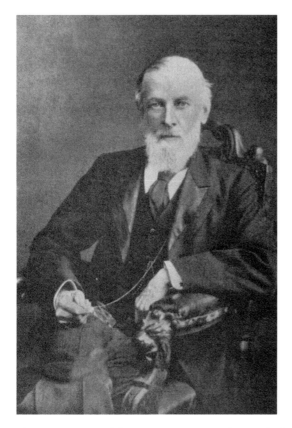

Figure 13 Sir William Gowers (1845–1915). His influential work *A Manual of Diseases of the Nervous System*, published in two volumes between 1886 and 1888, included a section on headaches. While he could accept that vascular factors might be involved in migraine headache, like Liveing he could not conceive how this could account for aura.

THE 20TH CENTURY

1900–1950

Ergotamine

The first blow in the new century was struck in favor of a primary vascular mechanism in migraine. The benefits of vasoconstriction induced by extracts of ergot in the treatment of "megrim" were by now well established, but it was not until 1916 that Arthur Stoll in Basel isolated "E," crystalline ergotamine (28,29). This drug, the first pure ergot alkaloid, was marketed under the trade name "Gynergen" and used mainly to control postpartum hemorrhage. In 1925, Rothlin confirmed Eulenberg's earlier observation of the successful treatment of migraine with subcutaneous ergotamine, and this was quickly confirmed by Tzanck in France, Maier in Switzerland, and O'Sullivan in the United States (29). These observational studies were followed by formal placebo-controlled clinical trials by Trautmann in Germany in 1928 (29) and Lennox in Boston in 1934, which confirmed the therapeutic effect (31). Then, in a pioneering study reported in 1938, John Graham and Harold G. Wolff in New York demonstrated, using a veritable "smoke and mirrors" technique

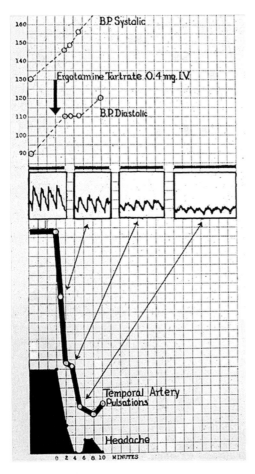

Figure 14 Graham and Wolff's "smoking drum" experiment. Tambours attached to a capsule were placed over palpable parts of the superficial temporal or occipital arteries and pulsations were recorded on moving bromide paper, by reflecting light from the capsule. In this recording from a subject during a migraine headache, intravenous ergotamine rapidly reduced the arterial pulsation amplitude, and there was a corresponding reduction in headache severity. As the effect of the drug wore off, the headache began to return. *Source*: Graham JR, Wolff HG. Mechanisms of migraine headache and action of ergotamine tartrate. Arch Neurol Psychiatr 1938; 39:737–763.

of extraordinary ingenuity (Fig. 14), that intravenous ergotamine exerted a vasoconstrictor affect on the dilated branches of the external carotid artery during migraine headache and that the headache was ameliorated in direct relation to this effect (32). There were no consistent changes in systemic blood pressure or pulsation of intracranial arteries (at least as reflected by CSF pulsation—some of these patients had lumbar cannulas placed during the attacks!), and the headache could be precipitated once again by vasodilatation using intravenous histamine, with a corresponding increase in arterial pulsation. Thus, migraine headache was associated with increased pulsation of extracranial arteries, sometimes accompanied by visible distension of these vessels, and ergotamine aborted the headache by causing vasoconstriction.

Subsequent studies by Wolff and colleagues provided further support for Latham's view that migraine headache was of vascular origin. Ray and Wolff (33) studied a series of patients undergoing neurosurgical procedures under local anesthesia, and found that the only intracranial structures that were pain sensitive were the venous sinuses and their tributaries, parts of the basal dura, and the dural and cerebral arteries at the base of the brain (particularly the middle meningeal artery). Although much quoted, in some respects these observations merely confirmed the conclusions reached by Thomas Willis 200 years earlier! Torda and Wolff (34) subsequently described edematous changes in the walls of the superficial temporal arteries excised from patients under general anesthesia during acute migraine attacks, although later observations challenged this observation (35).

Wolff's studies supported the view that dilatation of the cranial vasculature caused migraine headache. The observations and caveats of Liveing, Gowers, and others concerning the incompatibility of purely vascular mechanisms to account for many aspects of the migraine syndrome were largely forgotten. But although subsequent discoveries have negated some of his conclusions, Harold Wolff's influence and contributions to the furtherance of the scientific evaluation of headache in the early part of the 20th century cannot be overstated. His 1948 book *Headache and Other Head Pain* remains a classic (36), and he was instrumental in forming the Ad Hoc Committee for the Classification of Headache, which created the first modern headache classification in 1962.

Spreading Depression

In 1941, the neuropsychologist and phrenologist Karl Lashley (Fig. 15) wrote an account of his personal experience of visual aura, which he referred to as "scintillating scotoma" (37). By examining the progress of the visual disturbance over time, and from the knowledge that the anteroposterior length of the striate cortex is about 67 mm, he suggested that it resulted from a wave of intense excitation propagated from one pole of the occipital cortex and spreading at about 3 mm/min, followed by complete inhibition of activity, with recovery progressing at the same rate. He also noted that sometimes, the wave of inhibition could spread without an apparent

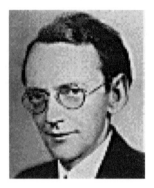

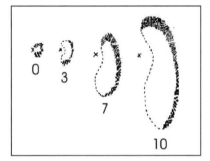

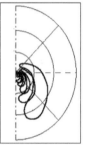

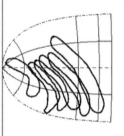

Figure 15 Karl Lashley (1890–1958). (*Bottom panel*) Lashley's illustration of his scintillating scotoma, with its advancing edge of "fortification figures." He mapped the advance over time (0, 3, 7, and 10 minutes) by fixing a mark on a sheet of paper and moving a pencil along different radiuses, marking the point at which the pencil disappeared into the scotoma. (*Bottom panel, right*) A spreading scotoma mapped onto the right visual cortical surface. The kidney shape is transformed to a wave front with constant width. *Source*: Copyright 2006 the Migraine Aura Foundation. Markus A. Dahlem, Modellierung gesichtsfeldbezogener. Phanomene bei der Migräne Aura auf der Grundlage von Erregungswellen in der primären Sehrinde. Diss. Otto-von-Guericke University, Germany, 2000.

preceding excitatory wave. The coincidental observations, in 1944, of the Brazilian neurophysiologist Aristides Leão, working in the Department of Physiology at Harvard, concerning a previously undiscovered and unexpected phenomenon that he called "spreading depression," provided a possible explanation (38). Leão noted that a mild traumatic or electrical stimulus to an area of the exposed dorsolateral neocortex of rabbits evoked a wave of depolarization that spread slowly outwards in all directions without regard to anatomical boundaries or vascular territories (Fig. 16). The rate of spread of the depolarization was commensurate with Lashley's

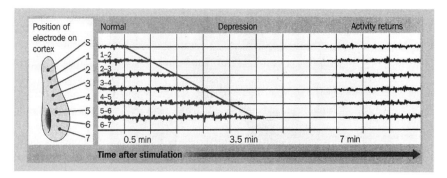

Figure 16 Leao's spreading depression. The recordings show the spread of electrical silence over time across the exposed cortex of a rabbit at around 3 mm per minute, following faradic stimulation. *Source*: From Silberstein, Stiles, Young. An Atlas of Migraine and Other Headaches. 2nd ed. Taylor and Francis, 56; J Neurophysiol 1994; 7:359–390.

description of visual aura. It was further shown that the leading edge of the wave of spreading depression was characterized by neuronal excitation (39). The neural excitation could thus account for the excitatory, positive aspects of visual aura (scintillations or phosphenes, the jagged edge of a teichopsia), while the depolarization could explain the "negative" symptoms of scotoma or hemianopia that usually followed in its wake. However, it was not until 1958, through the writings of the Canadian physiologist Milner (40), that this explanation was widely accepted.

The neural theory thus enjoyed resurgence. The major caveat to the hypothesis was that while spreading depression was relatively easy to evoke in the cortex of lower mammals, it proved very difficult to confirm in man until magnetoencephalography and new neuroimaging techniques became available (see Chapter 2, p. 52–53).

1950–1980

Serotonin and the Platelet Theory

In 1949, the potent vasoconstrictor serotonin [5-hydroxytryptamine (5-HT)] was isolated and characterized structurally by Maurice Rapport (41) and subsequently identified and isolated from blood in man in the early 1950s by Page and colleagues in the United States. In 1957, Gaddum and Picarelli identified the first 5-HT receptors on muscle and blood vessels—the "M" receptors on parasympathetic ganglia and the "D" receptors on smooth muscle (42). This simple classification sufficed for some three decades until it was realized that some effects of serotonin, in particular cerebral vasoconstriction, could not be accounted for on this basis.

This led to the identification of additional receptors and subtypes that proved essential to the eventual development of the triptans (see Chapter 7, p. 281). Chapman, in Wolff's group, isolated "neurokinin," later shown to be principally composed of substance P and bradykinin, from around extracranial vessel walls, establishing a potential link between head pain and blood vessel distension (43), and Kimball and Goodman showed that reserpine, which releases 5-HT, induced headache in most migraine patients (44).

The following year, Sicuteri reported that 5-hydroxyindoleacetic acid, (5-HIAA) the major metabolite of 5-HT, was increased in the urine of some migraineurs during an attack (45). This spawned a mass of research concerning vasomotor control and serotonin metabolism, particularly from Jim Lance's group in Sydney. In 1965, Curran showed that during most migraine attacks there is a release of 5-HT from platelets, resulting in a fall in blood serotonin levels (nearly all the blood serotonin is contained in platelets) (46), while Anthony et al. demonstrated that this acute reduction appeared to be specific to migraine attacks and was not seen following other painful or stressful events such as pneumoencephalography or angiography (47). Then, in 1967, Lance reported that intravenous injection of reserpine precipitated typical migraine headache in migraineurs (despite earlier publications that reserpine might actually be used to treat migraine!), but caused only a dull nonspecific headache in controls. This response was accompanied by a fall in platelet 5-HT (48), and Lance and Anthony then reported that intravenous 5-HT aborted both spontaneous and reserpine-induced headache (49). A few years later, Sicuteri confirmed his earlier observation that the serotonin antagonist methysergide could prevent migraine attacks (see Chapter 7, p. 302) (50).

As noted above, it was known that platelets were the principal repository of 5-HT, and it was subsequently reported in 1977 that the cyclical nature of migraine attacks was apparently reflected in periodic changes in platelet behavior (51). The following year, Damasio and Beck reported a relationship between autoimmune platelet destruction and migraine attacks (52), and Hanington subsequently proposed the *platelet hypothesis of migraine* (53), which stated that platelets were the prime mediators of migraine attacks. It was proposed that trigger factors acted on "abnormal" platelets in migraineurs to cause excessive aggregation and 5-HT release, leading to a migraine attack.

Therefore, by 1980, there was evidence that the migraine mechanism involved, to a greater or lesser degree, neural, vascular, platelet, and serotoninergic elements, although the primacy of each was disputed. As will be shown in this book, subsequent work has continued to implicate all of these elements, although a hierarchy of influence is emerging.

1980 to Present

> No anatomical changes are known to underlie the phenomena of migraine, and from the character of the symptoms, and the analogies of the disease, it is unlikely that any will be discovered.
> —*Sir William Gowers (1886)*

We would now be happy to dispute Sir William's assertion! The last 20 years have witnessed remarkable advances in our understanding of the migraine mechanism through technological developments. These have included measurements of cerebral blood flow during migraine attacks; an appreciation of the essential role of serotonin as a transmitter in both the central nervous system as well as the cerebral vasculature; studies on the unique innervation of the cerebral vasculature by the trigeminovascular system and its connections to the trigeminocervical complex in the brainstem; and most recently, the demonstration of cortical spreading depression by both magnetoencephalography, direct electrocorticographic recordings from the human brain and functional magnetic resonance (fMRI) imaging. The latter, in particular, has provided graphical confirmation of the processes underlying the progression of the visual aura across the occipital cortex.

"Migraine generator" sites at various locations in the brainstem have been demonstrated by both positron emission tomography (PET) and fMRI, and there have also been important advances in our understanding of the genetic predisposition to migraine. Several migraine susceptibility genes have been discovered, including genes encoding neural ion channel proteins that determine familial hemiplegic migraine. Indeed, it is plausible that genetic variation in neural ion channel function underlies our varying individual susceptibilities to primary headache.

A parallel development of equal importance was the establishment, in 1983, of the International Headache Society (IHS), which evolved from Wolff's 1962 Ad Hoc Committee. This has played a major role in establishing diagnostic criteria for different types of headache and headache syndromes, which have proved invaluable for defining homogenous patient populations for clinical and experimental investigations.

These developments and our current understanding of migraine pathogenesis will be considered in detail in Chapter 2, but we will now recount briefly the fates of the three main theories of migraine pathogenesis as matters developed over the last two decades of the 20th century.

Studies of Cerebral Blood Flow in Migraine

As we saw, the vascular hypothesis, based on the early clinical observations of Parry, Möllendorf, Du Bois-Reymond, Latham, and others, and supported by the later experiments of Wolff and his colleagues, proposed in essence that migraine aura was the result of cerebral ischemia due to constriction of intracranial vessels, while the headache phase was mediated by cerebral vasodilatation. The development of methods for studying cerebral blood flow using radioisotopes of inert gases during the 1950s allowed direct observations of cerebral blood flow changes during migraine attacks, both with and without aura.

One of the earliest methods used was [133] Xenon SPECT (single-photon emission computerized tomography). This radioisotope could be given by carotid injection or inhalation, and the brain was then scanned to follow the washout of the tracer. Xenon is removed more quickly from brain areas with high blood flow than from areas of lower flow, so a semiquantitative assessment of regional cerebral blood flow (rCBF) could be made. Whilst this technique had the advantage of allowing a number of scans to be performed sequentially during a single migraine attack, the technique lacked adequate spatial resolution. Nevertheless, the 1981 paper by Olesen showing spreading oligemia in MA but not in MO was a landmark publication (54). Generally, studies during the 1960s and 1970s tended to confirm reduced cerebral blood flow in cortical areas during the prodromal and aura phases, with increased flow during the headache phase, in keeping with the vascular hypothesis. However, other studies reported blood flow to be normal (55,56), while one group suggested that the clinical manifestations of "common migraine" (without aura), "classical migraine" (with aura), and hemiplegic migraine, reflected different degrees of cerebral vasoconstriction (57).

Development of scanners with better detection arrays and acquisition times allowed more rapid sequential scanning during the 1980s. Further studies by Olesen's group in Copenhagen identified differences between classical migraine and common migraine. During MA, a transient unilateral hyperemia was followed by reduced blood flow (oligemia) in the occipito-parietal region, which spread anteriorly in a manner suggestive of spreading depression, without regard to anatomical boundaries or vascular territories while blood flow during common migraine attacks was usually normal (58,59). However, the oligemia was found to persist well into the headache phase of the attack, long after the aura had resolved.

Olsen's group, also in Denmark, then considered patients with hemiplegic migraine and found a similar pattern of blood flow changes, but this time originating from the frontal lobe appropriate to the motor and/or sensory deficits, and spreading posteriorly. They also identified rapid focal fluctuations in blood flow in the oligemic areas, which they interpreted as evidence of vasomotor instability (60). Subsequently, ^{133}Xe inhalation studies were combined with the use of a long half-life tracer using SPECT to study later blood flow changes in classical migraine (Fig. 17) (61). The sequence of transient focal hyperemia followed by oligemia was confirmed, but again the oligemia persisted into the headache phase. A subsequent hyperemia did develop in the same area, but this was delayed some three to eight hours after

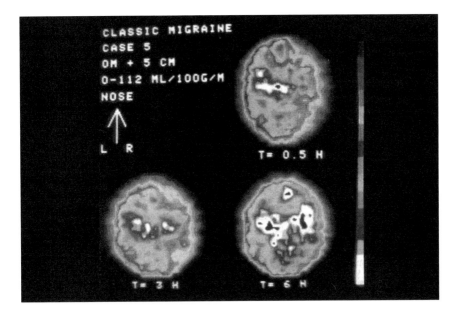

Figure 17 (*See color insert*) Study of regional cortical blood flow during spontaneous migraine with aura, studied using [133]Xenon inhalation and single photon emission computerized tomography. There is significant right hemisphere oligemia that persists for several hours, well into the headache phase (low blood flow values are blue, high blood flow values are white). *Source*: From Andersen AR, Friberg L, Olsen TS, et al. Delayed hyperemia following hypoperfusion in classic migraine. Single photon emission computed tomographic demonstration. Arch Neurol 1988; 45:154–159.

the onset of the attack in some patients and could persist for between 1 and 24 hours or more. Early PET studies tended to support these observations (62).

The introduction of the tracer hexa-methyl-propylene-amine-oxime (HMPAO) labeled with ^{99}Tc brought greater resolution to rCBF studies in migraine, and showed reduced cerebral blood flow in the cortex appropriate to the aura symptoms in MA, but no change in MO. These results were thus in keeping with Olesen's studies but the technique did not allow serial studies in the same attack. Figure 18 shows a typical result from one of the authors' studies.

Despite this lack of correlation between blood flow changes and the chronology of the aura and headache phases, the orthodox view that aura was the result of cerebral ischemia persisted (63). Heyck had earlier suggested a novel variant of the vascular hypothesis (64). He proposed, with evidence from just three subjects, that aura resulted from ischemia due to the shunting of blood through arteriovenous channels in the cerebral vasculature. The resulting high-pressure flow in the venous circulation was then responsible for the throbbing headache. This suggestion was later revived

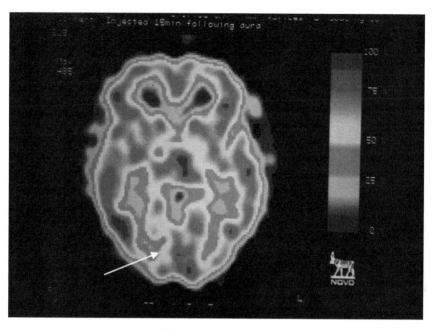

Figure 18 (*See color insert*) ^{99}Tc-HMPAO–single photon emission computerized tomography in acute migraine with visual aura. There is reduced blood flow in the right occipital cortex (*arrow*) appropriate to the aura symptoms. *Source*: With permission of The Princess Margaret Migraine Clinic, Charing Cross Hospital, London, England.

briefly as a possible mode of action of triptans, but it is not clear that such shunts exist (see Chapter 7, p. 282).

As noted, one of the oldest but perhaps most persuasive pieces of evidence in favor of a "vascular" component to migraine headache was the observation that extracranial arteries could become swollen and painful during attacks. However, the final nail in the coffin of the "vascular theory" came with the recent demonstration that cerebral blood flow velocity measured by transcranial Doppler was not significantly or consistently increased during migraine headache, either spontaneously (66) or when induced by the vasodilator sildenafil (67). It seems, therefore, that while vascular changes clearly occur in migraine attacks, and dilatation of extracranial vessels may contribute to the migraine headache, such changes probably represent delayed reflex vasodilatation secondary to more fundamental processes driving the attack, as will be discussed in Chapter 2.

The Platelet Theory

The relationship between the fall in blood (platelet) 5-HT and the increase in 5-HT metabolite levels in plasma and urine during migraine attacks, and the relationship between migraine attacks and abnormal platelet function indicated that platelets were important in migraine pathogenesis. Although the original contention that migraine was a primary platelet disorder (53,68) was considered unlikely (69,70), there is a consistent line of experimental evidence that shows that migraineurs have platelets that aggregate more readily and are more sensitive to factors that normally trigger platelet granule release. In addition, there seems to be a relationship between migraine attacks and platelet disorders (see Chapter 5, p. 241), and it is possible that platelet dysfunction might also play a part in migrainous infarction (see Chapter 4, p. 176).

Some 90% of the body's serotonin is contained in the enterochromaffin cells of the gut, with about 10% in platelets and 1% to 2% contained within the nervous system, particularly in the raphe nuclei and locus coeruleus of the brainstem, which are key loci in the migraine mechanism (see Chapter 2, Fig. 4, p. 58). Serotonin is released from the gut into the blood, but plasma levels are usually very low because of active uptake by platelets. The 5-HT system of human platelets comprises a specific 5-HT uptake mechanism at the plasma membrane, intracellular storage organelles (dense bodies or granules), a metabolizing enzyme (monoamine oxidase B), and 5-HT$_2$ surface receptors involved in the signalling processes that govern changes in protein phosphorylation and platelet shape. There is no synthesis or turnover of 5-HT in platelets, and it is suggested that the platelet system serves as a scavenger for free 5-HT (71).

A number of studies have shown that platelet 5-HT concentration appears to be constitutionally lower in migraine patients than normal control subjects (72–75). Kinetic analyses also suggest that platelet 5-HT uptake rates are reduced in migraineurs, not only during attacks but possibly also between attacks (72,74). In contrast, the ADP concentration and the size of the platelet dense bodies was found to be increased in migraineurs (76). Recent studies have shown that levels of platelet 5-HT are actually genetically regulated by polymorphisms of the serotonin transporter gene regulatory protein, but the observation concerning lower levels of platelet 5-HT in migraineurs was found to apply across all genotypes (77).

Revisiting her theory in 1989 (78), Hanington reiterated that platelets from migraineurs contain more ADP, have more (and larger) dense granules, aggregate more readily when exposed to 5-HT, have membranes with altered viscosity, and exhibit fibrinogen receptors with greater affinity. Triggers such as collagen and thrombin initiate the "platelet release mechanism," with resulting changes in platelet shape and release of ADP and 5-HT. This occurs more readily in platelets from migraineurs than controls. In addition, some drugs that inhibit platelet aggregation, such as methysergide, aspirin, and amitryptiline, prevent or relieve migraine. Subsequent research has not overturned these observations. Although the claim of primacy of platelet abnormalities in migraine pathogeneisis appears doubtful in light of the work now to be considered, these observations clearly have to be incorporated into any theory of pathogenesis. The possible relationship between platelet instability and the current interest in the relationship between patent foramen ovale and migraine is explored in Chapters 2 and 7.

The Neural Theory: "Nerve-Storms" Revisited

Liveing's hypothesis, later supported in principle by no lesser authorities than Hughlings Jackson and William Gowers, was that migraine was a neurogenic process and that vascular changes were secondary. Current evidence strongly supports this view. The deficiencies of the vascular theory revived interest in a primary neural process in migraine pathogenesis, especially with regard to aura. In particular, it was suggested that spreading oligemia might be secondary to spreading depression (79).

Following Leão's studies in the 1940s, spreading depression was demonstrated in a variety of experimental animals following stimulation of the cerebral cortex, not only by trauma but also by application of K^+ or excitatory amino acids. The phenomenon could also be elicited in the retina, brainstem, cerebellum, and most gray matter regions with the exception of the spinal cord. The processes underlying spreading depression will be discussed in Chapter 2, but the reason for the markedly greater susceptibility of the occipital cortex to this process remains unclear. One factor may be regulation of K^+ homeostasis. Sudden increases in extracellular potassium result in depolarization of synaptic terminals and release of neurotransmitters that in turn propagate the slowly advancing depolarization wave. K^+ homeostasis is largely maintained by the glia, so cortical areas with low glia-to-neuron ratios, such as the occipital cortex, might be particularly vulnerable (see Chapter 2, p. 51).

While spreading depression was clearly an attractive hypothesis for the basis of migraine, it proved frustratingly difficult to demonstrate in man. It could not be recorded during neurosurgical procedures using conventional electroencephalographic techniques. One author commented that he had not observed the phenomenon in nearly 1000 cases undergoing open operations for epilepsy and concluded that he doubted that spreading depression ever played a role in human cerebral pathophysiology, including migraine (80). It could be induced by microinjections of KCl into the hippocampus or caudate in patients, but it was not followed by focal symptoms or headache (81). However, early studies using magnetoencephalography, which detects the minute magnetic fluxes induced by cortically generated currents, showed a slow biphasic wave at the onset of migraine aura followed by generalized reduction of activity lasting about 10 minutes, compatible with spreading depression (82). More recently, as will be discussed extensively in Chapter 2, compelling neuroimaging studies have strongly supported the concept of spreading depression as the fundamental process underlying visual aura and spreading depression has also been recorded recently in the human brain by electrocorticography (see Chapter 2).

A neurogenic basis for the migraine mechanism therefore remains an attractive hypothesis, but it also raises a number of questions. What triggers the mechanism and where does it originate? Why are some individuals more susceptible than others? What is the link between the neural processes, the headache, the blood flow changes, and the changes in platelet behavior that occur during attacks? And what terminates attacks? These and other questions will be addressed in Chapter 2.

REFERENCES

1. Clower WT, Finger S. Discovering trepanation: the contribution of Paul Broca. Neurosurgery 2001; 49:1417–1425.
2. Finger S, Clower WT. Victor Horsley on "trephining in pre-historic times". Neurosurgery 2001; 48:911–917.
3. Rawlings CE, Rossitch E. The history of trepanation in Africa with a discussion of its current status and continuing practise. Surg Neurol 1994; 41:507–513.
4. Alvarez WC. Was there sick headache in 3000 B.C.? Gastroenterology 1945; 5:524.
5. Isler H, Clifford Rose F. Historical background. In: Olesen J, Tfelt-Hansen P, Welch KMA, eds. The Headaches. Philadelphia: Lippincott Williams & Wilkins, 2000:1–7.
6. Clifford Rose F. European neurology from its beginnings until the 15th century: an overview. J History Med 1993; 2:21–44.
7. Major RH. The Papyrus Ebers. Ann Med History (New Series) 1930; 2: 547–555.
8. Pearce JMS. Historical aspects of migraine. J Neurol Neurosurg Psychiatr 1986; 49:1097–1103.
9. Critchley M. Migraine from Cappadocia to Queen Square. In: Smith R, ed. Background to Migraine. London: Heinemann 1967:Vol 1:28–39.
10. Edmeads J. The treatment of headache: a historical perspective. In: Gallagher RM, ed. Therapy for Headache. New York: Marcel Dekker, 1990:1–8.
11. Sacks O. Migraine. Understanding a Common Disorder (Revised Edition). London: Duckworth, 1985.
12. Riley HA. Special article: migraine. Bull Neurol Inst NY 1932; 2:429–544.
13. Singer C. From Magic to Science. London: Ernest Behn:230–234.
14. Plant GT. The fortification spectra of migraine. Br Med J 1986; 293: 1613–1617.
15. Fothergill J. Remarks on that complaint, commonly known under the name of sick head-ach. In: Medical Observations and Enquiries by a Society of Physicians in London. London: T. Cadell, 1784:Vol. 6:103–137.
16. Wollaston WH. On semi-decussation of the optic nerves. Phil Trans Roy Soc Lond 1824; 114:222–231.
17. Herschei JFW. Familiar Lectures on Scientific Subjects. London: Alexander Strachan, 1866:406.
18. Airy H. On a distinct form of transient hemianopia. Phil Trans Roy Soc Lond 1870; 160:1247–1270.

19. Latham PW. On Nervous or Sick Headache, Its Varieties and Treatment. Two Lectures. Cambridge: Cambridge University Press, 1873.
20. Liveing E. On Megrim, Sick Headache and Some Allied Disorders. A Contribution to the Pathology of Nerve Storms. London: Churchill, 1873 (Available as Liveing: On Migraine. Nijmegen: Arts and Boeve, 1997).
21. Thomas L. La Migraine. Paris: Delahaye and Lecrosnier, 1887.
22. Adams F. The Seven Books of Paulus Aeginata. London: Sydenham Society, 1844:350.
23. Hughes JT. Eponymists in Medicine: Thomas Willis. London: Royal Society of Medicine, 1991.
24. Symonds CP. The Circle of Willis. Br Med J 1955; 1:119–122.
25. Knapp RD Jr. Reports from the past. Headache 1963; 3:112–122 and 143–155.
26. Koehler P, Isler H. The early use of ergotamine in migraine. Edward Woakes' report of 1868, its theoretical and practical background and its international reception. Cephalagia 2002; 22:686–691.
27. Eulenberg A. Subcutane Injectionen von ergotinin (Tanret): Ergotinum citricum solutum (Gehe). Deutsch Med Wochschr 1883; 9:637–639.
28. Silberstein SD, McCrory DC. Ergotamine and dihydroergotamine; history, pharmacology and efficacy. Headache 2003; 43:144–166.
29. Schiller F. The migraine tradition. Bull History Med 1975; 49:1–19.
30. Liveing E. Observations on megrim or sick headache. Br Med J 1872; i:364–366.
31. Lennox WG. Use of ergotamine tartrate in migraine. N Eng J Med 1934; 210:1061–1064.
32. Graham JR, Wolff HG. Mechanisms of migraine headache and action of ergotamine tartrate. Arch Neurol Psychiatr 1938; 39:737–763.
33. Ray BS, Wolff HG. Experimental studies on headaches: pain-sensitive structures of the head: their significance in headaches. Arch Surg 1940; 41:813–856.
34. Torda C, Wolff HG. Experimental studies on headache. Arch Neurol Psychiatr 1945; 53:329–332.
35. Adams CMW, Orton CC, Zilkha KJ. Arterial catecholamine and enzyme histochemistry in migraine. J Neurol Neurosurg Psychiatr 1968; 31:50–56.
36. Wolff HG. Headache and Other Head Pain. New York: Oxford University Press, 1948.
37. Lashley KS. Patterns of cerebral integration indicated by the scotomas of migraine. Arch Neurol Psychiatr 1941; 46:331–339.
38. Leão AAP. Spreading depression of cortical activity in the cerebral cortex. J Neurophysiol 1944; 7:359–390.
39. Leão APP, Morrison RS. Propagation of cortical spreading depression. J Neurophysiol 1945; 8:33–45.
40. Milner PM. Note on a possible correspondence between the scotomas of migraine and spreading depression of Leão. Encephalogr Clin Neurophysiol 1958; 10:705.
41. Rapport MM. The discovery of serotonin. Perspect Biol Med 1997; 40: 260–273.
42. Gaddum GH, Picarelli ZP. Two kinds of tryptamine receptors. Br J Pharmacol 1997; 120:134–139.

43. Chapman LF, Ramos AO, Goodell H. A humoral agent implicated in vascular headache of the migraine type. Arch Neurol 1960; 223–229.

44. Kimball RW, Goodman MA. Effects of reserpine on amino-acid excretion in patients with migraine. J Neurol Neurosurg Psychiatr 1966; 29:190–191.

45. Sicuteri F, Testi A, Anselmi B. Biochemical investigations in headache: increase in hydroxyindoleacetic acid excretion during attacks. Int Arch Allergy Appl Immunol 1961; 19:55–58.

46. Curran DA, Hinterberger H, Lance JW. Total plasma serotonin, 5-hydroxyindoleacetic acid and *p*-hydroxy-*m*-methoxymandelic acid excretion in normal and migrainous subjects. Brain 1965; 88:997–1010.

47. Anthony M, Hinterberger H, Lance JW. Plasma serotonin in migraine and stress. Arch Neurol 1967; 16:544–552.

48. Lance JW, Anthony M, Hinterberger H. The control of cranial arteries by humoral mechanisms and its relation to the migraine syndrome. Headache 1967; 7:93–102.

49. Lance JW, Anthony M. The effect of serotonin on cranial vessels and its significance in migraine. Proc Austr Assoc Neurologists 1968; 5:639–642.

50. Fanciullacci M, Granchi G, Sicuteri F. Ergotamine and methysergide as serotonin partial antagonists in migraine. Headache 1976; 16:226–231.

51. Deshmukh SV, Meyer JS. Cyclic changes in platelet dynamics and the pathogenesis of migraine. Headache 1977; 17:101–108.

52. Damasio H, Beck D. Migraine, thrombocytopaenia and serotonin metabolism. Lancet 1978; i:240–242.

53. Hanington E. Migraine: a blood disorder? Lancet 1978; ii:501–503.

54. Olesen J, Larsen B, Lauritzen M. Focal hyperemia followed by spreading oligemia and impaired activation of rCBF in classic migraine. Ann Neurol 1981; 9:344–352.

55. Edmeads J. Cerebral blood flow in migraine. Headache 1977; 17:148–152.

56. Hachinski VC, Olesen J, Norris JW. Cerebral haemodynamics in migraine. Can J Neurol Sci 1977; 4:245–249.

57. Skinhoj E. Hemodynamic studies within the brain during migraine. Arch Neurol 1973; 29:95–98.

58. Olesen J, Larsen B, Lauritzen M. Focal hyperemia followed by spreading oligemia and impaired activation of rCBF in classic migraine. Ann Neurol 1981; 9:344–352.

59. Lauritzen M, Olesen J. Regional cerebral blood flow during migraine attacks studied by Xenon-133 inhalation and emission tomography. Brain 1984; 107:447–461.

60. Friberg L, Olsen TS, Roland PE. Focal ischemia caused by instability of cerbrovascular tone during attacks of hemiplegic migraine. Brain 1987; 110:917–934.

61. Andersen AR, Friberg L, Olsen TS, et al. Delayed hyperemia following hypoperfusion in classic migraine. Single photon emission computed tomographic demonstration. Arch Neurol 1988; 45:154–159.

62. Herold S, Gibbs JM, Jones AKP, et al. Oxygen metabolism in migraine. J Cerebral Metab Blood Flow 1985; 5(suppl 1):445–446.

63. Olsen TS, Friberg L, Lassen NA. Ischaemia may be the primary cause of the neurologic deficits in classic migraine. Arch Neurol 1987; 44:156–161.

64. Heyck H. Pathogenesis of migraine. Res Clin Stud Headache 1969; 2:1–28.
65. Iversen HK, Nielsen TH, Olesen J, et al. Arterial responses during migraine headache. Lancet 1990; 336:837–839.
66. Limmroth V, May A, Auerbach P, et al. Changes in cerebral blood flow velocity after treatment with sumatriptan or placebo and implications for the pathophysiology of migraine. J Neurol Sci 1996; 138:60–65.
67. Kruse C, Thomsen LL, Birk S, et al. Migraine can be induced by sildenafil without changes in middle cerebral artery diameter. Brain 2003; 126:241–247.
68. Hanington E, Jones RJ, Amess JAL, et al. Migraine–a platelet disorder. Lancet 1981; ii:720–723.
69. Steiner TJ, Rose FC, Joseph R. Migraine is not a platelet disorder. Headache 1987; 27:400–402.
70. Joseph R, Welch KM. The platelet and migraine: a non-specific association. Headache 1987; 27:375–380.
71. Pletscher A. The 5-hydroxytryptamine system of blood platelets: physiology; pathophysiology. Int J Cardiol 1987; 14:177–188.
72. Waldenlind E, Ross SB, Saaf J, et al. Concentration and uptake of 5-hydroxytryptamine in platelets from cluster headache and migraine patients. Cephalalgia 1985; 5:45–54.
73. D'Andrea G, Welch KM, Riddle JM, et al. Platelet serotonin metabolism and ultrastructure in migraine. Arch Neurol 1989; 46:1187–1189.
74. Ferrari MD, Saxena PR. On serotonin and migraine: a clinical and pharmacological review. Cephalalgia 1993; 13:151–165.
75. Launay JM, Pradalier A, Dreux C, et al. Platelet serotonin uptake and migraine. Cephalalgia 1982; 2:57–59.
76. D'Andrea G, Welch KM, Riddle JM, et al. Platelet serotonin metabolism and ultrastructure in migraine. Arch Neurol 1989; 46:1187–1189.
77. Juhasz G, Zsombok T, Laszik A, et al. Despite the general correlation of the serotonin transporter gene regulatory region polymorphism (5-HTTLRP) and platelet serotonin concentration, lower platelet serotonin concentration is independent of the 5-HTTLPR variants. Neurosci Lett 2003; 350:56–60.
78. Hanington E. Migraine: the platelet hypothesis after 10 years. Biomed Pharmacotherapeut 1989; 43:719–726.
79. Lauritzen M. Cortical spreading depression as a putative migraine mechanism. Trends Neurosci 1987; 10:8–13.
80. Gloor P. Migraine and regional cerebral biood flow. Trends Neurosci 1986; 9:21.
81. Bures J, Buresova O, Krivanek J. The Mechanisms and Applications of Leão's Spreading Depression of Electroencephalographic Activity. New York: Academic Press, 1974.
82. Barclay GL, Tepley N, Simkins R, et al. Magnetometer studies of migraine patients. Cephalalgia 1989; 9(Suppl 10):127–128.

2

The Migraine Mechanism

INTRODUCTION

Until the twentieth century, opinion as to the cause and nature of migraine was speculative and based on symptom interpretation in the light of prevailing concepts of physiology and pathology. The idea that vasoconstriction caused aura through cerebral ischemia while headache was due to vasodilatation was generally accepted, and many of the current generation of doctors were taught this as medical students. We can now reflect, with the considerable benefit of hindsight, that this theory could never have accounted for the clinical picture of migraine, nor did it make any real sense on anatomical or physiological grounds. A number of studies, most particularly using functional imaging, have now shown that migraine is a pathophysiological neurogenic process originating in the brain.

From the outset, it must be said that our understanding is still rather rudimentary, and the evidence is at times confusing. A major challenge is to put the new observations within the framework of current ideas concerning the way the brain functions. The brain should not be thought of as a hierarchy of organized autonomous structures, each delivering its output to the next level in a linear function, but as a set of complex interacting networks that are in a state of dynamic equilibrium with the brain's environment. Migraine, as we shall see, can be considered as one result of an upset in this environment. We will speculate what biological purpose "migraine" may have at the end of this chapter. The challenge now is to better understand the complexities of the processes involved and, in particular, how the neural activity orchestrates vascular and neurotransmitter responses.

While migraine has been—and continues to be—discussed at a clinical level, technology of ever-increasing sophistication is being used to study brain behavior during attacks. This is not only giving us a better understanding of the migraine mechanism but also is contributing to the debate as to what we actually consider "migraine" to be. The clinical limits of the migraine spectrum are moving, and we wish to challenge them further in this book. For example, "chronic migraine" is a new and somewhat controversial clinical concept, but its introduction to the latest headache classification is supported by the results of cerebral blood-flow studies using positron emission tomography (PET) (1). Chronic migraine has the general phenotype of migraine but the symptoms are protracted and recurrent. Yet, the same pattern of brainstem activation that characterizes episodic migraine is also seen in chronic migraine. Again, in another newly recognized primary headache syndrome, "hemicrania continua," which has features of both cluster headache and migraine but is exquisitely sensitive to treatment with indomethacin, brainstem activation typical of migraine is seen alongside activation of the hypothalamus, the characteristic functional imaging feature of cluster headache (2). We will return to the implications of these brain imaging studies with regard to our understanding of the nature of primary headaches and their classification in Chapter 6, but will describe here the basic migraine mechanism as presently understood and review the evidence that supports current concepts. We will also consider the nature of migraine "triggers" and the factors that appear to determine susceptibility to attacks. This eclectic account is based on a number of authoritative reviews (3–8) colored by our own observations and conclusions from clinical experience.

WHAT IS MIGRAINE?

"Migraine," in terms of the clinical syndrome first defined by Arateus and his successors, is fundamentally a primary headache; that is, a headache for which no pathological cause can be defined. However, the migraine mechanism can—and frequently does—cause other neurological symptoms, quite often without headache. The diagnosis of "migraine," as with all primary headaches, depends entirely on the patient's description of symptoms, although it will be influenced by the clinician's conceptual framework and the diagnostic criteria of the day.

We will consider the classification of primary headaches in Chapter 5, but suffice to say here that migraine with aura (MA) and migraine without aura (MO) are now defined by the criteria of the International Headache Society (IHS). The first detailed definitions were published in 1988 (International Headache Classification, IHC-1) and were revised in 2004 (IHC-2) (9). We will outline these diagnostic criteria, because they are now universally accepted, but will then comment on their limitations. Table 1 shows the current IHC-2 classification of migraine.

Table 1 IHC-2 Classification of Migraine

IHC-2 code and syndrome

1.1 *Migraine without aura*

1.2 *Migraine with aura*
  1.2.1 Typical aura with migraine headache
  1.2.2 Typical aura with nonmigraine headache
  1.2.3 Typical aura without headache
  1.2.4 Familial hemiplegic migraine
  1.2.5 Sporadic hemiplegic migraine
  1.2.6 Basilar type migraine

1.3 *Childhood periodic syndromes that are commonly precursors of migraine*
  1.3.1 Cyclical vomiting
  1.3.2 Abdominal migraine
  1.3.3 Benign paroxysmal vertigo of childhood

1.4 *Retinal migraine*

1.5 *Complications of migraine*
  1.5.1 Chronic migraine
  1.5.2 Status migrainous
  1.5.3 Persistent aura without infarction
  1.5.4 Migrainous infarction
  1.5.5 Migraine-triggered seizure

1.6 *Probable migraine*
  1.6.1 Probable migraine without aura
  1.6.2 Probable migraine with aura
  1.6.3 Probable chronic migraine

Note: Items under Code 1.5 concern "complications" of migraine, and are discussed in Chapter 4. Under IHC-2, *ophthalmoplegic migraine* has been reclassified under Code 13—"*Cranial neuralgias and central causes of facial pain*" and is discussed in Chapter 5.
Abbreviation: IHC, International Headache Classification.

Diagnostic Criteria for Migraine (IHC-2)

MO is a headache characterized by the following features:

- The headache attacks last 4 to 72 hours and occur for less than 15 days per month (this time line distinguishes migraine from "Chronic Daily Headache" to which chronic migraine is a key contributor, see Chapter 5).
- The headache has at least two of the following characteristics:
  - Unilateral location
  - Pulsating quality
  - Moderate or severe pain intensity

♦ Aggravation by, or causing avoidance of, routine physical
   activity (e.g., walking or climbing stairs)

• During headache at least one of the following occurs:

♦ Nausea and/or vomiting
♦ Photophobia and phonophobia

MA is diagnosed when headache is associated with "neurological symptoms consistent with aura," as described below, in at least two attacks. It is accepted that the headache in such cases can be either

• MO headache as defined above, or
• "Non-migraine" headache, that is, headache not fulfilling the IHC-2 criteria for migraine headache.

Aura consists of at least one of the following but no motor weakness:

• Fully reversible visual symptoms, including positive features (flickering lights, spots, and lines) and/or negative features (scotoma)
• Fully reversible sensory symptoms including positive features (pins and needles) and/or negative features (numbness)
• Fully reversible dysphasic speech disturbance

At least two of the following should occur:

• Homonymous visual symptoms and/or unilateral sensory symptoms
• At least one aura symptom that develops gradually over five minutes or more and/or different aura symptoms that occur in succession over five minutes or more
• Each symptom lasts between 5 and 60 minutes.

The duration is important because it helps to distinguish migrainous aura symptoms from epileptic auras and the neurological symptoms of transient ischemic attacks, which usually develop more rapidly.

Advantages and Disadvantages of "International Headache Society Migraine"

These definitions are deliberately restrictive and designed to characterize homogenous patient groups to ensure conformity in clinical description and to aid research. A recent study has shown that a specific group of MA patients can indeed be identified using the IHC-2 criteria with a high degree of diagnostic sensitivity and specificity (10). However, we believe that the clinical spectrum of MA, and migraine in general, extends well beyond the strict confines of the IHS diagnostic criteria. In "real life," many patients do not fall into these neat categories. Indeed, the recognition of the origin of symptoms as migrainous may depend to some extent on specialist knowledge and insight. For example, as we will discuss in Chapter 3 and Chapter 7, the incidence of migraine and migraine auras among physicians, neurologists, and headache specialists is significantly higher than in the general population (11,12). The IHC-2 categories concede that migraine headache can vary to such an extent that it may not be categorized as migraine, and that headache may even be absent. Indeed, the diagnostic category "probable migraine" means that migraine can be diagnosed even when a patient's symptoms do not meet the diagnostic criteria!

Any hypothesis concerning the migraine mechanism has to account for the wide variation in manifestations that can be encountered in practice. For example, aura usually precedes headache, but can occur during and even after headache; headache can be ipsilateral or contralateral to the aura; or be bilateral; and aura can occur without headache, and so forth. Patients who suffer recurrent headaches will often distinguish their migraine headaches from their "ordinary ones." We will argue in Chapter 6 that all primary headaches stem from the same migraine mechanism and that nearly everyone gets, or will get, primary headaches or some other manifestation of the migraine mechanism sooner or later.

In this chapter, however, we will concentrate on IHS-defined migraine with and without aura.

"Hemiplegic migraine" is a special case and will be considered both in this chapter in the context of migraine pathogenesis and again in Chapter 3 with regard to the general issue of "auras." We consider "basilar type migraine" and "retinal migraine" to be migraine "variants," and these conditions will be discussed in Chapter 5.

ARE WE ALL POTENTIAL MIGRAINEURS?

What is a migraineur? The defining process or processes that determine migraine are unclear but we would argue that it is a symptom generated by normal brain structures and that everyone is effectively hard wired to suffer a migraine attack. Most people don't experience symptoms that are clearly identifiable as "migraine" as defined above during their lifetime, but many probably experience migrainous events unwittingly. Like a photograph developing in the dark room, the realization that a patient's symptoms stem from the migraine mechanism may only be understood when, at a critical moment, the condition becomes recognizable.

A single migraine attack does not make an individual a migraineur any more than a single seizure constitutes epilepsy. The IHS has arbitrarily deemed that a migraineur must have had at least five migraine headache attacks without aura to have MO and at least two with aura to have MA. It is not stated over what period they should have occurred. On this basis, it is estimated that 5% to 15% of women and 6% to 8% of men suffer from migraine and that 5% of people have at least 18 days of migraine attacks per year. Approximately 20% of migraine attacks are associated with aura (3). The 2003 U.K. Epidemiological Survey of 4007 households estimated that 5.8 million people aged 16 to 65 in the United Kingdom were current migraine sufferers, using IHC criteria (13). The epidemiology of migraine is explored further in Chapter 7.

THE MIGRAINE MECHANISM

We envisage that the migraine mechanism can be triggered at any time in any person. Moreover we believe that an individual's susceptibility or "threshold" for attacks is genetically determined, most likely by genes that regulate the sensitivity of brain cell ion channels or possibly specific integrated neural pathways or modules to particular activation mechanisms. This inherent threshold can be modified by constitutional factors such as age, sex, and hormonal activity. Triggers initiate a cascade of events that, if sufficient to exceed threshold, result in a migraine attack.

The activation pathway for the attack is usually well defined in an individual subject because particular neural networks are affected preferentially; symptoms tend to be stereotyped. However, the pathways can change on occasions and at different times of life, resulting in different symptoms or even a different form of primary headache. Once the migraine mechanism is engaged it usually has to "run its course," although interventions may terminate particular manifestations such as headache or nausea. It is possible that repeated interventions might actually prolong the timeframe of the process in some individuals, transforming a periodic disorder into a chronic condition.

Five clinical phases of a migraine attack can be identified (Fig. 1).

- Premonitory symptoms (or *prodrome*)
- Aura
- Headache
- Resolution
- Recovery (sometimes with "postdrome")

In many attacks, only one or two of these phases may be apparent; and although they usually follow this sequence, we will later illustrate that this is not always the case. It now seems possible that the aura and headache phases are independent. The duration of each phase is also variable, and phases may be temporally distinct or can overlap. Between migraine attacks, the neural networks may or may not return to normal, and this presumably determines the risk of a further attack in the short term.

Premonitory Symptoms

Some 20% to 30% of migraine sufferers are said to experience vague vegetative symptoms and behavioral changes before the migraine attack proper (14,15).

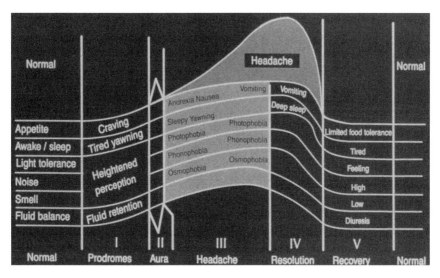

Figure 1 Symptoms and signs during a full house migraine attack. Most migraine attacks have less than these five stages. *Source*: Reprinted from Blau JN. Migraine: theories of pathogenesis. The Lancent vol. 339. 1202–1207. Copyright 1992, with permission from Elsevier.

These premonitory symptoms, previously called prodromes, are rare in our experience but they appear to be unique to the migraine phenotype. They can begin hours or even days before a migraine attack but may then blend with the symptoms of the attack proper.

Mood, Emotional, and Sensory Threshold Changes

During the premonitory phase, the sufferer feels "different." At the outset, there may be a period of arousal with heightened awareness with evidence of increased sensitivity, such as enhanced appreciation of visual contrast and colors, presumably reflecting "neuronal excitation." Other symptoms can then develop, such as elation or depression, hunger, thirst or cravings, fatigue, difficulty concentrating, yawning (considered to be generated from the paraventricular nucleus of the hypothalamus), and neck stiffness. Photophobia, phonophobia, and osmophobia may then evolve and usually become increasingly prominent as the attack progresses.

During the attack, the patient often seeks quiet and seclusion in the dark to limit the sensory aggravation. As the migraine attack subsides, there may be a postdrome during which symptoms may develop in the opposite sense, with lethargy, drowsiness, and "neurological depression" ("hebetude"). The migraineur may become drowsy, exhibit repeated yawning, and may even become confused or delirious. A short period of sleep may terminate an attack.

Patients who experience prodromal symptoms seem to be more susceptible to external triggers and generally experience more protracted aura and headache.

Very little is known of the underlying mechanisms, but some premonitory symptoms are consistent with dopaminergic activation. Between attacks, migraineurs demonstrate increased susceptibility to dopaminergic drugs such as apomorphine and bromocriptine, which can induce profound hypotension in migraineurs (16). Other premonitory symptoms suggest hypothalamic dysfunction, again possibly due to increased dopaminergic sensitivity. For example, L-deprenyl, which increases central dopamine, was found to produce a greater reduction in prolactin secretion in migraine patients than controls (16). In passing, it is noteworthy that the trigeminal autonomic cephalalgias (TACs), such as cluster headache, show hypothalamic activation during attacks (see Chapter 5) and that glyceryl trinitrate (GTN) may trigger migraine attacks with premonitory symptoms (17), an observation to which we will return later.

Fluid Balance

There may be significant changes in fluid balance during a migraine attack, presumably reflecting hypothalamic influences. Prior to the attack there is sometimes increasing thirst and fluid retention, with weight gain, tightness of clothes, rings, and shoes, and reduced urine output. However, fluid retention is not the cause of the headache, because it is not prevented by prophylactic diuresis (18). As Thomas Willis first observed (see Chapter 1), once the attack subsides, there is sometimes a phase of polyuria.

Gastrointestinal Symptoms

A number of gastrointestinal ("visceral" or "splanchnic") symptoms may evolve and subside during a migraine attack. Nausea may range from minimal to incapacitating, with repeated vomiting. Even if no nausea is experienced, there is usually at least anorexia. Waterbrash and other upper gastrointestinal symptoms, such as belching and hiccuping, may occur occasionally. These gastrointestinal symptoms can develop at any time during an attack. If nausea occurs early, it may prevent adequate absorption of oral rescue medication. This probably helps explain the common complaint of migraineurs that "nothing works" for the headache. Vomiting, like sleep, may terminate an attack.

Abdominal pain can also feature, and in "abdominal migraine" it may be the only manifestation (see Chapter 5). The pain may be intense, steady, and boring in quality, and examination may reveal gut distension with absent bowel sounds. Such attacks probably account for a proportion of surgical "acute abdomens" and "appendicitis with normal appendix." As the attack subsides, there may be colic followed by diarrhea and vomiting.

Autonomic Symptoms and Vasomotor Instability

Premonitory symptoms can also include manifestations of hyperactivity of both the sympathetic and parasympathetic nervous systems. Skin pallor, especially of the face, is common and often precedes the headache phase, although facial flushing may occur rarely. As we saw in Chapter 1, Du Bois-Réymond and Möllendorf, respectively, referred to "white migraine" and "red migraine" to describe these phenomena. The eyes may seem sunken (enophthalmos) or there may be periorbital edema due to transudation and sterile inflammation. The extracranial blood vessels may become swollen and extravasation can occur, with local edema, ecchymoses, or even skin hemorrhages. Signs characteristic of the TACs (see Chapter 5), including epiphora, conjunctival injection and edema, ptosis, miosis, and nasal blockage or discharge may be observed rarely prior to and during typical migraine attacks, as the following case illustrates.

CASE 1 MIGRAINE WITH PROMINENT TRIGEMINAL AUTONOMIC REFLEX

[Note that the features in this case are not compatible with a diagnosis of short-lasting unilateral neuralgiform headache with cranial autonomic symptom (SUNA) (see Chapter 5), chiefly because of their protracted duration]

A 22-year-old woman was referred by an otorhinolaryngologist because of troublesome recurrent facial and nasal symptoms that had not responded to treatment for "sinus headache." She described stereotyped attacks on either side, comprising a sudden piercing pain in the eye and supraorbital area, associated with ipsilateral nasal blockage, and sometimes ptosis, but without reddening or watering of the eye or pupillary changes. The head pain would then spread over the ipsilateral hemicranium. The headache often had a throbbing or even stabbing quality and would typically last all day. She would feel nauseous but did not vomit. She had a previous personal and family history of MO.

There may also be significant bradycardia. As will be discussed in Chapter 4, migraine is a common cause of otherwise unexplained syncope, which may occur in either the premonitory or headache phases. It can also occur in isolation as a migrainous equivalent. Sacks reported that 4% of migraineurs have syncope associated with aura on a frequent basis, but occasional syncopal attacks in isolation were recorded in 60 of 360 patients (19). Selby and Lance reported that 18 out of 60 of their cases had profound syncope, some with "seizure" features ("reflex anoxic seizures") (20).

Aura

As discussed in Chapter 1, the detailed description and characterization of migrainous visual aura and the subsequent proposal that cortical spreading depression (CSD) was a putative explanation for the phenomenon, put neural mechanisms to the forefront as the basis for migraine. We will now consider CSD in the context of its clinical expression.

What Is Cortical Spreading Depression?

In Chapter 1, we described how Karl Lashley first drew attention to the characteristics and temporal evolution of his own visual auras. He postulated that the scintillating edge of a teichopsia represented a wave of neural excitation, that propagated across the visual cortex, to be followed by neural depression, causing the scotoma. Three years later, while studying for his Ph.D. on epilepsy mechanisms, the Brazilian neurophysiologist Aristides Leão described cortical spreading depression (CSD), a hitherto unrecognized neural phenomenon observed in the electrocorticogram (ECoG) following stimulation of the exposed rabbit cortex by mild trauma or electrical stimulation (21,22). He observed a transient, complete suppression of neural activity at the focus of stimulation, with subsequent spread of the depression as a wave across the cortex at about 3 to 5 mm/min (see Chapter 1, Fig. 16). Milner later proposed CSD as the basis of visual aura (23).

The likely association between visual aura and CSD is immediately compelling. CSD comprises a short-lived positive wave of neural excitation, which traverses the cortex to a depth of about 5 mm, without regard to vascular boundaries, followed by a negative phase of neural depression. The unfolded human primary visual cortex is about 60 mm long and such a wave would take about 20 minutes to traverse it. This time interval fits very nicely with the typical duration and characteristics of aura.

The rate of expansion and size of the teichopsic arc in a spreading scintillating scotomatory migraine aura increases as it becomes more peripheral—as first beautifully illustrated by Hubert Airy (see Chapter 1, Fig. 7). This is not because the speed of CSD increases during propagation, but is a consequence of the retinotopic representation on the striate cortex from posterior to anterior. Thus, the cortical volume representing the fovea at the calcarine pole is large, and while the CSD spreads outwards the scintillation moves little in the visual field until the CSD enters more anterior cortical areas where retinotopic representation is smaller. Here, the progression of the CSD will cause an arc that accelerates away to the periphery of vision. Otto-Joachim Grüsser studied this in great depth. He examined the shape and position of his own migrainous phosphenes over time and found that the expansion of the hallucination conformed to an exponential function—the product of the first-order linear differential of the retinocortical magnification factor across the visual field and the presumed constant speed of the wave of CSD. The size of the phosphene pattern and extent of the trailing scotoma could also be predicted from the model. He showed that the phenomenon could be accounted for by an increase in extracellular K^+ and decrease in extracellular Ca^{2+} within the primary visual cortex, with a constant rate of ionic diffusion across the extracellular space (24).

Recent evidence indeed, suggests that the propagating CSD wave front is followed by an astrocytic Ca^{2+} wave that continues to propagate after CSD has terminated. The Ca^{2+} wave can cross gap junctions between astrocytes and the pia arachnoid, providing a direct link between CSD and structures mediating headache (7).

It is now well established in experimental models, that CSD is a common response to a variety of stimuli, including electrical stimulation, trauma, K^+, the excitatory neurotransmitter glutamate, and, importantly, nitric oxide donors such as glyceryl trinitrate (GTN). It can also be precipitated by carotid dissection and cerebral angiography, suggesting that an endothelial factor may be involved. Interestingly, topical application of endothelin-1, a potent vasoconstrictor, induced CSD in a rat model without causing ischemia (25).

Why Are "Typical" Auras Typical?

There would appear to be preferential pathways for the propagation of CSD, because certain auras, defined under IHC-2 as "typical" (visual hallucinations somesthetic and dysphasic symptoms) are more common than other forms of aura. Motor auras, for example, are distinctly uncommon. It seems likely that CSD is normally triggered by a critical increase in interstitial K^+ concentration. The control of interstitial K^+ concentration depends on glia. Neurons are a source of K^+, while glia represent a K^+ "sink," so it would therefore be expected that CSD would occur more readily in cortical sites with a low glia-to-neuron ratio. In Chapter 1, we mentioned that the susceptibility of brain areas to CSD probably depends on local glia-dependent K^+ homeostasis, and that the occipital cortex might be a "hot spot" for CSD because of its relatively low glia-to-neuron ratio compared, for example, to the frontal cortex (Table 2). It is also clear that CSD is more readily observed in lissencephalic than gyrencephalic animals such as primates, which have larger cortical glia-to-neuron ratios; and it cannot be elicited at all in the spinal cord, which has comparatively few nerve cell bodies (28).

Table 2 Crude Glia-to-Neuron Ratios in Different Cortical Regions: In Broad Terms, the Glial Content Is Greater in More Anterior Cortical Areas, Which Are Therefore Less Susceptible to Cortical Spreading Depression

Cortical area	Glia-to-neuron ratio
Left area 9	0.54
Right area 9	0.57
Left area 39	0.52
Left area 39	0.49
Area 17	0.49

Note: Area 9 is in the frontal cortex and area 39 is inferior parietal. Area 17 is calcarine cortex. Reference 26 except Area 17 which is reference 27.

Does Cortical Spreading Depression Account for the
Migraine Aura?

In Chapter 1, we noted that experimental CSD could be elicited readily in
the brains of lower animals and could also be provoked in several different
forms of neural tissue. However, it proved difficult to demonstrate this in
humans. It was not observed using conventional electroencephalogram
(EEG) recording during neurosurgery; and although it could be elicited in
the hippocampus or caudate nucleus during stereotactic surgery by ionto-
phoretic application of K^+, this was not followed by headache. However,
later magnetoencephalography studies of migraine with visual aura attacks
showed long-duration decrements and large-amplitude direct current (DC)
shifts suggestive of CSD, similar to observations in animal models (29,30).

In 1996, Mayevsky et al. reported that 1 of 14 patients undergoing
brain monitoring with a multiparametric system after head injury exhibited
a succession of spontaneous repetitive cortical EEG depressions that they
proposed. They suggested that this represented CSD, although their recording system did not allow mapping of the propagating wave (31). Tony
Strong and colleagues at Kings College Hospital in London subsequently
reported similar observations using electrocorticography (ECoG) in patients
undergoing open neurosurgical procedures for head injury and intracranial
hemorrhage (32). They observed episodes of spontaneous suppression of the
ECoG followed by recovery of the tracing after a period of complete silence,
as in Leão's original report Fig. 2 (22). Using sequential recordings from
the strip electrode, they were able to show that the locus of the electrical suppression spread from the initial site of origin at a rate consistent with CSD
in the majority of instances.

Studying Aura in Man Through Functional Brain Imaging

A number of brain scanning methods have been used to study brain function,
particularly aura, in migraine. It is notoriously difficult to recruit and study
patients who are in the throes of an acute migraine attack, and the recent use
of GTN as a trigger for the migraine mechanism has been an important
advance (see below). In Chapter 1, we discussed the early blood-flow studies
using single photon emission computed tomography (SPECT) reported by
the Danish schools. These generally showed that visual aura was associated
with occipital cortex oligemia but there was a rather poor correlation
between symptoms and the duration of the abnormality, which usually persisted well into the headache phase. Over the last decade, PET has been
used to study migraine; the timeframe parameters and spatial resolution of
this technique are much better than for SPECT. Still more recently, functional magnetic resonance imaging (fMRI), which allows dynamic studies of
cortical neuronal activity, has also been used. These newer techniques have
provided the best insight yet into regional cerebral blood flow (rCBF) changes in migraine. A brief outline of the results of these studies is given below.

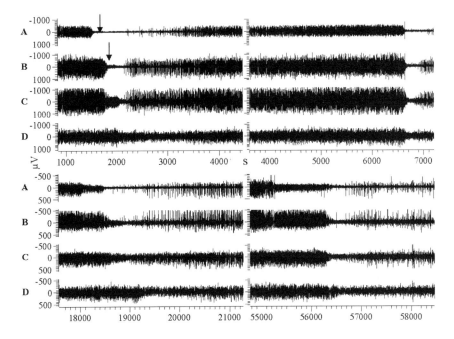

Figure 2 The first demonstration of cortical spreading depression by electrocortico-graphy (ECoG) in man. Time-compressed ECoG traces from subdural strips placed on the middle temporal gyrus after evacuation of a traumatic intracerebral haematoma (*upper*), and in a second patient (*lower*) after similar surgery (right frontal lobe). Each channel (A, B) shows the differential signal between a pair of adjacent electrodes 1cm apart on the strip (bipolar montage: A = 6/5, B = 5/4 etc). Scales: voltage = microvolts, time = seconds. Several periods of markedly depressed ECoG activity evolved over 10–30 seconds and lasted for 6–20 minutes (*arrows show two examples*). In channel C (*upper*), amplitude reduction occurs in two stages as the wave affects the first and later the second electrode in the pair. In the upper right trace, depression is synchronous in all channels, suggesting simultaneous arrival of SD at the strip from a lateral rather than end-on approach. Calculated propagation rates were 2.3 and 2.4 mm/minute in the upper traces, and ranged between 1.0 and 5.0 mm/min. in the lower trace consistent with that described by Leão and many others subsequently. Variation in velocity can be expected to result from variations in gyral anatomy underlying the ECoG strip in the gyrencephalic brain. *Source*: With permission from Strong AJ, Fabricus E, Boutelle MG, et al. Spreading and synchronous depressions of cortical activity in acutely injured human brain. Stroke 2002; 33:2738–2743.

Blood oxygen level–dependent functional magnetic resonance imaging, perfusion-weighted imaging, and diffusion-weighted imaging: The best evidence supporting CSD as the basis of aura in man comes from dynamic brain imaging during migraine aura (5,6). The sudden neuronal depolarization of CSD causes a secondary increase in rCBF lasting seconds ("neurogenic vasodilatation"), followed by neural suppression lasting minutes, accompanied by reduced rCBF. Many studies have now been published using blood oxygen level–dependent (BOLD) fMRI to study the sequence of events in visual aura, during both spontaneous and visually triggered attacks. During CSD, less oxygen is extracted from the activated, hyperperfused areas of the cortex and the proportion of deoxygenated hemoglobin therefore decreases. This reduces the paramagnetic effect on the transverse relaxation rate of protons, resulting in increased signal on T2-weighted images relative to baseline. Images can be collected rapidly to depict the sequence of neural activation during visual aura, and Margarita Sanchez del Rio and colleagues have produced dramatic illustrations of this process (Fig. 3) (7). These changes are unique to CSD.

Similar conclusions have been reached using perfusion-weighted imaging (PWI) (5). This technique examines MRI signal loss in brain regions during first-pass transit of a paramagnetic contrast medium, such as gadolinium, as an index of the total area of hypoperfusion. PWI studies

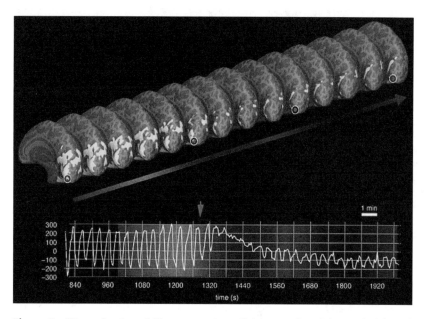

Figure 3 (*See color insert*) Demonstration of the neural activity underlying visual aura using BOLD-fMRI. A visual stimulus has triggered a teichopsic aura in a subject. The background signal oscillations are replaced with a steady initial signal increase, indicative of a temporary hyperaemia (*gray arrow*) that lasts about 3 to 4.5 minutes, spreading anteriorly at 3.5 mm per minuted and followed by hypoperfusion that lasts one to two hours, associated with reduced response to visual activation of the occipital cortex. *Abbreviation*: BOLD-fMRI, blood oxygen level–dependent functional magnetic resonance imaging. *Source*: Hadjikhanani N, Sanchez del Rio M, Wu O, et al. Mechanisms of migraine aura revealed by functional MRI in the human cortex. Proc Natl Acad Sci 2001; 98:4687–4692.

have shown a reduction in rCBF and cerebral blood volume, with an increased transit time of about one-third, confined to the affected occipital cortex during the aura phase and persisting up to 2.5 hours into the headache phase—similar to the timeline observed in earlier xenon studies. The resulting images can be compared with diffusion-weighted imaging (DWI), which defines areas of ischemic brain injury. Most importantly, such studies did not disclose a mismatch between PWI and DWI maps, showing that the oligemia associated with CSD is normally much less than the ischemic threshold (more than 50% decrease in rCBF) (33). Thus, the migraine mechanism "in isolation" does not normally cause ischemic brain injury—which is just as well!

The case for CSD as the mechanism of aura is convincing but there are phenomena that are difficult to reconcile. For example, auras can have a time course that is much shorter or much more prolonged than the "Lashley model." Some auras are only negative, others only positive; some do not seem to expand and not all are of the classical "scintillating scotoma" or teichopsia type that best conforms to the predicted consequences of CSD. As we will discuss later, the relationship between the aura and headache phases, both in terms of chronology and lateralization, is also challenging.

Pathophysiological Effects of Cortical Spreading Depression

Recent studies in animal models have shown that CSD results in activation of a number of genes in glia and neurons, which affect, among other things, neuroprotective responses to oxidative stress and the integrity of the blood–brain barrier (34). The result is a battle between potentially toxic and protective forces.

Neurotoxic and Protective Responses

Many potentially toxic agents, including K^+, H^+, and nitric oxide (NO) are released by CSD (35). These include galanin, which is known to promote the release of transmitters involved in nocioception (36). However, CSD also stimulates a number of neuroprotective mechanisms to counter these potentially neurotoxic effects. For example, cyclo-oxygenase 2 (COX2) expression is increased, encouraging local prostaglandin synthesis and thus reducing the risk of ischemia. In addition, there are local increases in the levels of tumor necrosis factor (TNFα), interleukin 1, and clusterin, a sulfated glycoprotein produced by neurons and activated astrocytes that has a protective function in response to brain injury (7).

Vascular Responses

CSD seems to produce both potentially deleterious and protective responses. As we will see in Chapter 4, stroke can be an occasional consequence of migraine, yet the migraine mechanism does not normally induce ischemia. What prevents this from happening? We do not know as yet, but CSD results in downregulation of the vasoconstrictor neuropeptide Y, while the vasodilatory atrial naturetic peptide is upregulated, consistent with the observed brief initial hyperperfusion of CSD (7). High K^+ levels and blockade of nitric oxide synthase (NOS) appear to abolish this hyperperfusion phase, resulting in more severe hypoperfusion during the oligemic phase with consequent cortical infarction in experimental models (37). It is possible that the vasodilatatory response might fail on rare occasions, leading to vasospasm and consequent infarction. Indeed, severe diffuse migrainous vasospasm leading to extensive cerebral infarction has been recorded (38). As we will discuss in Chapter 5, localized vasospasm may also be found in some instances of paroxysmal primary headaches, although it is not thought to be responsible for the headache per se.

Breach of the Blood–Brain Barrier

Extracellular proteinases can degrade intracellular matrix components, causing tissue injury. Michael Moskowitz has reported a marked increase in matrix metalloproteinase (MMP)-9 mRNA during CSD (39). This enzyme targets collagen IV and laminin, components of the zona occludens of capillary tight junctions. Upregulation was associated with breach of the blood–brain barrier in his model. This might allow potassium, nitric oxide, adenosine, and other products released by CSD to reach and sensitize the dural perivascular afferents. This process probably underlies the phenomenon of plasma protein extravasation (PPE) observed during experimental activation of the trigeminovascular system (TVS), which we will discuss shortly.

HEADACHE

Migraine headache can occur anywhere in the head and also in the neck or face. It is classically hemicranial but may be focal, bilateral (in about one-third of patients), or holocranial. It generally builds up over 30 minutes or so, lasts 4 to 72 hours (IHS definition, although in "real life" it may be much shorter, particularly in children, or indeed much longer), and is typically worsened by sensory inputs such as movement, light, sound, and odors. This suggests that sensitization of "sensory neural networks" is a key component—an increased afferent firing rate for an unchanged stimulus, resulting in a reduced threshold for transmission of nociceptive inputs.

There are a number of defined neural networks that mediate and modulate cranial pain (5). These include the following:

- Primary modality lateral pain pathway—trigeminal system, ventral posterior thalamus, and somatosensory cortex
- Autonomic and anti-nociceptive pathways—hypothalamus, periaqueductal grey (PAG), and ventral tegmentum
- Amygdala and hippocampus—emotional and affective responses
- Anterior thalamus—arousal and attention networks

- Basal ganglia and cerebellum—motor response preparation
- Anterior cingulate cortex and insula—integration and evaluation of pain

These brain areas have been shown to be activated in a number of pain paradigms studied by neuroimaging, including migraine, but migraine headache is also associated with other specific activation sites, as we will discuss.

Headache Mechanisms in Migraine

The headache phase seems to involve three main neural activation processes, but these may occur in any sequence or combination and the primacy of each in the overall headache mechanism is unclear and probably variable. These processes are:

- Activation of the TVS, leading to "neurogenic inflammation"
- Activation of the trigeminocervical complex (TCC) and consequent activation to variable extent of the trigeminal-autonomic reflex,
- Activation of cortical and brain stem regions involved in nociceptive transmission and modulation and the vomiting reflex

Neuroimaging studies using PET and BOLD-fMRI have demonstrated activation of certain brainstem regions, referred to as the "migraine generator," in association with the headache phase. Most importantly, unlike other areas activated as a general feature of head pain, the migraine generator regions remain activated after the headache has stopped. The relationship between CSD, brainstem activation, and the aura and headache phases is the subject of continuing interest. Figure 4 shows the main players in the headache mechanism, as we currently understand it.

Activation of the Trigeminovascular System— "Neurogenic Inflammation"

In Chapter 1, we described the evolution of the vascular theory of migraine. Evidence for the involvement of the cerebral vasculature in migraine is very clear from clinical observation alone, but blood vessel involvement now appears to be secondary to neural processes. With regard to the intracranial circulation, for example, we noted that there is no significant change in blood flow in the major intracranial arteries during typical migraine attacks. As measured by transcranial doppler, and as explained above, the changes in brain rCBF observed during aura are not independent but reflect neural activity. However, as known for centuries, prominent vascular changes affecting the extracranial circulation occur during a migraine attack. We now recognize that these result from both "peripheral" and "central" processes. In particular, changes in the meningeal vessels resulting from activation of the TVS may be an important factor in the headache phase.

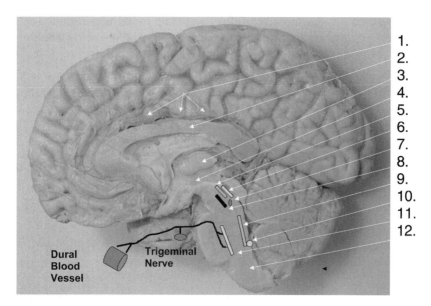

Figure 4 (*See color insert*) Sagittal section of the human brain, showing key components of the migraine mechanism. *Source*: Courtesy of Dr. Federico Roncaroli, Imperial College, London, U.K. *Key*: 1. Cingulate gyrus; 2. corpus callosum; 3. thalamus; 4. hypothalamus; 5. dorsal raphe nucleus; 6. periaqueductal grey; 7. red nucleus; 8. substantia nigra; 9. raphe nuclei; 10. area postrema; 11. trigeminal nucleus caudalis; 12. medulla oblongata.

Peripheral Activation and Sensitization

Surrounding the large cerebral vessels, venous sinuses and blood vessels of the pia and dura mater, is a plexus of largely unmyelinated fibers that arise

---

Figure 5 *(Figure on facing page)* The migraine mechanism. (*Upper panel*): Schematic representation of a typical attack of migraine with aura. CSD is initiated in the occipital cortex, resulting in a visual aura. Brainstem activation also occurs, with stimulation of the trigeminovascular reflex, possibly also the trigeminal autonomic reflex, and subsequent modulation of nociception from descending inputs. (*Lower panel*): Moskowitz's trigeminovascular hypothesis. (**A**) Meningeal vessels receive innervation from the first division of the trigeminal nerve. The nerve endings are uniquely characterised by axonal varicosities that contain a number of potentially nociceptive transmitters and peptides, including serotonin, histamine, bradykinin, prostaglandins and substance P. (**B**) CSD (or antidromic inputs from the brainstem) causes activation of the perivascular trigeminal axons, resulting in the release of these effector molecules. Nociceptive signals are transmitted orthodromically to the brainstem, while antidromic conduction results in the release of substance P into blood vessel walls. (**C**) Released substance P is thought to cause vessel dilatation and increased vascular permeability ("neurogenic inflammation," see Figure 6). It also causes thromboxane synthesis by macrophages, lymphocyte activation, and mast cell degranulation, with the release of histamine. *Abbreviation*: CSD, cortical spreading depression. *Source*: From Ref. 40.

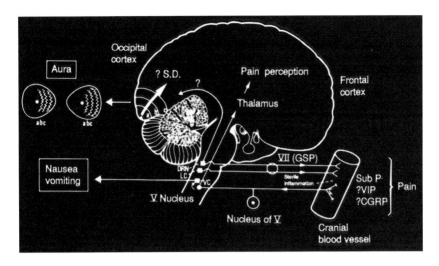

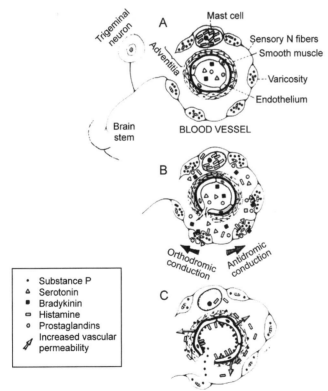

Figure 5 *(Caption on facing page)*

from the first (ophthalmic) division of the trigeminal nerve. The terminals of these nerve fibers bear varicosities that contain neurotransmitters and neuropeptides that are released into the walls of the vessel when the nerves are activated (Fig. 5). In a migraine attack, it seems that both peripheral and central processes are involved in the activation of these trigeminal fibers. The peripheral mechanisms are reasonably well understood.

Evidence of peripheral vascular activation in migraine headache comes from a number of observations. Calcitonin gene–related peptide (CGRP), one of the peptides contained in the trigeminal varicosities, was shown to increase in the jugular venous blood ipsilateral to the side of the headache during migraine attacks, and both the increase in CGRP and the migraine headache were inhibited by sumatriptan (3). There is good evidence that CGRP is released from meningeal afferent nerve fibers that are activated during the attack, and infusion of CGRP, one of the most potent vasodilators known, causes a migraine-like headache (3).

In a series of important experiments in animal models, Michael Moskowitz's group showed that the "neurochemical ferment" caused by spreading depression can activate meningeal primary sensory afferents, resulting in the release of effector molecules, including CGRP, substance P, and neurokinin A, into meningeal vessel walls, provoking "neurogenic inflammation" (Fig. 5). As a result, there is degranulation of mast cells in the vessel walls, releasing histamine and bradykinin, activating nitric oxide synthase (NOS) with the generation of nitric oxide (NO), and releasing prostaglandins. These events are thought to underlie PPE (3).

Consequent to the activation there is orthodromic transmission of nocioceptive signals to the brain stem, resulting in activation of the TCC. In keeping with this, as mentioned in Chapter 1, Doppler studies have shown that the walls of the middle meningeal artery ipsilateral to the headache swell during a typical migraine attack, while blood flow does not change.

Central Sensitization

In contrast to the peripheral mechanisms, the central processes involved in migraine pathophysiology are poorly understood. Thus far, we have largely considered the paradigm in which CSD initiates the headache phase by orthodromic stimulation of the brainstem via the TVS. However, it may be more often the case that the headache phase is initiated in the brainstem. Interestingly, hyperemia and extravasation of contrast medium from meningeal vessels, consistent with PPE secondary to neurogenic inflammation, has been demonstrated in an animal model by intrinsic brain stem activity (Fig. 6) (41,42).

Again, it has not yet been possible to image the activation of the TCC during migraine but indirect evidence of sensitization of the second-order neurons in the complex has come from the demonstration of reduced latency of nocioception-specific blink reflex responses (43) and from the

(A)

(B)

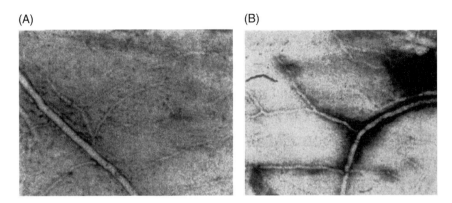

Figure 6 Plasma protein extravasation imaged. Trigeminal stimulation in the rat produces plasma protein extravasation. (**A**) Control (**B**) Stimulated. Triptans and other antimigraine drugs block this effect. *Source*: Reprinted from Brain Res. vol. 583, Buzzi MG, Dimitriadou V, Theoharides TC, et al. 5-Hydroxytryptamine receptor agonists for the abortive treatment of vascular headaches block mast cell, endothelial and platelet activation within the rat dura mater after trigeminal stimulation, 137–149. Copyright 1992, with permission from Elsevier.

demonstration by BOLD-fMRI of delayed nonpropagating blood-flow increase in ipsilateral meningeal vessels after initiation of CSD in an experimental model (44).

Moskowitz considers the trigeminal nerve/blood vessel interface as key to understanding migraine headache. In keeping with this, a number of drugs known to be effective in acute migraine treatment, such as triptans, have been shown to be capable of abolishing both headache and neurogenic inflammation. But there are inconsistencies. For example, whereas CGRP infusions cause migraine-like headache with associated vasodilatation, sildenafil causes migraine-like headache without vasodilatation (45), and a variety of agents that inhibit neurogenic inflammation but do not act centrally, such as conformationally restricted triptan analogues, have no effect on migraine headache (3). Conversely, while the 5-hydroxy tryptamine (5-HT)-selective agonist LY334370 was effective in stopping migraine headache in clinical trials, it lacks vasocontrictive properties and has no effect on neurogenic vasodilatation. It did, however, inhibit the second-order neurons of the TCC in an experimental model (3). Furthermore, from a purely clinical perspective, if CSD induces headache exclusively by neurogenic inflammation in meningeal vessels, how is aura without headache explained?

Activation of the Trigeminocervical Complex and the Trigeminal Autonomic Reflex

The trigeminal nerve afferents terminate on the ipsilateral principal trigeminal nucleus, which mediates general somatic sensation, and on the spinal trigeminal nucleus ["trigeminal nucleus caudalis," (TNC)]. The latter is analogous to (and indeed contiguous with) the ipsilateral dorsal horn of the spinal cord, together comprising the TCC. This complex is the origin of the second-order neurons that comprise the trigeminothalamic tract, which relays nocioceptive information to the thalamic nuclei and ventrolateral caudal periacqueductal gray matter (PAG) (Fig. 4).

Trigeminal autonomic reflex: The orthodromic trigeminal nocioceptive input to the brain stem may also result in delayed extracranial vasodilatation through activation of a parasympathetic reflex. The efferent arm of the reflex originates in the superior salivatory nucleus in the pons. Some 20% of the effect is mediated by antidromic activation of the trigeminal nerve and the remainder via the parasympathetic outflow of the facial nerve, through the greater superficial petrosal nerve to the pterygopalatine and otic ganglia. Neurogenic inflammation and reflex vasodilatation can be blocked by ipsilateral trigeminal nerve section, while the vasodilatation can be selectively blocked by a section of the ipsilateral parasympathetic fibers (3).

Stimulation of the trigeminal autonomic reflex results in parasympathetic symptoms and signs, which vary in magnitude in different primary headache syndromes (see Chapter 5). The most common clinical manifestations include changes in the external carotid vasculature, such as skin flushing ("red migraine"), sweating, and painful dilatation of blood vessels (which, as noted above, can rarely cause swelling and bruising), and sometimes nasal blockage or discharge, epiphora, and eyelid edema. Such features are not commonly experienced in typical migraine attacks but are defining symptoms of the TACs.

Facial pallor during attacks is much more common in typical migraine ("white migraine"). This presumably results from the general sympathetic stress response, which would cause bilateral affects.

Pupillary abnormalities in migraine: Occasionally, features of ocular sympathetic hypofunction can develop during headache attacks, resulting in partial Horner's syndrome (chiefly ptosis and miosis). This is thought to be a result of injury to sympathetic fibers investing the distended carotid vessel walls. Horner's syndrome is not uncommon in cluster headache and can be persistent, but can also occur rarely in migraine (46). Indeed, a variety of pupillary changes reflecting these autonomic disturbances can be seen during migraine attacks, as the following cases illustrate.

CASE 2: HORNER'S SYNDROME IN MIGRAINE

A 50-year-old man was referred with a history of stereotyped headaches dating back 10 years. In the previous six months, the attacks had been associated with prominent blurring of vision in the right eye. A typical attack would occur without warning or precipitant, and comprised either a dull discomfort in the right periorbital area or a more severe bifrontal headache spreading to the temples and then the neck. Photophobia was prominent but there was only mild nausea. During the attacks, his wife noted that he would develop a mild right-sided ptosis but there was no history of ipsilateral nasal symptoms or conjunctival injection. At the outset, the ptosis would recover between attacks but had recently become fixed. On examination, he was found to have a typical right-sided Horner's syndrome. No alternative cause was found on investigation.

CASE 3: ADIE'S PUPIL IN PRESUMPTIVE MIGRAINE ATTACKS

A 43-year-old woman developed a severe headache during the night. It was still present on waking the next morning, and she was aware of visual blurring. She noticed that her left pupil was markedly dilated but there were no other symptoms. She was seen in a local Emergency Room. The pupil showed the typical light-near dissociation of Adie's pupil. CT brain scan was normal and the pupil returned to normal over the course of a day. She was asymptomatic for a year, but then suffered an exact recurrence. Imaging by MRI on this occasion, including MR angiogram, was normal and she recovered fully within a day. She had no previous or family history of migraine.

Activation of Brain Stem Nuclei

Edward Liveing first mooted the brainstem rather than the cerebral cortex to be the source of migraine attacks. The observation by Bruyn and Ferrari that involuntary movements such as chorea could rarely be migraine auras also suggested brainstem involvement (47) and further support for the concept came from reports that brainstem stimulation during treatment of intractable pain could produce symptoms very similar to migraine (48,49). There are also case reports of tumors and vascular lesions in the brainstem producing migraine-like symptoms (50–52). These observations are considered further in Chapter 5, in connection with the phenomenon of "symptomatic migraine."

The migraine generator: Several imaging studies using PET and BOLD-fMRI during spontaneous and provoked headache attacks have demonstrated neural activation in brainstem nuclei. In 1995 Weiller et al. were the first to demonstrate such activation, in the region of the dorsal raphe nucleus, peri-aqueductal grey (PAG), and locus coeruleus, during spontaneous right-sided MO attacks (53). However, the resolution of their scanner prevented precise localization. Subsequent studies using PET and BOLD fMRI have confirmed these findings, although the sites of activation have been reported variously to also include the dorsal rostral pons (54) and the red nucleus and substantia nigra (Fig. 7) (55). These studies usually showed activation of the cingulate gyrus, insula, thalamus, and cerebellum ipsilateral to the headache, and sometimes bilaterally. It was later shown that these other activation sites were not integral to the migraine mechanism but were involved in general cranial pain perception because they were activated independent of the brainstem nuclei by application of capsaicin to the forehead (56). It has also been a general observation that when sumatriptan was used to abolish the migraine headache, activity was no longer evident in the "nonspecific"

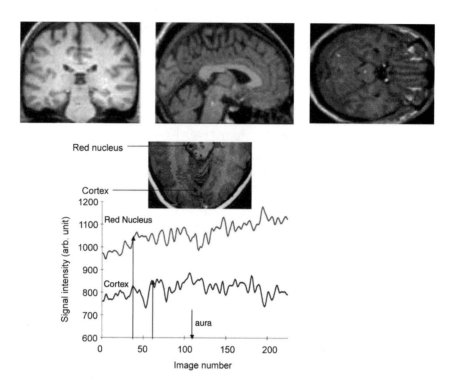

Figure 7 (*See color insert*) Neuroimaging of brainstem in migraine. (*Upper panel*): PET activation study. A migraine-without-aura attack has been triggered in a patient, who normally suffered from cluster headache, using glyceryl trinitrate. There is migraine-specific activation of the dorsal pons. (*Lower panel*): BOLD-functional magnetic resonance imaging study of a migraine with visual aura attack. A visual stimulus has triggered an attack, which in this case resulted in increased regional cerebral blood flow in the appropriate visual cortex followed by activation of the brain stem in the region of the red nucleus and substantia nigra. *Abbreviations*: PET, positron emission tomography; BOLD, blood oxygen level–dependent. *Source*: (*Upper panel*) Reprinted from Bahra A, Matharu M, Buchel C, et al. Brainstem activation specific to migraine headache. The Lancet, vol. 357:1016 1017. Copyright 2001 with permission from Elsevier. (*Lower Panel*) From Cao Y, Aurora SK, Nagesh V, et al. Functional MRI-BOLD of brainstem structures during visually triggered migraine. Neurology 2002; 59:72–78, with permission.

activation sites whereas the brainstem activation persisted. We will describe and illustrate some recent neuroimaging experiments of this type below.

It is not yet established how long this brainstem activation persists in typical migraine attacks, but ongoing activation has been observed in chronic migraine. When this condition was treated with an occipital nerve stimulator, headache was abolished but the brainstem activation persisted, and there was immediate recurrence of headache when the stimulator was turned off (1). This supports the concept that failure of the migraine mechanism to "switch off" for whatever reason, is likely to be a common cause of chronic daily headache.

It seems, therefore, that activation of brainstem structures plays a crucial part in the genesis of migraine headache and that aggravating factors that preserve activation might determine the transformation of episodic migraine to chronic migraine. However, although these brainstem activation sites have been referred to as the "migraine generator," it is possible that they are, in fact, part of the pain-modulating pathways rather than the site of "migraine initiation" (3). A descending inhibitory network extends from the frontal cortex and hypothalamus through the PAG to the rostral ventromedial medulla (including the raphe nuclei and reticular formation), down to the medulla and dorsal spinal horn (Fig. 4). Trigeminothalamic connections to other midbrain nuclei are involved in pain modulation and also in the activation of the vomiting reflex, via the tractus solitarius (see below). One suggestion is that different brainstem structures might participate in headache pathogenesis by either lowering the "migraine threshold" or decreasing the inhibitory nociceptive drive (5).

Allodynia

A series of important clinical and experimental studies by Rami Burstein's group have focused on central neural processing in the migraine mechanism. They reported that a majority of patients experience "allodynia," the appreciation of pain in response to normally nonpainful stimuli, during migraine attacks (57,58). Allodynia is thus the clinical expression of peripheral (afferent) and central sensitization.

"Peripheral" sensitization results in lowered sensory thresholds to all external stimuli. Neural firing rates are increased, and there is expansion of nociceptive receptor fields. Sensitization of trigeminovascular afferent nerve endings to mechanical stimuli would explain the throbbing quality of vascular headache and the worsening of headache by factors that increase intracranial pressure, such as coughing and stooping. Burstein's group reported that allodynia affected initially the distribution of the first division of the trigeminal nerve as a result of sensitization of the TNC (the rostral TCC), which receives afferent inputs from the meninges and periorbital skin. Subsequently, more extensive areas over the head and beyond are affected as a result of sensitization of third-order trigeminal thalamic neurons (57,58).

"Central" sensitization is the response in the brainstem to this increased sensory input. Manifestations include upregulation of *c-fos*, an early response gene, in the TNC neurons. There is also increased excitability of nociceptive neurons in the brain stem, which outlasts the duration of input, such that normally subthreshold inputs to the second-order neurons reach threshold, causing a protracted increase in sensitivity of cranial thermal and mechanoreceptors. Even anesthetic block of the primary dural afferents in rats did not diminish the protracted cutaneous allodynia in an animal model (59). It is of interest with regard to our later discussion, that the sensitization mechanisms underlying allodynia appear to be mediated by nitric oxide (NO), which in experimental animals increased nNOS and *c-fos* in TNC neurons, with protracted effects (3).

RESOLUTION AND POSTDROME

The processes involved in terminating a migraine attack are even less clearly understood than the events underlying initiation or the attack itself. Many patients find that a period of sleep can help, possibly by reducing sensory input; but why does vomiting sometimes also bring relief? Indeed, why does the headache usually stop? Better understanding could lead to better migraine treatments.

Nausea and Vomiting in Migraine

Anorexia, nausea, and vomiting are cardinal manifestations of the migraine mechanism and can occur at any time during an attack. Early-onset nausea and vomiting may reduce the effectiveness of oral antimigraine drugs while, paradoxically, the development of these symptoms late in the attack may herald resolution.

The structures comprising the vomiting center mark the caudal end of the migraine mechanism (see below and Fig. 4). The vomiting reflex is driven by efferent output from the vomiting center in the medulla, relaying to the vagus and motor neurons that supply the abdominal muscles and diaphragm, and can be triggered as a response to a variety of inputs—both internal and external. In migraine, the reflex is presumably activated as part of the brainstem activation intrinsic to the headache phase. The likelihood of nausea and vomiting occurring in an attack is closely related to headache severity. These symptoms are not typical features of acephalalgic migraine attacks, although the reflex can also by triggered by psychological insults such as certain unpleasant sights and odors to which migraineurs are more sensitive during attacks.

The vomiting mechanism comprises the following:

- The vomiting center—a diffuse network of neurons in the dorsolateral reticular formation of the medulla, which controls and coordinates the vomiting reflex through complex interactions between the parvicellular reticular formation, the nucleus tractus solitarius, autonomic nuclei and visceral and somatic nuclei, particularly the vagus nerve. The vomiting center also receives a wide range of afferent inputs from receptors in the gastrointestinal tract, peripheral pain receptors (responsible for the nausea that may accompany trauma), the nucleus tractus solitarius (involved in the gag reflex), vestibular system (involved in motion sickness), and the cerebral cortex (emotional triggers and possibly vomiting due to raised intracranial pressure). A large number of neurotransmitters are active in this region, with acetylcholine and histamine being particularly important.

- The chemoreceptor trigger zone (CTZ, area postrema)—a group of cells lying at the obex on the floor of the fourth ventricle. This area is extremely vascular and lies outside the blood–brain barrier, which makes it vulnerable to circulating drugs and toxins. The CTZ is also an integration center for baroreceptor function and the control of food intake and sleep. The two important neurotransmitters here are dopamine and 5-HT.

We will consider this again when we discuss the issue of the management of nausea and vomiting in migraine in Chapter 7.

Postdrome

There was a widely held belief among physicians in a bygone era that migraine "has to run its course." This could well be true. Even after the migraine headache has resolved, many patients remain unwell and although able to return to work or other activities, they may function suboptimally. As noted above, the postdrome may include symptoms that are, in a sense, the obverse of the prodrome.

What is going on in the brain at this time is unclear. Although there is no spontaneous headache, movements may produce headache and the sensory system remains hypersensitive. Another manifestation is rebound headache, which seems to be more common in patients who have experienced initial relief with triptans compared with other rescue medications, possibly because triptans work more quickly. Repeated interventions with rescue medications might be one factor in the pathogenesis of chronic migraine.

Neuroimaging studies that include this phase of the migraine attack are somewhat contradictory. Previous blood-flow studies showed persisting oligemia in cortical areas involved in aura, while more recent neuroimaging studies have shown ongoing brainstem activation, for example, in chronic migraine (1).

MIGRAINE MODELS

In the absence of a biological marker for "migraine," a great deal of interest has focused on factors that seem to precipitate migraine attacks in some individuals in a reproducible and predictable fashion. Patients sensitive to identifiable triggers have been invaluable in research into the migraine mechanism. The common triggers used in research have included visual stimuli, such as the alternating checkerboard, and a number of drugs and chemicals.

In Chapter 1, we noted that the antihypertensive reserpine had been notorious in its tendency to cause headache, and observations on this drug have provided important insights into the role of 5-HT in migraine.

Histamine was also found to readily induce headache and was used experimentally in the 1950s (60). Migraine sufferers were found to be more sensitive to subcutaneous histamine than controls, and the character of the headache was more likely to be "migrainous." This effect was later shown to be mediated through arterial endothelial histamine H_1 receptors and was prevented by the H_1 receptor blocker mepyramine.

It had been known since the late nineteenth century that glyceryl trinitrate (GTN) could precipitate both migraine and what we now interpret as cluster headache (60). Moreover it was suggested that GTN might be used as a diagnostic test (62). Olesen and Iversen in Denmark later revived this idea (63). It seems that histamine stimulates NO production from the vascular endothelium, and intravenous GTN was found to cause a very similar headache. But because mepyramine did not inhibit GTN headache, in contrast to its effect in histamine headache, it was reasoned that NO was the common headache effector (64). Sumatriptan was then shown to abort GTN-induced headache in a clinical trial, independently of any effect on cerebral blood flow, although the drug did cause a modest reduction in the diameters of superficial cranial vessels (65). Olesen's group subsequently showed that a specific NOS inhibitor blocked the GTN effect (66). In further studies, NO caused an immediate and reproducible dilatation of meningeal blood vessels, which was partially blocked by sumatriptan and indomethacin (which inhibits trigeminal activation and CGRP release), while flunarizine, and histamine H_1 and H_2 receptor antagonists, were unable to prevent the dilatation (67).

Triggering of Migraine by Intravenous GTN

GTN certainly seems to be a compelling model for migraine attacks. It has been established that GTN produces a headache that fulfils the IHS migraine criteria in all respects and faithfully reproduces the characteristics of individual patients' attacks. The intravenous GTN test has been rapidly adopted as a tool for studying the migraine mechanism. The consistency and relative ease with which migraine can be induced in this way has obvious logistical advantages over the study of patients during spontaneous attacks or attacks triggered by other means.

It is suggested that up to 80% of migraineurs are susceptible to triggering by GTN. For example, in a recent study by Shazia Afridi and colleagues in Peter Goadsby's group, at Queen Square intravenous GTN 0.5 mcg/kg/min was administered to 44 migraineurs (23 MO and 21 MA) and 12 controls. All subjects experienced a mild or modest drug-related headache over the period of infusion, but while this resolved in the controls, 33 of the 44 migraine patients subsequently developed a typical migraine attack after a delay of about two hours. Thirty-two of the provoked attacks were MO but one patient had typical migraine with visual aura. Intriguingly, 12 of the migraineurs also described premonitory symptoms, never before reported in chemically triggered migraine. In addition, repeat attacks were triggered using GTN in all but one patient, including visual aura in the patient who had also experienced this the first time (68).

In a follow-up study, Afridi and colleagues examined brain activation by PET in this model and, in particular, the relationship between headache lateralization and brainstem activation. They found that brainstem activation was invariably located in the dorsal pons and was always ipsilateral to the headache, or bilateral in cases with bilateral headache (Fig. 8). As in earlier studies noted above, the brainstem activation persisted after the headache had been terminated with subcutaneous sumatriptan (69).

One criticism of this GTN model is that it seems difficult to induce aura in patients who habitually experience it with their migraine attacks. Thus, only one patient in each of Afridi's two studies, which included a significant number of MA cases, experienced a triggered aura. This seems to be a common experience although greater success has been claimed (70,71). However, Afridi went on to further study one of her cases who had experienced GTN-induced MA, and for the first time was able to demonstrate both occipital cortical and brainstem activation appropriate to the visual aura using PET, supporting observations from fMRI studies (Fig. 9) (72).

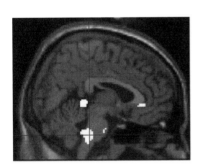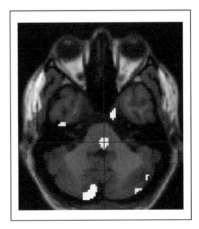

Figure 8 (*See color insert*) PET studies in GTN–triggered migraine. Dorsal pontine activation. Nonspecific activation also seen in the cerebellum and anterior cingulate. *Abbreviations*: PET, positron emission tomography; GTN, glyceryl trinitrate. *Source*: With permission from Afridi S, Matharu MS, Lee L, et al. A PET study exploring the laterality of brainstem activation in migraine using glyceryl trinitrate. Brain vol. 128, 2005; 128: 936.

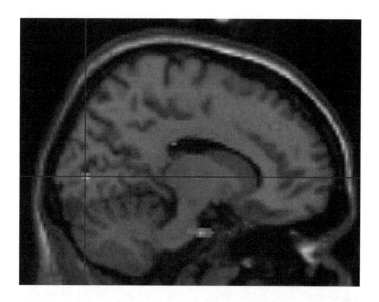

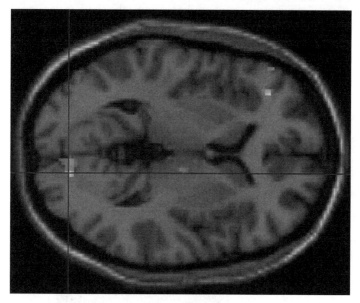

Figure 9 (*See color insert*) GTN-triggered PET activation study, showing both occipital cortex and brainstem activation during migraine with visual aura. *Abbreviations*: GTN, glyceryl trinitrate; PET, positron emission tomography. *Source*: Afridi S, Kaube H, Goadsby PJ. Occipital activation in glyceryl trinitrate induced migraine with visual aura. J Neurol Neurosurg Psychiatr 2005; 76:1158–1160; with permission from the BMJ Publishing Group.

It has, therefore, been suggested that NO might, in fact, be the chemical mediator of the migraine mechanism in both the brainstem and cortex. NO is generated in the vascular endothelium and circulates in blood, and its levels are increased by estrogen, possibly relevant to the well-recognized relationship between migraine attacks and menstruation. Typical attacks of migraine can be triggered by exogenous NO donors, and migraine headache can be blocked by drugs such as sumatriptan, indomethacin, and specific NOS inhibitors. We will return to the implications of these observations with regard to future migraine treatments, in Chapter 7.

HOW DO MIGRAINES START?

How do the components of the migraine mechanism link to produce the clinical features of a migraine attack? In the foregoing account, we have alluded to the issue of the temporal relationship between the different phases of migraine, and the question now arises as to the extent that these are dependent on each other. Individual migraine attacks are characteristically stereotyped, which might imply a link between the different phases. But do these phases occur in series; or are they only loosely connected, with their temporal sequence determined by parallel but dissociated processes? One immediately relevant issue in this discussion is the relationship between CSD and brainstem activation. Does CSD always cause brainstem activation via the TVS? This is current orthodoxy, at least in the case of MA (3–5), but one alternative view is that the headache phase in migraine is not the result of increased input to the brainstem as a result of CSD, but the consequence of impaired nociceptive regulation within the central nervous system (73).

Serial Processing? Aura Triggers Headache

In most episodes of typical MA, premonitory symptoms precede and blend with aura, and are then followed by headache, sometimes with a distinct intermission between the phases. It would be reasonable to infer, therefore, that this is a serial process in which aura triggers headache. However, while auras normally precede headache, they are occasionally perceived by patients to "follow" or at least intrude into the headache phase, as the following cases illustrate.

CASE 4: VISUAL AURA FOLLOWED BY SOMESTHETIC AURA
EVOLVING DURING THE HEADACHE PHASE

A 37-year-old woman presented with migraine with visual auras comprising typical central scintillating scotoma followed by migraine headache. These attacks could be precipitated by red wine, cheese, and chocolate; her mother also had migraine. On some occasions, the visual aura was followed by the headache phase in the normal manner but in other attacks, as the visual aura resolved, she would experience spreading parasthesia of the right arm over the subsequent 45 to 60 minutes, during the headache phase. The headache then continued for up to three days.

CASE 5: BASILAR TYPE MIGRAINE WITH AURA
FOLLOWING HEADACHE

The day before delivery of her first child, a 28-year-old woman suddenly experienced a "blinding" left frontal headache. The headache continued, and after 15 minutes, she experienced severe difficulty speaking, then tingling in the tongue and both periorbital areas, and then sequentially, in the left face, right arm and face, and then the left face and leg. The headache and sensory disturbances persisted until delivery and were associated with nausea and vomiting on two occasions. All the symptoms resolved rapidly after the birth. She had suffered very similar symptoms seven years earlier and had undergone extensive investigation, including MRI, brain scan, extracranial ultrasound studies, and transthoracic echocardiography, with negative results. Her mother suffered from migraine.

CASE 6: "HEMIPLEGIC MIGRAINE" WITH HEMIPLEGIA
FOLLOWING HEADACHE

A 25-year-old woman gave a history of episodic left-sided paralytic attacks dating from infancy. The first attack occurred at one year of age. While crawling, she suddenly became weak on the left side for 5 to 10 minutes, and then recovered fully. She had an identical attack at age 2, lasting two hours, but recovered after a short sleep. She had no further neurological symptoms until more than 20 years later, when she suddenly experienced several more attacks of left-sided paralysis over several weeks, some lasting only a few seconds. On a number of these occasions, episodes of paralysis were preceded by severe headache, lasting up to two hours. Her mother had typical MA attacks. MRI brain scan, magnetic resonance angiogram, extracranial ultrasound, and EEG were all normal.

   (In retrospect, this was possibly a case of familial hemiplegic migraine (FHM), but she was lost to follow-up).

   These three cases would suggest that the processes driving the aura and headache phases might run independently. It is also worth noting, from a historical perspective, that auras can recapitulate, as first illustrated by Dr. Hubert Airy (see Chapter 1, Fig. 7).

Parallel Processing? Aura and Headache Are Not/Only
Loosely Connected

Of course, a further problem with the serial processing theory is that most patients have neither premonitory symptoms nor aura, and, conversely, premonitory symptoms and auras sometimes occur without associated headache (74). Both clinical and experimental observations suggest that the situation is more complex than the simple serial processing model. For example, rCBF changes reflecting CSD should be seen on the same side as the headache due to ipsilateral activation of the TVS and TCC, whereas the aura symptoms should be perceived on the opposite side. However, headache and aura symptoms are sometimes experienced on the *same* side, and imaging studies have also occasionally shown rCBF changes contralateral to the side of headache. Furthermore, while rCBF gradually returns to normal toward the end of the aura phase and into the headache phase, patchy increases can occur subsequently without causing recurrent aura (3).

Silent Aura

One possibility, therefore, is that all migraine starts with cortical activation but this usually produces no symptoms—the concept of *silent aura*. We would presume that in such circumstances, CSD either fails to sensitize the nociceptive fields or involves noneloquent parts of the brain. There is some evidence to support this idea. In 1994, Woods et al. described a case in which changes compatible with bilateral CSD were observed during an attack of MO, using H_2O^{15} PET (75), and similar global hypoperfusion was reported in MO attacks by Bednarczyk et al. (76). Cao et al. (55) also found that visually triggered migraine attacks of both MA and MO could be associated with hyperemia of the occipital cortex on BOLD-fMRI, irrespective of whether visual aura occurred.

Modular Theory

Some 80% of migraine attacks are not associated with aura, so the alternative hypothesis is that CSD is not the initiation process for migraine headache. Rather, headache could be generated by direct activation of the "migraine generator" in the brainstem—a veritable black box solution! Peripheral sensitization could still occur through antidromic stimulation of the TVS. Recently, a modular theory has been proposed. This envisages a network of interacting neural networks (modules) that determine the nature and time course of the different migraine symptoms. During attacks, certain modular components are activated preferentially, explaining the habitual stereotypy of the symptoms in a particular patient, but other structures may become activated on occasions, resulting in variations (77). We will return to this rather attractive concept in Chapter 6.

WHY DO MIGRAINES START?

Triggers

Some 10% of migraine patients can identify particular agents or circumstances that will almost always induce their migraine attacks. Triggers may be "internal" or "external." Some are highly idiosyncratic, and it is difficult to discern a common theme. External triggers feed directly into the brain through the relevant cranial nerves (olfactory, optic, auditory, etc.), while internal triggers seem to relate to biological rhythms, such as the circadian cycle, length of daylight hours, and the menstrual cycle. Some triggers appear to act very quickly. The glare of the setting sun on the rippling sea, for example, may produce aura within seconds. Others seem rather slow. For example, chocolate consumption can trigger migraine in certain individuals but the trigger often takes several hours. Some triggers seem to set off one type of migraine only; menstrual migraine is almost never MA—but quite where or how they trigger is very poorly understood.

Internal Triggers

The most frequently cited internal trigger is "stress," or actually more often, apparent relief from stress, because a migraine attack is sometimes the "reward" for a prolonged period of hard mental work—the so called "weekend headache"! Perhaps this is the result of a sudden fall in circulating adrenaline levels, causing a reduction in 5-HT receptor stimulation, (adrenaline has agonist actions at $5-HT_2$ receptors). Other notable internal stimuli include sleep deprivation or poor sleep quality, starvation, and hormonal fluctuation in women, as the following cases illustrate.

CASE 7: STARVATION INITIATES MIGRAINE-TRIGGERED SEIZURES

A 19-year-old woman was admitted electively for appendectomy because of recurrent episodes of abdominal pain dating from childhood for which no cause could be found. Six days after discharge her mother heard her cry out and the patient was found on her bed unconscious. She had probably had a generalized seizure and was markedly amnesic for some time afterward. She had eaten very little in the previous 24 hours.

She had a protracted history of intermittent headaches, usually located around one or other eye, with associated nausea. On one occasion, an attack had been associated with a brief syncope. Two years earlier, while on a diet, she had suddenly developed a severe headache. She had slept for a short period but on waking developed uncontrolled generalized jerking, presumably myoclonic, without impairment of consciousness, and then suffered recurrences of these symptoms on waking on each of several subsequent days.

Baseline EEG was normal but bilateral frontal spike and slow wave discharges developed during hyperventilation. She subsequently had a further seizure early one morning. A finger prick blood sample indicated mild hypoglycemia but a 72-hour fast demonstrated normal, stable blood glucose levels throughout. She was advised to eat regularly and properly and had no further headaches, blackouts, or seizures on follow-up.

CASE 8: HORMONE REPLACEMENT THERAPY TRIGGERS MIGRAINE DE NOVO

A 43-year-old woman with no previous headache history underwent a hysterectomy and bilateral salpingo-oophorectomy and was treated subsequently with hormone replacement therapy (HRT). She was fine for four months but then began to have recurrent unilateral or more generalized headaches associated with nausea and occasional vomiting. The attacks occurred weekly. After three months, the HRT was stopped. The headaches gradually reduced in frequency, and on review a few months later, she had gone a month with no attacks at all. Subsequently, due to increasing menopausal symptoms, she restarted HRT and the migraine attacks returned. She then stopped HRT once more, and the migraine attacks stopped again.

Circadian rhythms and seasonal influences: A prominent feature of primary headaches is their diurnal variation and link with sleep; the "internal clock" has an important influence on primary headaches. For example, many patients report migraine onset as they wake, and as noted (somewhat paradoxically) returning to sleep can terminate attacks. Migraine is perhaps the only primary headache that can be stopped in this way.

Cluster headache attacks characteristically develop during sleep, waking the patient in the early hours of the morning, whereas hypnic headache occurs exclusively during sleep (see Chapter 5, p. 225). Cluster headache by definition shows periodic behavior, but migraine attacks can also "cluster" chronologically (see Chapter 5, p. 230). Cluster headache and migraine also show seasonal influences in some sufferers.

The suprachiasmatic nucleus (SCN) of the hypothalamus is the site of a "master circadian pacemaker" (78). It closely controls internal physiological, hormonal, and behavioral rhythms. Exposure to light, and physical and social activities, set these circadian rhythms to the 24-hour clock, which can be easily disrupted, for example, by sleep deprivation and jet lag. Light activates pathways that affect the pineal gland and the secretion of melatonin. Melatonin secretion occurs in darkness and modulates the neural activity of the circadian clock. The SCN projects to areas of the hypothalamus, such as the dorsomedial and preoptic areas, which then project to other areas concerned with sleep regulation, such as the ventral lateral preoptic nucleus, and to "wakening" centers in the brainstem. There are also projections to pain-modulating pathways.

There is now increasing evidence that changes in these hypothalamic sleep and wakening centers play a role in the mechanisms underlying at least some of the primary headache syndromes. The strongest evidence for hypothalamic involvement in primary headache is in the TACs. As noted above, PET studies show activation of the ipsilateral posterior inferior hypothalamus during attacks (see also Chapter 5). Further evidence for hypothalamic involvement in cluster headache comes from a number of neuroendocrine studies that show altered hormonal levels during acute attacks. Melatonin production is reduced in cluster headache patients (79). Whether these changes are primary or merely associations remains to be seen. The premonitory symptoms of migraine, as we have noted, suggest hypothalamic involvement but unfortunately there are no neuroimaging studies (to our knowledge) of this stage of the acute migraine attack.

Sleep: Sleep in the adult consists of four to six cycles, each of about 90 minutes duration. In each cycle there is a period of non–rapid eye movement (NREM) sleep followed by a shorter period of rapid eye movement (REM) sleep. NREM sleep is divided into four stages of increasing depth (stages I–IV). NREM predominates early and REM late in a normal night's sleep. REM is thought to be initiated by cholinergic neurons in the dorsolateral tegmental and pedunculopontine nuclei, while REM "off" cells have been found in the noradrenergic locus coeruleus and the serotonergic dorsal raphe nucleus.

As noted, sleep can both resolve and precipitate primary headaches, and sleep is particularly provocative in cluster headache, hypnic headache, and exploding head syndrome (see Chapter 5) (80). Cluster attacks often start about 90 minutes after the sufferer falls asleep, and this coincides with the first REM sleep of the night. However, attacks are also seen in NREM sleep. With advancing age, the function of the hypothalamic-pineal axis and the SCN declines. It is unclear how this might relate to hypnic headache, but this is a condition of elderly patients. It has been shown that these syndromes can respond to melatonin and lithium, both of which impact on the sleep–wake cycle (80).

We will consider the relationship between migraine, dreams, and nightmares in Chapter 3.

External Triggers

Particular foods and drinks are commonly said to "cause" migraine. These include alcoholic beverages, cheese, chocolate, and citrus fruit. Red wine and other alcoholic drinks have been studied with particular interest— arguably one of the more engaging fields of headache research! Patients may describe themselves as "allergic" to such triggers but there no convincing evidence that the effect is immunologically mediated.

Richard Peatfield and colleagues at Charing Cross Hospital studied the effects of the 5-HT_2 antagonists ketanserin and pizotifen in patients who typically developed migraine after drinking red wine. Both drugs effectively blocked the response, whereas mepyramine did not. No definite conclusions could be drawn concerning the mechanism of red wine–induced migraine but the findings suggested that the effect was mediated by different receptors in different patients (81).

Other external triggers include increased visual, auditory, or olfactory inputs such as intensely bright or flashing lights, patterns, loud noises, and perfumes. Use of such triggers in susceptible migraineurs has been invaluable in migraine imaging studies, as noted above. Physical triggers can also be identified in some cases. These can include head injury ("post-traumatic migraine") and exercise, as illustrated by the following cases. Note that exercise-triggered migraine needs to be distinguished from "exertional cephalalgia" (see Chapter 5).

CASE 9: EXERCISE-TRIGGERED MIGRAINE
A 13-year-old boy was referred with stereotyped headaches associated exclusively with sporting activities. Attacks would not occur with every such event and were quite unpredictable. He had no symptoms during the sporting activity; attacks would typically start one to two hours afterwards. Each began with a two-minute visual aura of blurred vision followed by shattering of the image. Shortly afterwards, he would experience headache, always in the right frontal region, lasting up to two hours. He was occasionally nauseous but rarely vomited. On two occasions he had also

experienced paresthesiae in his left arm during the headache phase, lasting about five minutes. His father was a migraineur. Neuroimaging showed no abnormality.

CASE 10: EXERCISE-TRIGGERED MIGRAINOUS VISUAL AURAS

A 26-year-old woman suffered two attacks of MA as a young teenager. On each occasion she remembered losing vision to the right for 30 minutes, and then experiencing a bad headache and nausea lasting 24 hours. She was then asymptomatic until a year prior to referral. Over that year, she experienced six attacks of loss of vision, each lasting 30 minutes, very similar to the visual auras in her earlier attacks, except that there was no headache. On each occasion, the attacks had occurred an hour or so after a workout at the gym.

Migraine attacks can sometimes be initiated by neck pain, presumably through C2–C4 cervical afferent inputs to the TCC. This observation links migraine to "cervicogenic headache," and there are anecdotal reports of interventions such as cervical foramenotomy ameliorating migraine attacks. Electrical stimulation of the occipital nerves is currently being explored as a treatment for chronic intractable migraine (1). The following case illustrates the association.

CASE 11: MIGRAINE TRIGGERED BY CERVICAL MANIPULATION

A 51-year-old woman presented with a history of MO dating back some 30 years. Attacks were heralded by nausea, fatigue, and watering of the right eye and she would often vomit repeatedly throughout the 24 hours of the attack. She had three or four attacks per year and both her father and sister had migraine. She began to be troubled by neck and shoulder discomfort and was referred for physiotherapy by her rheumatologist. She noticed that following each and every session of neck manipulation, she would suffer a typical migraine attack such that at the time of neurological referral she was having two to three attacks per week. She had also had two attacks of migrainous syncope (see Chapter 4). The attacks stopped when the physiotherapy was discontinued.

Recently, an apparent association between MA and patent foramen ovale (PFO) has also been recognized. This is discussed extensively in Chapters 4 and 7 but it is of interest that intravenous injection of air-agitated saline or gelofusin during contrast echocardiography to identify PFO will sometimes precipitate typical MA in migraineurs with significant right-to-left shunts (personal communication, Dr Michael Mullen, Consultant Cardiologist, Royal Brompton Hospital, London). The reason is not yet established but probably relates to platelet activation.

Threshold

Presumably, susceptibility to migraine attacks is related to cortical or at least neuronal excitability. Do migraineurs have more excitable neurons? There are several lines of evidence that suggest this is so.

Migraineurs experience more visual discomfort and experience more illusions when presented with particularly vivid geometrical patterns and such stimuli can induce migraine attacks in susceptible MA patients (82). From clinical experience, some migraineurs are generally photosensitive even between attacks, and may resort to using photoreactive lenses in their glasses to protect themselves.

Findings concerning "neuronal excitability" based on cortical evoked potential (EP) and transcranial magnetic stimulation (TMS) studies have been somewhat inconsistent (3) but most have reported reduced thresholds for the induction of elemental visual auras (e.g., phosphenes, see Chapter 3) by TMS, and reduced latencies and increased amplitude responses in visual and other EPs. A more consistent finding in migraineurs is an increased negativity of the initial contingent negative variation wave in the electroencephalogram (EEG), which normally precedes voluntary movement (3). Interestingly, this finding appears to be inherent, and migraineurs also show loss of the normal habituation of this potential to stimuli that evoke cortical potentials. This is consistent with the increased sensitivity to sensory inputs such as light and sound, characteristic of migraine. Of still greater interest is the observation that many of these neural threshold abnormalities return to normal during migraine attacks, paralleled by changes in the EEG power spectrum. It has also been shown that the defective habituation can be normalized in migraineurs by repetitive high-frequency cortical TMS (3). This raises the interesting philosophical concept that migraine might, in fact, be a restorative process in which sensory thresholds are reset (see below).

The variance of observations among migraineurs in these different studies might be technical, but could also be due to real changes in neural excitability over time. This has been referred to as "neurophysiological periodicity" (83). Thus, there might be regular (internal clock driven) or random fluctuations in the migraine mechanism threshold. Periodic lowering of threshold could result in increased susceptibility to triggering of attacks and the initiation of premonitory symptoms.

Cortical excitability has been related to a number of factors. Levels of the excitatory transmitter glutamate are said to be higher in cerebrospinal fluid in migraineurs (84), and brain levels of Mg^{2+}, which plays a part in the regulation of the activity of glutamate, are lower (85). The respective activities of transmitters such as 5-HT in the raphe nuclei (decreases cortical excitability), noradrenaline, in the locus coeruleus, and acetylcholine in the nucleus basalis of Meynert, (provoke arousal) are also important (3). However, current evidence suggests that the intrinsic sensitivity of neuronal ion channels to depolarization might be the prime determining factor for "threshold." This is presumably genetically determined.

MIGRAINE GENES

We suppose that each individual has a threshold for activation of the migraine mechanism and that this threshold is genetically determined.

The majority of the population has a high threshold, and typical migraine attacks affect only a minority. At the other extreme, migraineurs are afflicted by frequent and often disabling attacks.

Population Studies

As noted in Chapter 1, the hereditary tendency to migraine has been recognized for centuries, but the relative contribution of genetic and environmental factors to the familial aggregation of the disorder is unclear (86). Many older epidemiological studies suffered from methodological problems such as lack of homogenous diagnostic criteria for migraine and questionable ascertainment practices, resulting in wildly differing estimates of genetic risks. Using rigorous methods, Russell and Olesen found that compared with the normal Danish population, first-degree relatives of patients with MA had a three- to four-fold increased relative risk of migraine, whereas the risk for first-degree relatives of patients with MO was about 1.5- to 2-fold (87). However, a study involving a similar number of probands in Maryland found that the risk in first-degree relatives was not significantly greater than in controls, except among cases with disabling attacks where the risk was about twice as great (88). Such inconsistencies in observation between different patient populations may be the result of methodological differences but might also indicate that migraine is a complex polygenic disorder and that genetic background in different populations plays a part.

It would be expected that examining the concordance rates for migraine between monozygotic and dizygotic twins would clarify the respective roles of genetic and environmental factors, but even this approach has produced confusing results. Olesen's group compared 1013 monozygotic and 1667 dizygotic twin pairs in Denmark, and found the concordance rate for both MA and MO was significantly higher among the monozygotic twins (89). The effect was somewhat higher in MA; but a further analysis of this data indicated that liability to MO resulted from additive genetic effects, together with individual-specific environmental effects (90). This confirmed a strong genetic influence on susceptibility but raised the question as to whether or not MA and MO are genetically distinct. Olesen's group therefore looked for evidence that these conditions share genes. If they do, then both MA and MO should occur more commonly together in twins than in the general population. However, in a study of 5360 Danish twins, they found that the observed cooccurrence of MA and MO using IHS diagnostic criteria did not, in fact, differ from that expected from the prevalence in the population. Moreover, twin pairs with MA had no increased risk of MO, and twins with MO had no greater risk of MA. This suggested that the conditions have a different genetic basis (91). However, an equally large study from Australia involving 6265 twins, but using quite different methods, came to precisely the opposite conclusion! Overall, 13% of female and 6%

of male twins had MA, and 20% of female and 9% of male twins had MO according to IHC-1 criteria, consistent with other studies. However, an analysis based on headache severity and other headache symptoms using "latent class analysis" showed a continuum, with MA being more severe but not etiologically distinct from MO. In addition, many more individuals were identified as having migraine using latent class analysis than were identified by the IHC-1 criteria, and this increased the observed apparent genetic contribution to the condition. It was concluded that some common genes probably underlie all primary headache subtypes, but that modifying genetic and environmental factors leads to differential expression (92).

Familial Hemiplegic Migraine

While most forms of migraine are presumably polygenic, several specific "migraine genes" have been identified (Table 3) (3,86,93). The first such gene to be identified was in families with the very rare condition familial hemiplegic migraine (FHM), an autosomal dominant disorder characterized by severe migraine attacks preceded by a true hemiplegic aura. We will discuss the clinical features and unique neuroimaging characteristics of this interesting condition in Chapters 3 and 4, but will consider here its genetic basis in the general context of migraine genetics.

Familial Hemiplegic Migraine 1 (FHM1)

The CACN1A1 gene on 19p13 codes for a pore-forming alpha1 subunit of $Ca_{v2.1}$, a voltage-gated P/Q type Ca^{2+} channel gene. Mutations in this gene account for about half of all FHM cases, referred to as FHM1. The resulting alteration of calcium influx and calcium currents in neurons could be an important factor in predisposing to spreading depression, which as noted above is carried by a Ca^{2+} current. For example, a knock-in mouse model expressing a human FHM1 *CACN1A1* mutation showed a reduced threshold

Table 3 Migraine Genes Reported up to End of 2005

Condition	Chromosome	Gene (if known)
Familial hemiplegic migraine		
FHM1	19p13	*CACNA1A*
FHM2	1q21-23	*ATP1A2*
FHM3	2q24	*SCN1A*
Migraine without aura	4q21	*MGR1*
Migraine with aura	15q11-13	*GABA-A*
Migraine	1q31, Xp22	?
	Xq24-28, 19p13	?
CADASIL	19p13.2	*notch 3*

to induction of CSD (94). $Ca_{v2.1}$ channels are present on neural presynaptic and somatodendritic membranes throughout the brain, including all the structures known to be involved in the migraine mechanism and expression of migraine headache. These channels are also particularly densely expressed in the cerebellum, and about half of all FHM1 cases develop a progressive cerebellar syndrome and suffer severe hemiplegic attacks and coma. This is the most common FHM1 phenotype and is caused by a T666M mutation with very high penetrance. In contrast, the S218L mutation is associated with cerebral edema and coma triggered by minor head injury (see Chapter 4).

Mutations in *CACNA1A* also cause episodic ataxia type 2 (EA2) and spinocerebellar ataxia type 6 (SCA6), both conditions in which migraine headache can be prominent. For example, migraine headaches occurred frequently in more than half of EA2 patients in one study but there did not seem to be any clear relationship between the type and location of the mutations and the clinical phenotype (95). Indeed, individuals with FHM, EA2, and SCA6 phenotypes were reported in a single large family with a unique mutation in exon 13, suggesting that the three conditions are in fact allelic (96).

Familial Hemiplegic Migraine 2 (FHM2)

FMH2, which accounts for a further 15% of cases of FHM, is caused by missense mutations in the alpha-2 subunit of a neuronal Na/K ATPase (ATP1A2, 1q23) (97). Haploinsufficiency of the gene has been hypothesized to result in an increase in extracellular potassium because of faulty Na^+/K^+ exchange, with consequent depolarization and increased liability to spreading depression. Another possibility is that mutations lead to abnormal local calcium levels because of the concomitant activation of the Na^+/Ca^{2+} exchanger, with consequences comparable to that in FHM1.

Familial Hemiplegic Migraine 3 (FHM3)

Recently, mutations in a voltage-gated *SCN1A* neuronal sodium channel gene on 2q24 have been reported in two FHM pedigrees (98). Mutations in this gene have also been associated with epilepsy, and it is homologous with the muscle sodium channel gene commonly involved in hyperkalemic periodic paralysis. The mutations identified were predicted to affect fast inactivation of the channel.

Genetics of "Ordinary Migraine"

So, which genes cause or predispose to "ordinary migraine?" FMH1, FMH2, and now FMH3 account for the majority of FHM cases, but other FHM families and some families with non-hemiplegic migraine have shown linkage to loci on 1q, Xp22, and Xq24–28. A locus for MA on 19p13 distinct from *CACNA1A* has also been reported (93). In fact, the 19p13 region seems to be something of a "hot spot" for migraine genes. In addition to FHM1, it should be noted that this region also includes the *notch 3* gene, mutations of which cause cerebral autosomal dominant arteriopathy with subcortical infarcts and leucoencephalopathy (CADASIL), a condition in which MA is a prominent feature. This condition is considered further in relation to migrainous infarction in Chapter 4 and as an example of "symptomatic migraine" in Chapter 5. However, mutations in *CACNA1A* and *ATP1A2* do not seem to be associated with the "common" forms of migraine, nor with sporadic hemiplegic migraine (99). A gene for MO has been identified at 4q21 (100) and a susceptibility locus for MA containing three GABA-A receptor genes has been found at 15q11–13 (101). Genetic polymorphisms of several other genes, including the dopamine D_2 receptor, angiotensin converting enzyme, serotonin transporter, dopamine β hydroxylase, endothelin type A receptor, insulin receptor, TNF-β, and methylene-tetrahydrofolate reductase, have been found to be more common in migraineurs (94).

Finally, some studies have reported reduced mitochondrial phosphorylation potential in brain and muscle in migraineurs. Patients with mitochondrial encephalopathy with lactic acidosis and stroke-like episodes (MELAS) typically suffer migraine-type headaches (see Chapter 5, p. 253) (102), but there is no increased incidence of any of the common mitochondrial DNA mutations among patients with migraine (93).

THE BIOLOGICAL SIGNIFICANCE OF MIGRAINE

Ideas concerning migraine and its pathophysiology come from many directions and pose many questions. For example, are migraineurs a specific group, or are migraine headache and other manifestations of the migraine mechanism something we will all experience at some point in our lives? We favor the latter and suggest that it is simply a question of threshold variation; some individuals are more prone to "migraine" than others by virtue of their genetic constitution. Certainly, the migraine mechanism appears to be a function of the normal brain rather than a disease state, and despite the rather alarming pathophysiological changes that occur in CSD, there is no indication that the brain is injured by the process, except in rare instances (see Chapter 4).

Does the "migraine mechanism" truly have to run a course irrespective of the apparent effects of therapeutic intervention? Many patients say that they can "feel an attack building up" and often experience a sense of relief and well-being after recovery from the attack, echoing Liveing's nineteenth century concept that "megrim" represented the tendency of the nervous system to *"periodically resolve the accumulation of nerve-force in paroxysmal or sometimes truly explosive symptoms."* So, since migraine is extremely common yet pathologically benign, and, generally speaking, a profound nuisance at worst, does it have a purpose in terms of brain homeostasis?

Concept 1. Migraine Is a Consequence of Disordered Sensory Control

If we consider migraine symptoms, divided as they are into premonitory, aura, and headache phases, we see that they are mostly disturbances in sensory awareness. The most common aura symptoms are visual and somesthetic, while motor symptoms are rather uncommon. As we will discuss further in Chapter 6, this is the converse of epilepsy, where motor manifestations are more common. We take in a lot of sensory information, and sensory inputs are common migraine triggers. During a migraine attack, levels of light, sounds, and smells that would normally be tolerated comfortably may become overpowering. Cranial allodynia, representing increased tactile sensibility, was well appreciated by physicians in earlier times but had been largely forgotten until Burstein's more recent work.

One could suggest then, that the migraine mechanism is engaged to reset a temporary fault in the control of sensory input. If so, what structures modulate sensory inputs?

As noted above, the reticular formation is an area in the brainstem, which receives diverse inputs and sends out widely branching axons to distant parts of the brain, where they modulate brain function (Fig. 4). A number of neurotransmitter-specified neuronal groups lie in the reticular formation, in particular, the noradrenaline neurons of the locus coeruleus in the pons and medulla and the serotoninergic neurons of the raphe nuclei in the midbrain. The most rostral neurons of the locus coeruleus project to the mesencephalon, hypothalamus, and basal forebrain, whereas the caudal group projects to the lower brainstem and spinal cord. From its projection patterns, the locus coeruleus appears to be involved in regulating sensory input and cortical activation. The raphe neurons project rostrally, innervating nearly the entire forebrain in a pattern suggesting a role in the regulation of behavioral states. Thus, we have a neuronal framework for theories of migraine pathogenesis that involves alterations in sensory control relating to disturbances in central serotonin and noradrenaline activity.

Concept 2. Migraine Is a Protective and Restorative Process

A migraine attack often develops after a period of sustained stress, sometimes combined with factors such as lack of sleep, missed meals, menstruation, and so forth. Once an individual's migraine threshold is crossed, potentially noxious external and internal triggers can initiate the attack. In response, the sufferer typically withdraws to a quiet, dark place to reduce provocative inputs. This behavior provides some justification for considering migraine as a "restorative" process.

We noted above that some parameters of heightened neural excitability are normalized as a result of a migraine attack. In rats, CSD seems to protect the brain against ischemic damage, and Tony Strong's findings (see p. 52) suggest that spreading depression may occur spontaneously in the normal human cortex much more often than we realize (32). Might migraine in humans, therefore, have some protective role when the cortex is "threatened" by a migraine trigger? It may be a process to protect an "overloaded cortex." Thus, visual systems may be "protected" by photophobia, olfactory systems by osmophobia, and so forth.

CONCLUSION: A BROAD CONCEPT OF MIGRAINE

We suppose that the migraine mechanism is set in motion when one or more triggers exceed an individual's genetically determined activation threshold. The consequence may be a neurological manifestation of cortical activation in isolation (an aura, possibly preceded by premonitory symptoms), aura associated with headache (MA), or headache in isolation (MO). The headache may sometimes be accompanied by features of cranial afferent sensitization (allodynia) and occasionally by symptoms resulting from activation of the trigeminal autonomic reflex ("red migraine," parasympathetic signs), although generalized pallor, ("white migraine,") reflecting sympathetic affects, is more common. In response, the affected individual will usually seek to reduce sensory inputs, allowing resetting of the sensory modulation mechanisms.

We believe that the cortical activation that produces aura is independent of activation of the brainstem, which is probably the seat of migraine headache, although migrainous vertigo aura seems to be generated in the brainstem (see Chapter 3). The fundamental process underlying activation in both sites is probably spreading depression. It would seem that the threshold for triggering CSD is significantly higher that that for brainstem activation in most migraineurs, as shown by the GTN-triggering experiments in which it proved difficult to initiate aura even in patients with habitual aura. However, it may be that a subset of migraineurs have "cortical modules" with significantly lower thresholds, and therefore experience auras more often, sometimes or even frequently without headache. This hypothesis should be testable.

The issues of the role of "neurogenic inflammation" in the pathogenesis of migraine headache, and the concept of "silent aura," whereby all migraine attacks are initiated by cortical events, remain unresolved.

In this chapter, we have largely omitted reference to the role of serotonin and platelets in the migraine mechanism, although this was discussed in some detail in Chapter 1. This is because serotonin and its receptors are so intimately associated with the basis of the current treatment of migraine attacks and with migraine prophylaxis, that we have deferred further discussion of this topic to Chapter 7. Suffice to say here that central serotonin neuron systems and platelet 5-HT are probably key factors in attack initiation. Loss of serotoninergic "tone" may be the spark that ignites the migraine fire.

While our understanding of the migraine mechanism is now advancing rapidly, there is much to learn. Why do some patients with MO sometimes get aura in isolation? What determines the anatomical course of spreading depression and thus the symptoms of auras, and why are some auras more common than others? Why does migraine sometimes cause brain injury? And are all primary headaches actually caused by the same mechanism? These issues and others will be addressed in the following chapters.

REFERENCES

1. Matharu MS, Bartsch T, Ward N, et al. Central neuromodulation in chronic migraine patients with suboccipital stimulators: a PET study. Brain 2004; 127:220–230.
2. Matharu MS, Goadsby PJ. Functional brain imaging in hemicrania continua: implications for nosology and pathophysiology. Curr Pain Headache Rep 2005; 9:281–288.
3. Pietrobon D, Striessnig J. Neurobiology of migraine. Nat Rev Neurosci 2003; 4:386–398.
4. Oshinsky O. Pathophysiology of migraine. In: Silberstein SD, Stiles A, Young WB, eds. An Atlas of Migraine and Other Headaches. 2nd ed. Florida: Taylor and Francis, 2005:53–64.
5. Sanchez del Rio M, Linera JA. Functional neuroimaging of headaches. Lancet Neurol 2004; 3:645–651.
6. Cohen AS, Goadsby PJ. Functional neuroimaging of primary headache disorders. Curr Neurol Neurosci Rep 2004; 4:105–110.
7. Sanchez del Rio M, Reuter U. Migraine aura: new information on underlying mechanisms. Curr Opin Neurol 2004; 17:289–293.
8. Goadsby PJ. Trigeminal autonomic cephalalgias; fancy term or constructive change to the IHS classification? J Neurol Neurosurg Psychiatr 2005; 76:301–305.
9. Headache classification subcommittee of the International Headache Society. The International Headache Classification 2nd Edition 2004. Cephalalgia 2004; 24 (suppl 1):1–160.
10. Eriksen MK, Thomsen LL, Olesen J. Sensitivity and specificity of the new international diagnostic criteria for migraine with aura. J Neurol Neurosurg Psychiatr 2005; 76:212–217.
11. Alvarez WC. The migrainous scotoma as studied in 618 cases. Am J Ophthalmol 1960; 49:489–504.
12. Evans RW, Lipton RB, Silberstein SD. The prevalence of migraine in neurologists. Neurology 2004; 62:342.
13. Steiner TJ, Scher AL, Stewart WF, et al. The prevalence and disability burden of adult migraine in England and their relationships to age, gender and ethnicity. Cephalalgia 2003; 23:519–527.
14. Giffin NJ, Ruggiero L, Lipton RB, et al. Premonitory symptoms in migraine: an electronic diary study. Neurology 2003; 60:935–940.
15. Kelman L. The premonitory symptoms (prodrome): a tertiary care study of 893 migraineurs. Headache 2004; 44:865–872.

16. Fanciullacci M, Allessandri M, Del Rosso A. Dopamine involvement in the migraine attack. Funct Neurol 2000; 15(Suppl 3):171–181.

17. Stewart J, Kaube H, Goadsby PJ. Glyceryl trinitrate triggers premonitory symptoms. Pain 2004; 110:675–680.

18. Davidoff RA. Clinical manifestations of migraine. In: Davidoff RA, ed. Migraine: Manifestations, Pathogenesis and Management. Philadelphia: FA Davis, 1995:58.

19. Sacks O. Migraine. Understanding a common disorder (Revised Edition). Duckworth: London, 1985.

20. Selby G, Lance JW. Observations on 500 cases of migraine and allied vascular headache. J Neurol Neurosurg Psychiatr 1960; 23:23–32.

21. Leão AAP. Spreading depression of cortical activity in the cerebral cortex. J Neurophysiol 1944; 7:359–390.

22. Leão APP, Morrison RS. Propagation of cortical spreading depression. J Neurophysiol 1945; 8:33–45.

23. Milner PM. Note on a possible correspondence between the scotomas of migraine and spreading depression of Leão. Encephalography Clin Neurophysiol 1958; 10:705.

24. Grüsser O-J. Migraine phosphenes and the retino-cortical magnification factor. Vision Res 1995; 35:1125–1134.

25. Kleeberg J, Petzold GC, Major S, et al. Endothelin-1 induces cortical spreading depression via activation of the ETA receptor/phospholipase C pathway in vivo. Am J Physiol Heart Circ Physiol 2003; 125:102–112.

26. Diamond MC, Scheibel AB, Murphy GM, et al. On the brain of a scientist: Albert Einstein. Exp Neurol 1985; 88:198–204.

27. O'Kusky J, Colonnier M. A laminar analysis of the number of neurones, glia and synapses in the cortex (area 17) of adult macaque monkeys. J Comp Neurol 1982; 210:278–290.

28. Hansen AJ, Lauritzen M. Spreading depression of Leão. In: Olesen J, Edvinsson L, eds. Basic Mechanisms of Headache. Elsevier: Amsterdam, 1988:99–107.

29. Bowyer SM, Aurora KS, Moran JE, et al. Magnetoencephalographic fields from patients with spontaneous and induced migraine aura. Ann Neurol 2001; 50:582–587.

30. Bowyer SM, Tepley N, Papuashvilli N, et al. Analysis of MEG signals of spreading cortical depression with propagation constrained to a rectangular cortical strip. II. Gyrencephalic swine model. Brain Res 1999; 843: 79–86.

31. Mayevsky A, Doron A, Manor T, et al. Cortical spreading depression recorded from the human brain using a multiparametric monitoring system. Brain Res 1996; 740:268–274.

32. Strong AJ, Fabricius M, Boutelle MG, et al. Spreading and synchronous depressions of cortical activity in acutely injured human brain. Stroke 2002; 33:2738–2743.

33. Cutrer FM, Sorensen AG, Weisskoff RM, et al. Perfusion-weighted imaging defects during spontaneous migrainous aura. Ann Neurol 1998; 43:25–31.

34. Choudhuri R, Cui L, Yong C, et al. Cortical spreading depression and gene regulation; relevance to migraine. Ann Neurol 2002; 51:499–506.

35. Strassman AM, Raymond S, Burstein R. Sensitisation of meningeal sensory neurons and the origin of headaches. Nature 1996; 384:560–564.

36. Shen PJ, Larm JA, Gundlach AL. Expression and plasticity of galanin systems in cortical neurones, oligodendrocyte progenitors and proliferative zones in normal brain and after spreading depression. Eur J Neurosci 2003; 18:1362–1376.

37. Dreier JP, Korner K, Ebert N, et al. Nitric oxide scavenging by haemoglobin or nitric oxide synthase inhibition by N-nitro-L-arginine induces cortical spreading ischemia when K+ is increased in the subarachnoid space. J Cereb Blood Flow Metab 1998; 18:978–990.

38. Sanin LC, Mathew NT. Severe diffuse intracranial vasospasm as a cause of extensive migrainous cerebral infarction. Cephalalgia 1993; 13:289–292.

39. Moskowitz MA. Membranes, barriers and migraine. How intrinsic brain activity causes headache. Cephalalgia 2003; 23:566.

40. Moskowitz MA. The neurobiology of vascular head pain. Ann Neurol 1984; 16:157–168.

41. Buzzi MG, Dimitriadou V, Theoharides TC, et al. 5-Hydroxytryptamine receptor agonists for the abortive treatment of vascular headaches block mast cell, endothelial and platelet activation within the rat dura mater after trigeminal stimulation. Brain Res 1992; 583:137–149.

42. Bolay H, Reuter U, Dunn AK, et al. Intrinsic brain activity triggers trigeminal afferents in a migraine model. Nature Med 2002; 8:136–142.

43. Kaube H, Katsarara Z, Przywara S, et al. Acute migraine headache: possible sensitisation of neurones in the spinal trigeminal nucleus. Neurology 2002; 58:1234–1238.

44. Netsiri C, Bradley DP, Takeda T, et al. A delayed class of BOLD waveforms associated with spreading depression in the feline cerebral cortex can be detected and characterised using independent component analysis (ICA). Magn Reson Imaging 2003; 21:1097–1110.

45. Kruse C, Thomsen LL, Birk S, et al. Migraine can be induced by sildenafil without changes in middle cerebral artery diameter. Brain 2003; 126: 241–247.

46. Fields CR, Barker FM II. Review of Horner's syndrome and a case report. Optometry Vis Sci 1992; 69:481–488.

47. Bruyn GW, Ferrari MD. Chorea and migraine: "Hemicrania choreatica"? Cephalalgia 1984; 4:119–124.

48. Raskin NH, Hosobuchi Y, Lamb S. Headache may arise from pertubation of the brain. Headache 1987; 27:416–420.

49. Veloso F, Kumar K, Toth C. Headache secondary to deep brain implantation. Headache 1998; 38:507–515.

50. Afridi S, Goadsby PJ. New onset migraine with a brainstem cavernous angioma. J Neurol Neurosurg Psychiatr 2003; 74:680–682.

51. Goadsby PJ. Neurovascular headache and a midbrain vascular malformation—evidence for a role of the brainstem in chronic migraine. Cephalalgia 2002; 22:107–111.

52. Katsavara Z, Segelhof T, Kaube H, et al. Symptomatic migraine and sensitisation of trigeminal nociception associated with contralateral pontine cavernoma. Pain 2003; 105:381–384.

53. Weiller C, May A, Limmroth V, et al. Brainstem activation in spontaneous human migraine attacks. Nat Med 1995; 1:658–660.
54. Bahra A, Matharu MS, Buchel C, et al. Brainstem activation specific to migraine headache. Lancet 2001; 357:1016–1017.
55. Cao Y, Aurora SK, Nagesh V, et al. Functional MRI-BOLD of brainstem structures during visually triggered migraine. Neurology 2002; 59:72–78.
56. May A, Kaube H, Beuchel C, et al. Experimental cranial pain elicited by capsaicin: a PET study. Pain 1998; 74:61–66.
57. Burstein R, Yarnitsky D, Goor-Aryeh I, et al. An association between migraine and cutaneous allodynia. Ann Neurol 2000; 47:614–624.
58. Burstein R, Cutrer MF, Yarnitsky D. The development of cutaneous allodynia during a migraine attack. Clinical evidence for the sequential recruitment of spinal and supraspinal nociceptive neurones in migraine. Brain 2000; 123:1703–1709.
59. Burstein R, Yamamura H, Malick A, et al. Chemical stimulation of the intra-cranial dura induces enhanced responses to facial stimulation in brainstem trigeminal neurons. J Physiol 1998; 79:964–982.
60. Von Reis G, Lund F, Sahlgren E. Experimental histamine headache. Acta Med Scand 1957; 157:451–460.
61. Laws GL. The effects of nitroglycerine upon those who manufacture it. J Am Med Assoc 1898; 31:793–794.
62. Dalsgaard-Nielsen T. Migraine diagnostics with special reference to pharma-cological tests. Int Arch Allerg Immunol 1955; 7:312–322.
63. Olesen J, Iversen HK, Thomsen LL. Nitric oxide supersensitivity: a possible molecular mechanism of migraine pain. Neuroreport 1993; 4(8):1027–1030.
64. Lassen LH, Thomsen LL, Kruuse C, et al. Histamine-1 receptor blockade does not prevent nitroglycerin induced migraine. Support for the NO-hypothesis of migraine. Eur J Clin Pharmacol 1996; 49(5):335–339.
65. Iversen HK, Olesen J. Headache induced by a nitric oxide donor (nitrogly-cerin) responds to sumatriptan. A human model for development of migraine drugs. Cephalalgia 1996; 16(6):412–418.
66. Lassen LH, Ashina M, Christiansen I, et al. Nitric oxide synthase inhibition: a new principle in the treatment of migraine attacks. Cephalalgia 1998; 18(1): 27–32.
67. Akerman S, Williamson DJ, Kaube H, et al. The effect of anti-migraine com-pounds on nitric oxide-induced dilation of dural meningeal vessels. Eur J Pharmacol 2002; 452(2):223–228.
68. Afridi S, Kaube H, Goadsby PJ. Glyceryl trinitrate triggers premonitory symptoms in migraineurs. Pain 2004; 110:675–680.
69. Afridi SK, Matharu MS, Lee L, et al. A PET study exploring the laterality of brain-stem activation in migraine using glyceryl trinitrate. Brain 2005; 128:932–939.
70. Christiansen I, Thomsen LL, Daugaard D, et al. Glyceryl trinitrate induces attacks of migraine without aura in sufferers of migraine with aura. Cephalal-gia 1999; 19:660–667.
71. Sances G, Tassorelli C, Pucci E, et al. Reliability of the nitroglycerin provoca-tive test in the diagnosis of neurovascular headaches. Cephalalgia 2004; 24:110–119.

72. Afridi S, Kaube H, Goadsby PJ. Occipital activation in glyceryl trinitrate induced migraine with visual aura. J Neurol Neurosurg Psychiatr 2005; 76:1158–1160.

73. Goadsby PJ. Migraine, aura and cortical spreading depression: why are we still talking about it? Ann Neurol 2001; 49:4–6.

74. Ebersberger A, Schaibie HG, Averbeck B, et al. Is there a correlation between spreading depression, neurogenic inflammation and nocioception that might cause migraine headache? Ann Neurol 2001; 49:7–13.

75. Woods RP, Iacoboni M, Mazziota JC. Brief report: bilateral spreading cerebral hypoperfusion during spontaneous migraine headache. N Eng J Med 1994; 331:1689–1692.

76. Bednarczyk EM, Remler B, Weikart C, et al. Global cerebral blood flow, blood volume and oxygen metabolism in patients with migraine headache. Neurology 1998; 50:1736–1740.

77. Young WB, Peres MFP, Rozen TD. Modular headache theory. Cephalalgia 2001; 21:842–849.

78. Antle MC, Silver R. Orchestrating time: arrangements of the brain circadian clock. Trends Neurosci 2005; 28:146–151.

79. Bussone G, Waldenlind E. Tension-type headache, cluster headache, and miscellaneous headaches. Biochemistry, circannual and circadian rhythms, endocrinology, and immunology. In: Olesen J, Tfelt-Hansen P, Welch KMA, eds. The Headaches. New York: Raven Press, 1993:551–559.

80. Cohen AS, Kaube H. Rare nocturnal headaches. Curr Opin Clin Neurol 2004; 17:295–299.

81. Peatfield RC. Relationships between food, wine, and beef-precipitated migrainous headaches. Headache 1995; 35:355–357.

82. Chronicle EP, Mulleners WM. Visual system dysfunction in migraine: a review of clinical and psychological findings. Cephalalgia1996; 16:525–535.

83. Siniatchkin M, Gerber WD, Kropp P, et al. How the brain anticipates an attack: a study of neurophysiological periodicity in migraine. Functional Neurology 1999; 14:69–77.

84. Ferrari MD, Odink J, Bos KD, et al. Neuroexcitatory plasma amino acids are elevated in migraine. Neurology 1990; 40:1582–1586.

85. Mauskop A, Alutra BM. Role of magnesium in the pathogenesis and treatment of migraines. Clin Neurosci 1998; 5:24–27.

86. Ducros A, Tournier-Lasserve E, Bousser M-G. The genetics of migraine. Lancet Neurol 2002; 1:285–283.

87. Russell MB, Olesen J. Increased familial risk and evidence of genetic factors in migraine. Br Med J 1995; 311:541–544.

88. Stewart WF, Staffa J, Lipton RB, et al. Familial risk of migraine: a population-based study. Ann Neurol 1997; 41:166–172.

89. Ulrich V, Gervil M, Kyvik KO, et al. Evidence of a genetic factor in migraine with aura: a population-based Danish twin study. Ann Neurol 1999; 45:242–246.

90. Gervil M, Ulrich V, Kaprio J, et al. The relative role of genetic and environmental factors in migraine without aura. Neurology 1999; 53:995–999.

91. Russell MB, Ulrich V, Gervil M, et al. Migraine without aura and migraine with aura are distinct disorders. A population-based twin survey. Headache 2002; 42:332–336.

92. Nyholt DR, Gillespie NG, Heath AC, et al. Latent class and genetic analysis does not support migraine with aura and migraine without aura as separate entities. Genetic Epidemiol 2004; 26:231–244.

93. Sandor PS, Ambrosini A, Agosti RM, et al. Genetics of migraine: possible links to neurophysiological abnormalities. Headache 2002; 42:365–377.

94. Van den Maagdenberg AM, Pietrobon D, et al. A CaCNA1a knockin migraine mouse model with increased susceptibility to cortical spreading depression. Neuron 2004; 41:701–710.

95. Jen J, Kim GW, Baloh RW. Clinical spectrum of episodic ataxia type 2. Neurology 2004; 62:17–22.

96. Alonoso I, Barros J, Tuna A, et al. Phenotypes of spinocerebellar ataxia type 6 and familial hemiplegic migraine caused by a unique CACN1A missense mutation from a large family. Arch Neurol 2003; 60:610–614.

97. De Fusco M, Marconi R, Silvestri L, et al. Haploinsufficiency of ATP1A2 encoding the Na+/K+ pump alpha2 subunit associated with familial hemiplegic migraine type 2. Nat Genet 2003; 33:192–196.

98. Dichgans M, Freilinger T, Eckstein G, et al. Mutations in the neuronal voltage-gated sodium channel SCN1A in familial hemiplegic migraine. Lancet 2005; 366:371–377.

99. Jen JC, Kim GW, Dudding KA, et al. No mutations in CACNA1A and ATP1A2 in probands with common types of migraine. Arch Neurol 2004; 61:926–928.

100. Bjornsson A, Gudmundsson G, Gudfinnsson E, et al. Location of a gene for migraine without aura to chromosome 4q21. Am J Human Genet 2003; 73:986–993.

101. Russon L, Mariotti P, Sangiorgi E, et al. A new susceptibility locus for migraine with aura in the 15q11-q13 genomic region containing three GABA-A receptor genes.

102. Ohno K, Isotani E, Hirakawa K. MELAS presenting as migraine complicated by stroke: case report. Neuroradiology 1997; 39:781–784.

3

Aura

No one has given aura its due since Liveing.
—*W.C. Alvarez*

INTRODUCTION

In Chapter 1, we recalled that Hippocrates, Arateus, and other physicians of the ancient World had noted an association between a particular form of headache and visual disturbances. Pelops had referred to neurological symptoms that sometimes precede epileptic attacks as "aura" and, much later, this term was used to refer to similar symptoms that could occur in migraine. Visual symptoms are certainly the most common type of migraine aura, and it can take many forms. Although Le Pois described a case of sensorimotor aura as early as 1618, it was Liveing's work in the nineteenth century that first emphasized the broader range of auras that might be encountered.

Liveing noted that although "megrim" usually behaved in a stereotypic fashion in a particular patient, there was significant heterogeneity between individuals. He found that the neurological symptoms associated with headache could be simple—a single symptom such as teichopsia, vertigo, or hemianopia—or increasingly complex, with the sequential evolution of, for example, visual disturbance, then numbness on one side of the body, perhaps followed by speech disturbance and "confusion." Liveing recorded instances of "affectation of sight," "affectation of touch and general sensibility," "affectation of speech," "emotional and intellectual disorder," and "vertigo" among his cases. The tempo—the occurrence of positive as well as negative symptoms—and the characteristic evolution of migraine aura, crossing different vascular territories of the brain, is quite different from the typical history of a transient ischemic attack (TIA) and one of the strongest pieces of evidence that aura is a neurally generated phenomenon rather than a vascular one. Furthermore, the duration of migraine aura is usually much longer than that of epileptic aura, another hint that the mechanism underlying migraine aura is specific and unique.

Definitions

The syndrome of migraine with aura (MA) has been known by a variety of terms over the years, including *classic* or *classical* migraine, *migraine accompanée, complicated migraine*; and depending on the nature of the aura symptoms, *ophthalmic, hemiparesthetic, hemiplegic,* or *aphasic* migraine.

The current International Headache Classification (IHC-2) (1) defines aura as follows:

> A recurrent disorder manifesting in attacks of completely reversible focal neurological symptoms with a mix of positive and negative features, which usually evolve over 5–20 minutes, which may or may not be followed by headache.

This definition allows that the accompanying headache may be either of typical migraine type or another primary headache form, and also that aura may not necessarily be associated with headache at all [defined as *"typical aura without headache"* under IHC-2, and sometimes called *acephalalgic* or (erroneously) *acephalgic* migraine]. As we will see, this somewhat restrictive definition of aura belies the rich variety of phenomena and wide range of time course that auras may demonstrate.

Incidence

The incidence of neurological auras in the community is not known, but a recent study of 952 migraine patients attending a tertiary care center in Atlanta (2) found that just over one-third of migraineurs reported aura with about 20% of all migraine attacks being associated with aura. The average aura duration was about 27 minutes, and the headache phase began about 10 minutes after the onset of aura. More than 90% of auras were visual.

MA may affect only 5% to 10% of the population, but auras without headache are much more common and frequently go unrecognized or undiagnosed.

Knowledge of the characteristics of migraine headache and aura almost certainly influence the observed prevalence. For example, Alvarez recorded 618 instances of migrainous auras preceding headache in migraineurs. Overall, 12% of his male cases reported visual auras occurring in isolation, but among physicians (almost all male), 87% had experienced auras without headache (3). He concluded that aura without headache might be much more common than "classical" migraine.

In Chapter 2, we considered the basis of the migraine mechanism. We noted that it is probably driven by neural activation in the cortex or brainstem, or probably both. The headache phase involves brainstem systems, and available evidence supports the view that visual aura, and therefore probably all auras, results from cortical spreading depression (CSD). We also noted that some functional imaging studies had shown cortical activation during migraine *without* aura (MO). This raises the possibility that cortical and brainstem activation in migraine might be independent parallel processes. Aura (from CSD) might affect an eloquent area of the brain only infrequently so that aura symptoms would be perceived in only a minority of attacks. Conversely, some patients experience auras without headache for most of their lives before some event precipitates more typical attacks with headache (4).

Characteristics

Like epileptic auras, migraine auras usually begin with an excitatory phase with *positive* symptomatology, believed to reflect the advancing excitatory wave of spreading depression. For example, excitation of the visual cortex results in auras such as "flashing lights," whereas auras arising in the primary sensory cortex cause paresthesia on the opposite side of the body, and so forth. The neuronal inhibition and, possibly the associated oligemia that follows, cause *negative* symptoms such as scotoma, dysphasia, numbness, and paresis. Such symptoms are not a feature of epileptic auras, although Todd's paresis might be analogous. This neural inhibition phase lasts much longer than the excitatory phase, and indeed can sometimes persist for weeks or months—*persistent aura without infarction* and *migraine coma* are discussed in Chapter 4.

Migraine auras occur in clear consciousness and are perceived by patients as "real," although recognizing that they are not. They are generally considered to be hallucinations. A *hallucination* is the apparent perception of an external stimulus or object that is not actually present—perceiving things that are not there—as opposed to an *illusion*, the perception of an external object as a result of a "false belief" or misinterpretation of real events or inputs. As we will describe, however, migraine auras can also produce illusions, such as vertigo and metamorphopsias. The distinction is arguably an exercise in arcane semantics, but when interpreting visual symptoms, it is important to distinguish auras from *vivid imagery*, i.e., images that appear "in the mind's eye." Such perceptions are largely under voluntary control.

Migraine auras have typically "cortical" characteristics—visual experiences such as bright dots, flashes, lines and colors, and rarely more bizarre distortions and extracampine manifestations such as numbness and tingling—rather than the hallucinations encountered, for example in Parkinsonism, especially with dopamine-agonist treatment, such as the appearances of well-formed people and animals, or "shadow figures." These are thought to be of brainstem origin and principally cholinergic. We would suppose from this reasoning that migrainous visual auras would not occur in cortically blind persons, while the elaborate visual hallucinations typical of Charles Bonnet syndrome experienced by the visually handicapped can be encountered rarely in migraine (see section on "Peduncular Hallucinosis" below).

CLASSIFICATION OF AURAS

The International Headache Society classification defines the common visual, sensory, and dysphasic auras as *typical* auras. However, there are numerous other manifestations of aura. This diversity of expression of the migraine mechanism has been dubbed "the menagerie of migraine" (5). For clarity, we have developed a simple classification for auras that includes these *"atypical"* forms, which can be considered under three headings (Table 1).

- Other sensory auras
- Motor auras
- Auras affecting higher integrative function: mood, perception and ideation, and memory.

We will also speculate on the relationship between migraine and dreams and nightmares. Each category and item will be discussed with case illustrations from our practice.

In defining a neurological symptom as an aura, we have adopted the following criteria:

- The symptom is recurrent and stereotyped.
- Some of the auras are followed by, or associated with, primary headache, usually of migrainous type.
- Neuroimaging and other appropriate investigations fail to demonstrate an alternative explanation.

A previous personal or family history of IHC-2-defined migraine would also be supportive. Occasionally, we will diagnose visual symptoms as migraine auras when these criteria are not fulfilled, if there is no other rational explanation. We accept, however, that future developments may show that some of the entities we describe as "auras" may have an alternative explanation.

"Typical" Auras

Visual Auras

Visual auras originate in the visual cortex and are generated by CSD. Such auras are typically simple, involving the functions of the striate and

Table 1 Classification of Auras

"Typical" auras	
Visual	Simple
	Positive, e.g., phosphenes and teichopsia
	Negative, e.g., scotoma and hemianopia
	Complex
	e.g., visual metamorphopsia
Somesthetic	Simple
	Positive, e.g., tingling
	Negative, e.g., numbness
	Complex
	Somesthetic metamorphopsia
Aphasic	Expressive dysphasia
	Receptive dysphasia
	Dyslexia
"Atypical" auras	
Primary sensory	Olfactory
	Auditory
	Visceral
	Kinesthetic
	Limb pain
Vestibulocochlear	Vertigo
	Deafness
	Drop attacks
Motor	Chorea
	Dystonia
	Hemiplegia
Higher integrative functions	Memory
	Mood
	Perception and planning

extrastriate cortex. Complex auras, with symptoms suggesting involvement of visual and parietal cortical-association areas, are rare. It is characteristic of all visual auras that the images persist when the eyes are closed. The visual phenomena are often perceived as confined to one eye and described as such by the patient but are actually hemianopic. A classification of visual auras is given in Table 2.

Positive symptoms: Simple auras usually include "positive" elemental phenomena, such as dazzling stars, sparks, or flashes, which are usually white but sometimes spectral, occurring singly or in multiple showers. Patients usually describe them as "flashing lights." These primitive hallucinations are generally referred to as scintillations or phosphenes. Other descriptions of positive visual auras given by patients include "electric light bulb element"

	...ental (scintillations, phosphenes, kaleidoscopic)
	...ing, heat haze, "water on glass"
	...opsia (scintillating scotoma and fortification spectra)
	Hemianopia
	Tunnel vision
	Blindness
Complex	Visual metamorphopsia
	Agnosia
	Distortion of motion and space

and "like a wriggling snake." As noted above, the more formed auras sometimes have colored edges. Less commonly, they may become progressively more pronounced with kaleidoscopic effects. A common experience is of "shattering" of images into an irregular crystalline mosaic.

CASE 12: FRAGMENTATION OF IMAGE

A 53-year-old man presented with a one-year history of recurrent visual symptoms, preceded by nondescript malaise. These comprised, variably, a corona of colored sparkles in both hemifields and a degree of tunnel vision; "water running down glass" effect; and sudden fragmentation of the image, followed by a bright white scotoma. Each event lasted about 5 to 10 minutes. None was associated with headache, but he became mildly dysphasic in one attack. There was no previous or family history of headache and no abnormalities were found on ophthalmological or neurological investigation.

CASE 13: MULTIPLICATION OF IMAGES

A 56-year-old man was on holiday when he began to notice a church he was admiring split into two and then gradually begin to split further into four, eight, and so on, spreading across the visual field. He was not sure whether it was more to one side or to the other. The visual disturbance lasted five to ten minutes. He returned to his hotel room and went to bed but noticed that he had right frontal headache following this episode. There were no other associated features and he made a full and complete recovery. A few weeks later, at home in the kitchen, he was helping his wife by chopping some vegetables and then suddenly he realized that there were 'more fingers' on the worktop than he expected. Soon he noted that this was a similar phenomenon of splitting of the visual image. This event lasted five to ten minutes and was again followed by a headache. He developed a third episode while driving, when a blue car in front of him became two, four, eight, and so on. The periphery of this field was blurry and the cars seemed to move slightly, giving a shimmering effect. Vision was not completely obscured and he was able to 'see through' the shimmering haze. Again, this was followed by a frontal headache. MRI brain scan and an EEG were normal.

Negative symptoms: Negative visual aura symptoms are actually more common than positive symptoms and often occur in isolation. Typical impressions include "blurring" of vision, a rippling effect in the central fields like water running down glass, a "corona" around the image, or a heat haze. More dramatic negative symptoms include the classical expanding translucent *scintillating scotoma*. This may have a jagged edge, in which case the image is referred to as *teichopsia* or *fortification spectrum*, as first clearly illustrated by Hubert Airy (see Chapter 1, Fig. 6). The fortification spectrum, so called by Dr. John Fothergill (1712–1780) because of its similarity to the castellations of a battlement, such as surrounds the French town of Lille (Fig. 1) or the Dutch town of Naarden, starts as a zigzag figure near the fixation point and gradually spreads right or left (depending on which visual cortex is generating the image), assuming a laterally convex shape with an angulated scintillating edge (the *expanding angular spectrum of Gowers*), leaving variable degrees of absolute or relative scotoma in its wake. The zigzag edge, the positive part of the aura, may be colored.

Pathophysiology of aura. In Chapter 2, we noted that Otto Joachim Grüsser proposed that the incremental rate of expansion of a visual aura over time was a function of the retinotopic cortical magnification factor and the linear progression of CSD. We also noted that in the BOLD-fMRI studies by Mike Moskowitz's group at Harvard University, Cambridge,

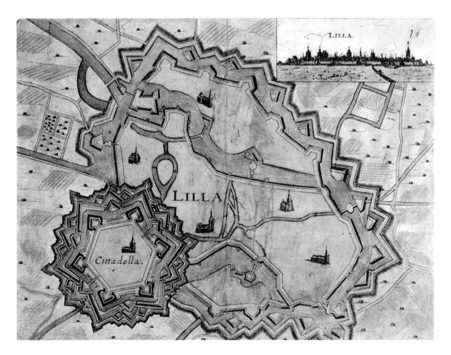

Figure 1 Aerial map of Lille in northern France. The castellations of the outer town wall and citadel are strikingly reminiscent of Airy's "sinistral teichopsia." *Source*: From Galeazzo Gualdo Priorato's *Teatro del Belgio*, 1673.

MA, U.S.A. and Margarita Sanchez del Rio in Madrid, Spain, the CSD underlying visual aura was found to start in the extrastriate visual cortex (areas V3A and then V3) and then spread posteriorly into areas V2 and V1 (the primary visual cortex, area 17) (Fig. 2 and see also Chapter 2, Fig. 4). V3A is particularly sensitive to motion and luminance contrast and is highly retinotopic to one complete hemifield, consistent with hemifield aura symptoms. It was suggested that the common elemental auras might result from neuronal discharge from this region and that other types of visual aura, such as the fortification spectrum, might be generated in V1, which is particularly sensitive to lines and borders (6). For example, the teichopsia experienced by Shazia Afridi's patient studied by positron emission tomography (PET) was associated with activation in V1. Other less common phenomena, such as colored illusions and distortions of time

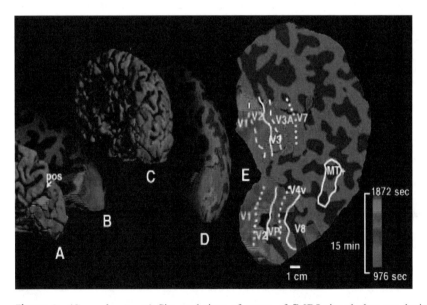

Figure 2 (*See color insert*) Site and time of onset of fMRI signal changes during visual aura. (**A**) and (**C**) represent the normal anatomy of the right hemisphere, (**B**) and (**D**) show the same data on an "inflated" cortical surface, and in (**E**), the surface has been "flattened." Activation data were not acquired from the extreme posterior tip of the occipital pole. The sites of earliest activation are shown in red, with subsequent times of cortical activations shown by the color scale. The aura-related changes appeared first in extrastriate cortex (V3A, closely followed by V3 and V2), then progressed into V1. The spread of the aura began, and was most systematic, in the representation of the lower visual field (*upper bank*), becoming less regular as it progressed into the representation of the upper visual field. *Abbreviations*: Pos, parieto-occipital sulcus; fMRI, functional magnetic resonance imaging. *Source*: From Hadjikhanani N, Sanchez del Rio M, Wu O, et al. Mechanisms of migraine aura revealed by functional MRI in the human cortex. Proc Natl Acad Sci 2001; 98:4687–4692.

and motion, would presumably indicate involvement of other extrastriate areas (V4, V8 for color, V5 for motion, etc.). It was also suggested that somesthetic auras might originate in the somesthetic cortex in an analogous way. When they occur, sensory auras commonly follow visual auras but because CSD was not seen to cross major sulci, such as the parieto-occipital, this might imply an independent cortical origin for the sensory symptoms (6).

Studies of the characteristics of teichopsia have contributed to our understanding of visual processing in the primary visual cortex. Following in the footsteps of many distinguished scientists and physicians (see Chapter 1), Richards analyzed the detailed drawings of the teichopsias experienced by his wife and other acquaintances (7). He noted that the edge of the expanding arc actually comprised *a pair* of scintillating zigzag lines oscillating at about 5 Hz in a "rolling" or "boiling" fashion, with all the "inside" lines "on" while the "outside" lines were off, and then vice versa. The edges of the fortification might be colored in part, most often in primary colors (red, blue, and yellow), while composite colors such as green were rare. He reasoned that this phenomenon represented reciprocal inhibition of the neural networks generating the hallucination, in which activation of neurons responsible for producing one set of lines would be followed by their disappearance (inhibition), and then their reappearance as the wave of depolarization advanced. He also reasoned that the arc was serrated, with the edge consisting of sets of discrete lines rather than smooth curve, because the visual neuronal elements were organised into columns, probably in the form of a hexagonal lattice or honeycomb.

As noted, patients frequently, describe an aura as affecting one eye only, but it is unusual for true monocular aura to occur. Monocular symptoms, including blindness, however, can occur in *retinal migraine*. The negative phase of visual aura may also cause hemianopia and tunnel vision, while bilateral central scotoma with temporary complete blindness may occur rarely in cases of basilar-type migraine.

Migrainous hemianopia and monocular blindness. The common visual aura symptoms of migraine that we have described so far are so characteristic that further evaluation may be unnecessary, although rare instances of typical visual auras due to carotid dissection, occipital meningiomas, and arteriovenous malformations have been reported (see Chapter 5). We present below some examples of less common simple visual auras.

CASE 14

A 65-year-old lady presented with an episode of bilateral "flashing lights" in the peripheries of the visual fields of both eyes. This lasted 30 minutes. There were no other symptoms, and she had never experienced migrainous symptoms previously. A week later, the "flashing lights" recurred and lasted all evening. Ophthalmological examination showed no abnormalities. She had no further problems until 10 months later, when she suddenly developed a right hemianopia followed an hour later by a nonspecific muzzy headache. The hemianopia resolved completely, but she subsequently began to have recurrent attacks of the flashing lights once more. Magnetic resonance imaging (MRI) brain scan and magnetic resonance angiography (MRA) were normal, and the attacks eventually settled without treatment.

CASE 15
A 67-year-old man suddenly developed a right hemianopia while visiting EuroDisney with his family. The obscuration was bright and shimmering. It was an extremely hot day. The symptom resolved in 15 to 20 minutes. There were no other symptoms, but he recalled that he had suffered an identical attack some 15 years earlier. No further investigations were undertaken. On direct inquiry three years later, he had no further symptoms. There was no other previous or family history of migraine.

CASE 16
A 54-year-old man suddenly developed a bright shimmering right-sided hemianopia while working. There were no other symptoms, and it gradually resolved over some 90 minutes. It was followed by a modest, nonspecific generalized headache. He had no previous history or known family history of headache (he was adopted). Examination was normal and investigation was considered unnecessary.

CASE 17
A 40-year-old woman had a long history of migraine with typical teichopsia. She also had occasional acephalalgic attacks, with primitive auras of flashing lights. Following one of these, she experienced total obscuration of vision in the left eye. She checked the right eye, and the acuity and field of vision seemed normal. The obscuration progressed to a unilateral tunnel vision, with a bright halo scotoma and an island of preserved vision in its center, which resolved after half an hour.

Cases of Bilateral Blindness in Basilar-Type Migraine

CASE 18
A 28-year-old man awoke after a normal night's sleep, completely blind. He remained blind for five minutes and then his vision slowly began to return although it remained fuzzy. Extraordinarily, he drove to work, but was later told to go home because he could not see the computer screen properly and his speech seemed slurred. He visited his doctor about seven hours after the onset and was found to have minimal meningism and mild horizontal nystagmus on looking to the right. When seen in the hospital, he had a reverse internuclear ophthalmoplegia. Later that day, he developed a severe bilateral headache with nausea and photo- and phonophobia, but there was no impairment of consciousness. All the symptoms resolved over a few days, and he recovered completely. He had no previous history of migraine but his maternal grandmother had suffered recurrent headaches. Subsequent MRI brain scan revealed no abnormalities.

CASE 19
A 28-year-old woman developed increasingly frequent attacks of MO, with headache beginning in the occipital area, over some nine months. She would sometimes also get typical attacks about half an hour after her gym workout. During one typical

attack, while traveling on a bus, she became increasingly sweaty and dizzy, then went completely blind for a number of minutes in clear consciousness. MRI brain scan was normal. The migraine attacks resolved when she stopped the oral contraceptive pill.

CASE 20

A 15-year-old schoolgirl was sitting in class when she suddenly experienced "colored spots in the eyes," and then became completely blind for about 40 seconds. She recovered completely, and there were no other symptoms. A several days later she had an identical attack and then began to have recurrences every several days. On one occasion, the visual disturbance was followed by a typical migraine headache. She also had an attack following a gym lesson, in which she went completely blind for five minutes. The clinical examination and neuroimaging were normal.

Crescendo visual auras. Sometimes the frequency of visual aura changes with age, or attacks may be precipitated by a change in situation such as an intercurrent illness or drug treatment (see p. 93). Some patients experience an alarming crescendo of auras for no apparent reason.

CASE 21

A 64-year-old man was referred because of an increase in the frequency of his visual auras. He had suffered migraine with stereotyped visual aura comprising a typical migrating scintillating scotoma about twice a year, since childhood. By the time he was seen, the auras were occurring daily, but were rarely associated with headache. They seemed to largely remit when he started on pizotifen. On inquiry four years later, however, he was still getting acephalalgic visual aura attacks about twice a month.

CASE 22

A 51-year-old woman presented with a two-year history of attacks in which print would suddenly become jumbled and jumpy, and then a classical fortification spectrum would evolve, usually migrating to the left. At the outset, the auras developed over 10 minutes or so and occurred monthly, but became progressively more frequent and prolonged until she was having attacks every three or four days, each lasting 30 to 40 minutes. On one occasion, she had two attacks in a single day. She never experienced headache or other symptoms apart from mild photophobia, and after six months, the attacks stopped completely. There was no previous or family history of migraine.

Acephalalgic visual auras. The symptoms of migrainous visual auras without headache cause particular concern and diagnostic difficulty. They are usually different from those of retinal detachment, which is typically characterized by images of dark spots or webs, although episodes of acute detachment may also be associated with bright flashes due to retinal nerve fiber stimulation ("floaters and flashes"). Acute glaucoma can produce concentric visual "halos" as part of the symptom complex, but severe pain—red eye and impaired acuity—are additional prominent symptoms. It should also be noted that the visual symptoms of these ocular disorders are almost always unilateral. Occipital epilepsy can also produce elemental visual auras, but these are rather different in kind, typically comprising multiple colored circles (8).

CASE 23
A 42-year-old woman was referred because of three visual disturbances, interpreted by her doctor as "transient ischemic attacks (TIAs)." On the first occasion, she had noticed a sudden brightness of vision and difficulty focusing, lasting some 15 to 20 minutes. She more carefully documented the features of the second event two days later, and was able to draw the obscuration, which was a typical right-hemifield teichopsia that migrated to the right over the next 10 minutes. There was no head-ache. MRI brain scan was normal.

CASE 24
A 34-year-old woman began to have recurrent attacks of stereotypic visual symp-toms, comprising a sudden appearance of a curved arc of light with a jagged edge, usually in the right hemifield but sometimes on the left. This would migrate outward and then disappear after about 20 minutes. There was no headache. She was not too concerned, even when she had several attacks in a single day on one occasion, because she remembered having had similar attacks 12 years previously when preg-nant. However, she was referred when she suddenly also began to get episodes of vertical diplopia lasting two minutes at a time, in addition to the previous symptoms. She had no personal or family history of migraine headaches. Computed tomogra-phy (CT) brain scan was normal.

Migraine Art

Visual auras can be so dramatic that a flourishing migraine art movement has evolved through which migraineurs illustrate and share their experiences (9,10). Several authors have also reviewed the influence of migraine experi-ences on artists (11,12). For example, it is suggested that Giorgio de Chirico, the originator of "metaphysical art," who strongly influenced the surrealists in Paris after the First World War, suffered from migraine, and that some of his work illustrated his own visual auras. The British artist Sarah Raphael (1960–2001) suffered from catastrophic migraine attacks that proved increasingly intrusive after the birth of her third daughter, to the extent that she became addicted to pethidine. At the time she was producing her signa-ture work, the "Strip!" paintings of the mid-1990s, she was frequently con-fined to bed and could work only for brief periods. It has been suggested that these pictures, comprising large numbers of small discrete images arranged in rows in the manner of a cartoon strip, provided a convenient way of working under such strictures. The pictures feature elements like car-toon speech and thought bubbles, and areas devoid of feature, which it has been suggested might represent fortification spectra (12), although they might equally represent "exclamatory" devices used in cartoons ("splat," "bang," and so on). Her "Time Travel" series (2000 onward) has similar structure but in a more three-dimensional form.

Complex Visual Auras

Visual auras are most often elemental, comprising little more than vague central visual blurring or scintillations. At the other extreme—and much less common—elaborate hallucinations and illusions can occur, with gross visual distortions presumably related to involvement of cortical centers for visual integration and visual memory. These auras can include distortions of color, shape, spatial resolution, and motion, referred to generally as *visual metamorphopsia*. It has been our experience that such auras often occur without headache.

Visual metamorphopsia: While typical visual auras are hallucinations, the most common visual metamorphopsias are illusions. These include distortions of size perception usually described, with reference to Swift's *"Gulliver's Travels,"* as "Lilliputian" (micropsia) and "Brobdingnagian" (macropsia). Images may also appear abnormally distant (teliopsia) or near (peliopsia), can increase and decrease in size sequentially (zoom effect), or may become flattened and appear two-dimensional. Entomopia refers to multiple copies of the image appearing in a grid-like pattern, as an insect might see. There can also be distortions of movement, with action appearing as a series of still "freeze frames," as if from a movie film (cinematic vision, a phenomenon also encountered in partial seizures and schizophrenic psychosis). Rarely, unusual consequences of visual aura can include curious agnosias, in which the affected individual is unable to interpolate the loss of visual field, or substitutes bizarre images that can sometimes be alarming or frightening.

Simultanagnosia, the inability to attend to more than one object presented simultaneously within both hemifields, although the fields are normal on testing, may also occur as a migraine aura, as a result of bilateral parietal or parieto-occipital dysfunction. *Prosopagnosia*, the specific inability to recognize faces, even of intimates, and also to fail to appreciate facial and bodily expressions may also occur. These complex visual auras are evidently rare, and we have encountered few examples.

CASE 25: MACROPSIA
A 37-year-old man presented after his third headache attack with associated visual disturbance. In the first of these episodes, some 5 months previously, he was reading when he noted loss of his ability to see the words on the page clearly. Within minutes he could see zigzag lines in his field of view. After about 25 minutes, the visual symptoms settled and he developed increasingly severe right-sided headache with nausea, which settled after about 8 hours. In the second episode, he was driving his car when he again experienced visual problems. The writing on the side of a truck to his right became broken up. Then, as he looked ahead, his right hand appeared enormous for several seconds. His initial thought was that the hand was a lot nearer to him than it was, and he felt, briefly, that it would hit him in the face. He moved his head to one side to avoid the anticipated blow and pulled up at the

roadside. After some minutes his vision returned to normal and he experienced a right-sided headache. His third migraine attack was very similar to the first.

CASE 26
A 60-year-old woman, with a long history of frequent migraine attacks with and without typical visual auras, including hemianopia, presented with a four-year history of recurrent episodes of visual and somatosensory illusions in which the shape, size, and orientation of objects seemed distorted. They occurred about twice monthly, without headache or other migraine symptoms. For example, during one attack, when she looked at a table, it seemed twice as wide as it should. In another, the room she was in suddenly increased in size in the horizontal plane and appeared "flattened." On another occasion, when standing, she felt she was kneeling, because the floor seemed to have risen three feet. These distortions would persist for up to two days, but she did not seek medical attention until one day when, while walking, the floor suddenly "appeared in the wrong place," and she collapsed. A witness said, "She leapt into the air and her legs looked as though she was cycling." She recovered and continued walking, even though the distortions persisted.

Peduncular hallucinosis. Our colleague, Nick Silver, has encountered two patients with migrainous visual hallucinations suggestive of peduncular hallucinosis (presented at the 3rd Oxford Headache Symposium, September 2005). This interesting clinical syndrome, first described by Jean Lhermitte in 1922 and named by Ludo van Bogaert two years later, comprises the occurrence in clear consciousness of vivid, usually colored, often bizarre and very detailed ("formed") hallucinations. As noted, these symptoms are similar to those of Charles Bonnet syndrome. Typically, the patient is not alarmed by the apparitions, knows that the phenomena are not real, and may even find them engaging. Lhermitte and van Bogaert postulated from clinical and pathological observations that these visual hallucinations were unique in that they were generated in the midbrain (*pédoncule*), remote from the visual pathways. This proposition has been supported subsequently by clinical observations such as Caplan's "top of the basilar syndrome" (13) and by autopsy and MRI studies demonstrating lesions in the mesencephalon in typical cases. It has been suggested that involvement of the pars reticulata of the substantia nigra is a key component in the pathogenesis (14). It is interesting to note in this context, the reported localization of brainstem activation in migraine attacks, as discussed in Chapter 2.

In the following cases extensive investigation failed to provide an alternative to migraine as an explanation for the symptoms.

CASE 27
A 29-year-old woman was referred with a six-week history of persistent "tension" headache. She had suffered from typical MO since her teens. She described three episodes of hallucinations in the two months prior to consultation. In the first, she stopped her car to let an old lady cross a deserted road. The old woman seemed to move very slowly, and when she turned to face the patient, the woman had a badly distorted face "like a goblin." She continued to cross the road, but when the patient

checked her rear view mirror a few seconds later, the old woman had vanished. In the second event, a month later, the patient was at a dance when she saw a friend she had not seen for two years. Strangely, he was dressed in exactly the same clothes he had been wearing when they had last met. Another person walked between them, and when she looked again, he had vanished. She then remembered that he had actually died sometime ago. In the third event, she suddenly saw a huge tarantula crawling up a radiator. None of these hallucinations were specifically associated with headache, but she had developed the persistent daily headache problem prior to the last hallucination. This was a constant background headache with mild photo-phobia, punctuated by episodes of more severe bitemporal headache with nausea, photo- and phonophobia, relieved by rest, and accompanied on occasions by additional typical stabbing headaches. Over this period, she had also experienced other unusual visual auras, including persistent coronas, zoom effects, and other image distortions.

CASE 28
A 26-year-old man was referred with a two-year history of severe recurrent head-aches. He had suffered "white migraine" attacks and marked travel sickness in childhood, and in his late teens, had rare attacks of disabling MO. His current attacks were more frequent and severe, and on occasions, he had experienced sen-sory and vertiginous auras.

He also described very brief, but vivid, visual hallucinations on five occasions. In the first, he had been cycling along when he suddenly saw a train coming towards him. It seemed so real that he swerved off the cycle track and fell, fracturing his wrist. He had a recurrence of this "train hallucination" sometime later, and also had hallucinations of children dressed in Victorian costumes, and of a crouching girl whose face suddenly "went runny, like a ghost." These events were not associated with headache. However, on another occasion, he suddenly became aware of "yel-low gunge" on his hands. He found he could run it through his fingers, and it smelled of dog excrement. He immediately washed his hands, and the apparition vanished, but he then developed diarrhea and vomiting. The following day, he had a severe migraine attack. On yet another occasion, he suddenly saw a church pulpit appear, and then developed vertigo, nausea, and vomiting.

Somesthetic Auras

Simple somesthetic auras: Somesthetic auras are the second most common form of aura. If the dominant hemisphere is involved, dysphasia may accompany or follow the sensory symptoms. Positive symptoms, such as tingling or vibration, are followed by numbness, reflecting the negative phase of CSD but the symptoms may sometimes be negative from the out-set, with numbness or "deadness," which is often misinterpreted by the patient as "weakness."

The sensations affect mainly those areas that have the largest represen-tation on the sensory homunculus (the lips, tongue, mouth, and hands), and spread centripetally. They are usually unilateral (*hemisensory aura*), but may be bilateral in migraine of basilar type. Again, the diagnosis of acephalalgic migraine manifest as sensory disturbance in isolation can be difficult but is probably common.

CASE 29

A 32-year-old woman was referred with a four-year history of stereotyped attacks. These would begin with sudden tingling of the right hand, spreading up the arm to the right face, mouth, and tongue over about two minutes, followed by numbness. On some occasions, she would also experience a shimmering sensation in the right hemifield, during which she was able to read words but was unable to understand them. The aura would usually, but not invariably, be followed by a generalized headache, without nausea or vomiting. Attacks could last anywhere from an hour to a whole weekend. She had no previous or family history of migraine.

CASE 30

A 23-year-old man suddenly developed dizziness and unsteadiness followed within a minute by paresthesia affecting the whole of the right side, which also felt weak. Vision and speech were unaffected. A nonspecific generalized headache followed shortly afterward. MRI brain scan, extracranial ultrasound, and echocardiograph were normal. There was a strong family history of migraine, but no prior personal history of attacks.

CASE 31

An 18-year-old girl awoke feeling nauseous. Thirty minutes later, on the way to work on the bus, she began to feel tingling and then numbness spreading slowly up the left arm. Eventually, she was unable to pick things up or use her fingers properly. She got off the bus and promptly vomited. She then became aware of a thumping headache in the right frontotemporal area. She experienced increasing difficulty in walking, due to loss of feeling in the left leg. On admission, mild objective sensory loss on the left was confirmed, with equivocal weakness. CT brain scan and cerebrospinal fluid (CSF) examination were normal. The sensory symptoms recovered within a day, but the headache persisted for three days, and full recovery took three weeks. Both her mother and paternal grandfather suffered from migraine.

CASE 32

A 29-year-old man presented with a year's history of stereotypic attacks of left-sided hemisensory disturbances, two or three times monthly. These would begin in the face, arm, or leg, and migrate to affect the whole left side over a number of hours. This feeling would then last about two days, and then resolve, leaving no deficit. There was no associated headache but he had subsequently experienced a number of accidental minor head injuries, that were often followed by holocranial headache and photophobia, lasting two days to a week.

CASE 33

A 35-year-old woman developed acute back pain and took analgesics. On waking from a short sleep, she developed a severe left frontal and periorbital headache with marked sensory impairment down the left side, affecting particularly the arm and hand, but sparing the face. She also felt mildly nauseous. The symptoms began to recede, but as they were still present three days later, she was referred to the emergency room. There were no objective abnormalities on examination, and CT brain scan was normal. She arranged an MRI brain scan herself, which was also normal. There was no previous personal or family history of headache. She stopped taking the oral contraceptive pill (OCP). On review six months later, she had two further mild left-sided hemisensory attacks without headache, and also episodes of nonspecific headache and more severe hemicranial headache with nausea, but without aura. On inquiry, these attacks had persisted over the following year and had become increasingly frequent and severe, often lasting three to four days, despite treatment with β-blockers.

CASE 34

A 45-year-old lady was shopping when she suddenly found that the left side of her face had become numb and immobile. This sensation spread rapidly to her left arm and leg. There was no headache. There were no abnormalities on examination, and the symptoms gradually resolved over about four weeks. She gave a history of headaches lasting from a few hours to a week, mainly in the left occipital region. She had been seen two years earlier, because of recurrent episodes of "weakness" affecting either side of the body, sometimes associated with difficulty of speech, dating back some six years, and her son had suffered from similar symptoms associated with headache. Extensive imaging and other studies disclosed no abnormalities.

CASE 35
A 21-year-old woman was referred with recurrent stereotyped sensory symptoms in the right arm and face. The first had occurred at a party. She suddenly experienced pins and needles in the right side of the face that spread rapidly to the arm, which seemed to be weak. The right hand developed a cramp-like feeling, but speech and legs were unaffected. The symptoms persisted for three hours but then resolved completely, only to be followed about an hour later by a severe right-sided headache and nausea, which lasted until she slept that night. Five days later, she had a recurrence of the right-sided sensory symptoms, but without headache, and had two such acephalalgic attacks each week from then on, with full recovery on each occasion. There was a strong family history of migraine. MRI brain scan was normal.

Somesthetic metamorphopsia: More complex somesthetic auras can also occur. Body parts can feel unusually small or large, and kinesthetic auras in which a feeling that a limb has spontaneously moved to a new posture has also been described.

Caro Lippman first described the relationship between migraine and bizarre hallucinations of this type. In a series of papers (15–17), he described a number of patients who would experience sudden distortions of body image, in which they felt that certain parts or even the whole body had altered in size and shape, or even that they had two bodies (*"physical duality"*). Some patients would then suffer their familiar headache, before, during, or after the illusion, confirming to them that such sensations were merely part of their habitual migraine syndrome. Often the symptoms would occur in isolation, in which case a patient might well not volunteer such information, fearing that they might be considered "mad."

Lippman drew an analogy between such symptoms and the experiences of Lewis Carroll's immortal heroine, Alice. Subsequently, Dr. J. Todd, writing from Menston in Wharfedale, England in 1955, described six cases of somesthetic metamorphopsia under the title of *"The Syndrome of Alice in Wonderland"* (18). It will be recalled that Lewis Carroll's character had dreams in which she imagined herself to be remarkably tall or remarkably

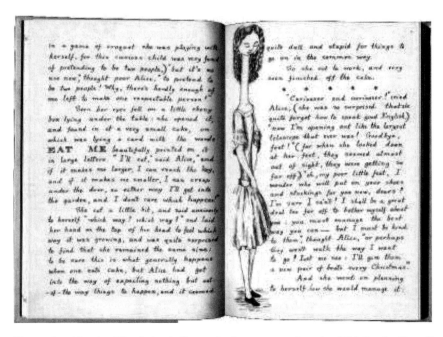

Figure 3 *Alice in Wonderland*. Somesthetic metamorphopsia. Did Lewis Carroll draw inspiration from migraine auras?

short, and would also experience depersonalization and derealization (Fig. 3). Because Carroll is known to have suffered migraine, it has been suggested that he was describing his own migraine aura experiences. For example, the disappearance of the Cheshire cat (all but for the smile!) might have been based on experience of a migrainous scotoma. Although Carroll probably did not develop migraine attacks until some 20 years after the publication of "Alice" (19), this would not exclude the possibility that he had experienced auras without headache earlier in life.

The most common experiences reported by these patients were of being much taller or shorter than normal, and a feeling that body parts were enlarged, reduced, or missing. In some cases, there were also visual metamorphopsias such as a distorted perception of room shape and size. These feelings were often accompanied by extreme fear or even *angor animi* (feeling of impending death). Todd's patients had been referred to a psychiatric clinic and had several other comorbid neuroses, and although they had personal or family histories of migraine, none described associated headache. However, a convincing example of somesthetic illusions, with shrinking of the body or growing taller and gross magnification of both hands sometimes associated with "typical" aura symptoms and followed by migraine headache, was reported and illustrated by Kew et al. in 1998 (Fig. 4) (20).

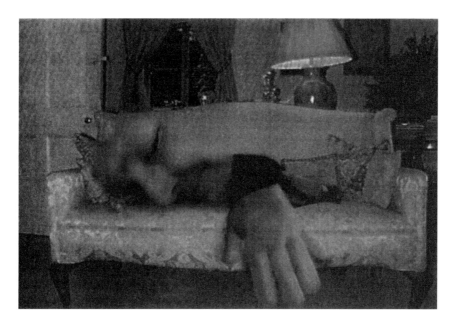

Figure 4 (*See color insert*) Macrosomatognosia. The drawing is based on the description of symptoms by the patient. *Source*: Reprinted with permission from Elsevier, Kew J, et al. Somesthetic aura: the experience of "Alice in Wonderland". Lancet 1998; 351:1934.

Although we have rarely encountered such phenomena among our patients, it is said that people may often not volunteer such descriptions, because they are often distressing and may raise the fear of impending insanity.

CASE 36
A 49-year-old woman consulted with regard to the management of her migraine headaches. During the consultation, it emerged that she had occasionally experienced auras without headache throughout her life. These were most often typical teichopsias and scintillating scotomas, and she had also rarely suffered presyncope during the headache phase. However, she also recalled a number of episodes in childhood, in which, just before waking or falling asleep, she would feel that one of her hands had increased in size or was disproportionately large. On waking, she would then feel that the bedroom looked strange and distorted in shape. However, these episodes were not associated with headache. She did experience "sick headaches" from time to time, and her first and worst attack of migraine headache with aura occurred at age 13, shortly after her first menstrual period. She subsequently experienced frequent lucid dreams.

Dysphasic Auras

Hemisensory auras are often associated with dysphasia if the dominant hemisphere is involved, and occasionally migrainous dysphasia can be an isolated manifestation. The dysphasia is typically expressive in type, with impoverishment of verbal output but preserved comprehension. Speech is typically slurred. Migrainous receptive aphasia is said to result in speech sounding like white noise to the sufferer, with loss of phonemic structure, while the observer perceives a typical fluent dysphasia pattern. The cases that follow are typical example of migrainous dysphasia and also include an example (Case 40) of isolated *dyslexia* as a migraine aura. Dysarthria and speech apraxia have also been described as migraine manifestations, and dysarthria may be a feature of migraine of basilar type.

CASE 37
A 46-year-old woman suddenly felt faint and then developed numbness down the right side of her body, with mild dysphasia. These symptoms began to resolve after about 20 minutes, to be succeeded by a dull headache that persisted for two days, during which she felt nauseous. There was no previous or family history of headache. She had been started on aspirin, but CT brain scan and extracranial ultrasound studies were normal, and the drug was stopped. She was later found to have iron deficiency anemia with associated thrombocytosis of 550×10^9/L (arguably an example of secondary migraine). On review a year later, she had continued to experience similar hemisensory attacks, often with mild dysphasia, lasting 40 to 45 minutes, but without further headaches.

CASE 38
A 62-year-old man was referred following an episode of dysphasia. He had been talking to his wife when he suddenly stopped and stared into space for an instant. He then began to talk, but his speech was irrelevant and sometimes incomprehensible. After half an hour he began to make sense again and complained of a headache over the right eye. There was no nausea or other symptoms. He recovered after a short sleep. He remembered a similar event some 20 years earlier while sitting in a restaurant, he had suddenly begun sweating profusely and became unable to move or talk for some five minutes. He then recovered, but the following day he had an identical event, again with complete recovery. He had had no further symptoms until two years prior to referral, when another similar event occurred, this time lasting 15 minutes, followed by a long period of sleep. He had recovered completely the next day. Electroencephalograph (EEG) and MRI brain scan were normal. His mother had suffered from severe migraine attacks.

CASE 39
A 59-year-old woman with a 14-year history of MO suddenly experienced a very frightening illusion of movement, in which she felt that cuboidal shadows were whirling around her head. She felt that she was moving her head to follow the shadows, but whenever she did, they moved away. In fact, her husband observed that she sat completely still, looking calm, and apparently in full consciousness. He tried to talk to her, but after a number of minutes it was clear that although she was speaking very fluently, the speech was nonsensical. The patient believed she was speaking normally throughout the event. After some minutes she began talking appropriately again, but appeared to have lost her autobiographical memory. By the time she was seen in hospital about an hour later, she had largely recovered, but then began to experience a left frontal headache with mild nausea and photophobia, typical of her migraine episodes.

CASE 40

A 39-year-old man was referred by his general practitioner, with the complaint that he had suddenly experienced an attack of "loss of comprehension" of the contents of a book, while reading in the gym. It transpired that after a workout, he was having a drink and reading a novel, when he had suddenly become aware of some wavy distortion of vision in the right hemifield. In addition, while he could clearly see the words on the page and knew they were words, he was completely unable to interpret their meaning. He did not attempt to speak, so it is not known if he was also dysphasic. He eventually got the train home, but while his vision returned to normal over the next hour, the dyslexia persisted. He slowly began to recognize individual words, but could not understand sentences. He retired to bed feeling dizzy and slept for a short period. On waking, he began to experience a severe frontal headache and slept again. His reading function had recovered by the following day, although he continued to have vague problems with interpretation and had further headache attacks. He had had only one significant headache previously, the previous year, and there was no family history of headache. MRI brain scan was normal.

"Atypical" Auras

Other Primary Sensory Modalities

Auras involving other primary sensory modalities have also been described in migraine but are much less common than their counterparts in epilepsy. We classify these auras with reference to the topography of the sensory organ or modality involved.

Olfactory auras: Olfactory auras occur rarely in migraine. The symptoms are said to be like those of uncinate seizures, typically producing cachosmia. *Gustatory auras* are said to be rare, and we have not encountered examples.

Auditory auras: Auditory auras, with hissing, growling, or rumbling tinnitus followed by impairment of hearing, can occur as migraine auras, but are, again, very rare. These symptoms are the auditory equivalents of the positive elemental visual auras of scintillations or phosphenes, followed by scotomas. Hallucinations of stereotypic music themes, as in musicogenic epilepsy, may also be encountered. Complex auditory auras, such as loss of appreciation of tonality or even the concept of music have been described, as has loss of voice perception and recognition (the auditory equivalent of prosopagnosia).

The possible relationship between migraine and sudden unilateral deafness is noted briefly below in the section on "Migraine and deafness," and discussed further in Chapter 4.

Abdominal aura: Abdominal aura, with a rising sensation from the abdomen to the throat and intense nausea, is a rare feature of migraine attacks, but extremely common in focal and complex partial seizures (often referred to as *epigastric aura*). Other recurrent abdominal symptoms may also be due to the migraine mechanism. These are most often encountered in childhood as *abdominal migraine*, but abdominal aura symptoms may rarely occur in adults, as described below.

CASE 41

A 52-year-old man with a three-year history of recurrent stereotypic abdominal symptoms was referred by a gastroenterologist. These attacks seemed to occur most commonly when the patient was relaxing and comprised sudden nausea and lightheadedness, followed by retching. He would also experience mild photophobia. He would then feel suddenly fatigued and would have to go to sleep in a darkened room. He might also feel pain and numbness in the left groin during the event. At no time did he experience headache, and he had no personal or family history of migraine. Extensive imaging of the gut and abdomen had disclosed no abnormalities. At referral, the attacks were occurring once or twice monthly and would last several hours. However, they gradually stopped of their own accord, without intervention.

Thirst: Thirst is a more common component of migraine aura. As noted in Chapter 2, it may be a premonitory symptom but is occasionally more typical of an aura.

CASE 42

A 22-year-old woman gave a two-year history of frequent migrainous headaches. These would begin with an aura of unquenchable thirst lasting for up to an hour, which was relieved by the onset of headache, usually accompanied by nausea and vomiting, and lasting up to two days. There was a family history of migraine in a sister and paternal uncle. Her attacks seemed to be hormonally related, occurring just prior to menstruation, and she became entirely free of attacks during pregnancy.

CASE 43

A 40-year-old woman was referred with recurrent headaches preceded by "insatiable thirst," over the previous year. These attacks seemed to occur in clusters on a more or less daily basis for several days, followed by several weeks without symptoms. Typically, the symptoms would be present on waking. She would experience a dull holocranial headache, together with a raging thirst that could not be slaked by drinking, lasting hours. There was no subsequent polyuria. She noted minimal nausea but no other migrainous symptoms, and the attacks were not disabling. She gave a history of recurrent nondescript headaches dating back to childhood, and five years earlier had experienced a typical attack of migraine with visual aura. There was also a strong family history of migraine.

CASE 44

A 65-year-old woman gave a history of stereotyped "spells" dating back some 25 years. The attacks would begin with a premonitory feeling of insecurity and agitation, followed by quite severe migraine headache. Sometimes, the headache was preceded by a brief syncopal attack. Recovery was accompanied by migraine headache, drowsiness, and severe thirst. On other occasions, she would experience migraine attacks with typical visual auras. Eating cheese or chocolate or drinking red wine could precipitate attacks. Her mother and her daughter both had a history of migraine. At first consultation, she had a typical attack under observation. She complained of a strange feeling in the upper abdomen accompanied by thirst, and then rapidly lost consciousness and slumped in her chair. She was unconscious for less than a minute. There was no jactitation, and she recovered quickly without any postictal symptoms, apart from raging thirst. Neuroimaging and EEG showed no abnormalities. On inquiry 13 years later, she had continued to have these attacks, but they were much milder, and infrequent.

CASE 45
A 57-year-old lady suddenly felt strange while cooking, and rapidly developed an expressive dysphasia. She recovered within minutes, but then felt intensely thirsty and began drinking copious amounts of water. Over the next few weeks, she began to experience episodes of right-sided homonymous visual auras described as a "spinning wheel." She had a previous history of occasional attacks of MO that could be precipitated by eating chocolate, and her mother had experienced numerous episodes of migraine with expressive dysphasia, diagnosed as "TIAs," and extensively investigated, with negative results. Without our knowledge at that time, our patient's 38-year-old sister had recently been investigated elsewhere, following an attack comprising sudden loss of central vision, lasting 40 minutes, followed by short-term memory loss for events earlier that day and loss of semantic memory for common words and facial recognition, accompanied by feelings of fear and general malaise. She had also developed a hemisensory aura as the visual aura receded. Headache was not prominent at the time, but she was troubled with headache the following day. Over the succeeding few days, she continued to have problems such as misspelling words. She had a history of migraine with dyschromatopsic visual auras during her teens.

Pain: Pain in the limbs can also result from the migraine mechanism. This was described by many authors in the past but is not widely known as an occasional manifestation of migraine. Sometimes such pains will radiate to the chest, presenting as so-called "cardiac migraine" (21). Guiloff and Fruns reported an association between limb pain and migraine and also cluster headaches (22). The limb pain, which was usually ipsilateral to the headache, most commonly affected the upper limbs, but was always on the same side as sensory or motor symptoms if they occurred. In some cases, a slow and progressive evolution of the phenomenon typical of aura would follow. While we have included this phenomenon among the auras because it usually precedes the headache, it may well represent extension of allodynia, which is a typical feature in migraine attacks (see Chapter 2).

Vestibulocochlear Auras

Migrainous vertigo: While the atypical auras described thus far are uncommon or rare in practice, vertiginous aura is very common indeed. It will be recalled from Chapter 1 that the various terms used for what we now recognize as "migraine" were also used in the sixteenth century A.D., to describe vertigo and motion sickness. Arateus, in the first century A.D., referred to "scotoma" in association with migraine but he was not describing a feature of visual aura. The Greek word "scotoma" is actually translated as "vertigo" in Latin, and Arateus noted that "heterocrania" could progress to "scotoma." Caelius Aurelanius, translating Soranus of Ephesus from the second century A.D., stated that "scotoma" could be distinguished from epilepsy because it did not deprive the patient of his senses, and from cephalea (chronic headache) because it did not cause pain (23). Edward Liveing also included "vertigo" as one of his cardinal features of megrim. Yet, curiously IHC-2 does not include vertigo in its rubric for migraine, except in the context of "migraine of basilar type," which demands additional symptoms of brainstem or bilateral hemispheric dysfunction. What then is the relationship between migraine and episodic vestibular symptoms in isolation?

Vertigo, in modern parlance, is an illusion of motion, often rotatory, most commonly caused by vestibular dysfunction, whereas *dizziness* denotes light-headedness, faintness, or unsteadiness of nonvestibular origin. Such symptoms can coexist but can usually be distinguished. Both can be migrainous phenomena. Vertigo and dizziness are extremely common symptoms, affecting one-quarter of the population in some surveys (24); so an observed association with migraine, which is also very common, might therefore be simply by chance. However, there is good epidemiological evidence that migraineurs are over-represented among patients with a variety of vertigo syndromes, including nonvestibular dizziness, motion sickness, and psychiatric conditions such as depression and panic disorder. Can recurrent vertigo therefore be caused by migraine, or are individuals prone to migraine attacks just more susceptible to episodic vertigo and dizziness?

A recent expert review suggested that migrainous vertigo (MV, sometimes referred to as *vestibular migraine*) could prove to be the most common cause of spontaneous recurrent vertigo (25). The proposed diagnostic criteria for migrainous vertigo can be broadly summarized as follows:

- Recurrent episodic vestibular symptoms of at least moderate severity, interfering with but not necessarily precluding normal activity
- Current or previous history of migraine
- One or more of the following migrainous symptoms during at least two of the vertigo attacks: headache, photophobia, phonophobia, or visual or other auras
- Exclusion of other causes (including migraine of basilar type)

Additional supportive evidence would include precipitation of vertigo by known migraine triggers, a family history of migraine, and response of attacks to antimigraine drugs.

The pathogenesis of MV is not fully understood. Rare reports of patients examined during attacks have described eye movement abnormalities consistent with vestibular disturbance of central origin, although features of peripheral vestibular dysfunction have also been observed in some cases. Lempert and colleagues recently reported a prospective study of 20 MV patients studied shortly after an acute attack (26). They noted that vertigo usually began some twenty years after the onset of migraine, which could be with or without other types of aura. In half of the cases studied, the attacks began with vertigo, with the migrainous elements (commonly head-ache and photophobia), developing subsequently as is typical of the usual sequence of events in migraine with aura. However, in other patients, the attack began with the headache phase, or the headache and vertigo devel-oped simultaneously. Occasionally patients also experienced visual and somesthetic auras with vertigo and on other occasions the habitual vertigo could also occur in isolation (acephalalgic MV). The most unusual feature of the syndrome, however, was the duration of the vertiginous aura. While it is said that perhaps a third of MV cases have vertigo lasting up to an hour—typical of migraine aura—in this group of patients, the vertigo lasted much longer (often for a week and sometimes up to a month).

Spontaneous or positional nystagmus was present in 14 patients (70%) when examined during the acute attack, but voluntary saccades were rapid and accurate in all cases. Two-thirds of the patients had mid-line ataxia and Rombergism. Overall, the vestibular disturbance in MV was heterogeneous, being classified as "central" in half the patients, "peripheral" in 15%, and indeterminate in the remainder. The character of the nystagmus in different patients indicated possible disturbances at the pontomedullary junction, midbrain, vestibulocerebellum, or medulla. The postural instability indi-cated vestibulospinal dysfunction, while testing of neocerebellar function proved normal and ocular motor signs such as saccadic pursuit and gaze-evoked nystagmus were present only in a few instances. The authors concluded that the vestibulocerebellum is not the predominant site of involve-ment in MV.

As we will discuss in Chapter 6, these observations have important implications for our views on the pathogenesis of migraine. If we accept that vertigo is a common migraine aura and that aura results from spreading depression, is MV generated in the cerebral cortex? Vertigo can rarely be a symptom of focal epilepsy originating in areas of cortex, which represent the vestibular system, including the superior lip of the intraparietal sulcus, the posterior superior temporal lobe, the temporoparietal border regions, and V5. Vertiginous aura in epilepsy is momentary, much briefer than in migraine, but it is conceivable that some instances of MV might result from cortical spreading depression involving these cortical regions. The weight of evidence, however, favors the *brainstem* as the origin of MV. Does this imply that spreading depression occurs in the brainstem? As noted in Chapter 2, brainstem spreading depression can be demonstrated experimen-tally but has not been recorded in man to our knowledge. The duration of the process also seems unusually long compared to typical cortical spreading depression, but the activation of various brainstem regions during migraine attacks shown by recent neuroimaging studies would be compatible with the hypothesis, because the locus coeruleus and dorsal raphe nucleus project to the vestibular nuclei and could affect vestibular processing.

Cases of Migrainous Vertigo

CASE 46
A 43-year-old woman had suffered severe and frequent attacks of headache since the age of 11. The attacks comprised spontaneous rotatory vertigo unrelated to head or body movement or position, associated with severe nausea and vomiting, and followed 30 to 60 minutes later by a typical migraine headache. The headaches would usually last up to three days. These attacks continued throughout her life, and despite extensive investigation and vigorous treatment strategies suggested by several neurological centers, the attacks remained disabling to the extent that she became unemployable. She eventually found the combination of rizatriptan followed later by naratriptan, together with prochlorperazine suppositories, to be reasonably helpful in reducing the severity of the attacks.

CASE 47
A 25-year-old woman suddenly began to experience "funny turns." These were composed of light-headedness followed by rotatory vertigo and difficulty with visual focussing. Within half an hour, she would experience a progressively severe headache in the retro-orbital area, with nausea and vomiting, and mild photophobia. She had suffered quite frequent nonspecific but stereotyped headaches previously, and her mother suffered from migraine with visual aura.

CASE 48
An 18-year-old man presented with a two-year history of stereotyped attacks of sudden, unprovoked rotatory vertigo followed by severe headache in the orbital and occipital region. The attacks were of such severity that he would be rendered bed bound. Nausea was not prominent, and he did not vomit. The symptoms would typically last three to four days and would recur every two months or so. Between attacks, he was entirely well. His father had suffered from severe migraine without aura.

CASE 49
A 17-year-old college student was referred following several stereotyped attacks of unprovoked, rotatory vertigo, with nausea and vomiting, each rapidly followed by a severe headache in the fronto-vertical area, and marked photophobia. In some attacks, she would feel her eyes being forced to the left and would sometimes experience diplopia, but there were no other brainstem symptoms. Attacks would last about two hours, with complete recovery. At the outset, she was having attacks almost daily but they became progressively less frequent over 18 months. Neuroimaging and EEG were normal. She did not find sublingual prochlorperazine useful but there was some response to pizotifen.

CASE 50
A 37-year-old woman, with a long history of occasional nonspecific headaches, presented with attacks of vertigo. On each occasion, the symptoms were present on waking. She would immediately be aware of an illusion of rotation and this was followed by nausea and repeated vomiting. After about an hour, she would develop a severe headache that could then persist for anything up to four days, during which

she was unable to function. At presentation, she had been having the attacks every two months. Neurological examination, including positioning maneuvers, was normal.

CASE 51

A 25-year-old woman presented with a four-year history of stereotyped attacks, usually precipitated by stress. Without warning, she would suddenly develop severe rotatory vertigo rapidly followed by intense bitemporal headache with photo- and phonophobia, lasting 15 to 20 minutes and followed by tinnitus for a further 30 minutes. She would have to stop all activities during such attacks, and lie down. Between episodes, she was entirely well. MRI brain scan was normal, and extensive neuro-otological studies showed no evidence of auditory or vestibular dysfunction. The attacks resolved on using topiramate.

CASE 52

A 44-year-old woman was referred because of apparently separate problems of recurrent vertigo and headaches. For years she had experienced recurrent rotatory vertigo, that on occasions had postural components; but if attacks occurred at the time of menstruation, they were typically followed by severe headache. Audiogram was normal. Two years earlier, she had been admitted after an episode of right-sided hemiplegia followed by a similar headache. CT brain scan at the time was normal and she recovered fully. (This was probably an episode of true sporadic hemiplegic migraine.)

CASE 53

A 68-year-old woman presented with a two- to three-year history of recurrent vertigo, sometimes rotatory, with nausea and vomiting. On occasions, there was a feeling of "deafness" in her right ear during attacks, but no tinnitus. Independently, she also suffered attacks of migraine headache preceded by left-sided hemianopic aura, and she had noted that the same type of headache could precede the vertigo on occasions.

As noted, in some instances, attacks of migraine and spontaneous recurrent vertigo appear to be unrelated but the similarity of the symptoms to attacks of migrainous vertigo is consistent with acephalalgic MV, as in the following case.

CASE 54

A 58-year-old man was referred because of recurrent vertigo. Four years earlier, he had suffered a severe rotatory vertigo attack with nausea and vomiting, lasting 10 hours. Full recovery took six weeks, during which he suffered occasional nonspecific headaches. MRI brain scan was normal. Six months later, he had a similar but milder attack lasting three weeks. He began to notice mild, fluctuating bilateral tinnitus but no impairment of hearing. He had two further episodes of vertigo in the six months prior to referral, both associated with a feeling of fullness in the left ear. None of these attacks of vertigo were associated with significant headache, but he began to experience episodic left-sided headaches, sometimes associated with mild dizziness, and he had attacks of migraine with typical teichopsia about once a year. Full neuro-otological examination (optokinetics, calorics, eye tracking, and positional studies) was normal and he had a normal audiogram and tympanogram.

Other vertigo syndromes: There is also a statistical association between migraine and other causes of dizziness and vertigo (24,25). Positioning vertigo can be a feature of migrainous vertigo and was the presenting or predominant feature in a third of Lempert's series (see above). This can be distinguished from benign paroxysmal positioning vertigo (BPPV), which is characterized by recurrent, brief (10 seconds to one minute), stereotyped attacks of vertigo provoked by particular head movements and usually accompanied by torsional nystagmus. Surprisingly, however, migraine was found to be twice as common in patients with BPPV than in controls, and three times more common in patients with idiopathic BPPV than in BPPV secondary to trauma or surgical procedures (25). The syndrome of benign paroxysmal vertigo of childhood is also likely to be a migrainous equivalent. This syndrome resolves as the child grows older, often to be replaced by more typical migraine attacks (24).

Hearing loss, tinnitus, and sensations of aural fullness compatible with Ménière's disease have been reported in MV and, indeed, Prosper Ménière suggested a link between migraine and the syndrome he described in 1861. The lifetime prevalence of migraine is significantly higher in Ménière's disease patients than the general population and migrainous symptoms are commonly reported during vertigo attacks. In Lempert's series none of the patients developed hearing impairment during attacks of MV, although four did report "bilateral aural pressure for up to a minute at the beginning of the attack."

We have encountered cases in each of these categories, and patients with mixed vertigo syndromes can also be encountered, as in Case 58.

Migraine with positioning vertigo

CASE 55
A 38-year-old woman was referred because of a change in her migraine symptoms. For two years, she had experienced infrequent left-sided thumping headaches with photophobia and nausea, lasting up to two days. Her mother had suffered from migraine. Five months before referral, she had suffered a six-week period of frequent disabling, recurrent migraine attacks, sometimes with vomiting and diarrhea. In many of these, she would experience positioning vertigo after about 24 hours of headache, with rotatory illusion provoked by head or body movement in the saggital plane. Investigations showed no abnormalities. On follow-up a year later, she continued to experience frequent episodes of migraine but without vertigo.

Migraine with Ménière's syndrome

CASE 56
A 60-year-old woman was referred because of recurrent headaches. She had developed tinnitus and episodic vertigo in her mid-50s, and her mother had developed similar symptoms in middle age, and also had recurrent headaches. The patient's headaches were typical of migraine, with a visual aura of haloes and associated nausea. Her audiogram showed bilateral symmetrical hearing loss. Neuroimaging was

normal. On follow-up three years later, her symptoms had gradually improved, with only occasional vertigo attacks lasting hours to one day.

CASE 57

A 52-year-old woman was referred because of stereotyped attacks of headache in the left temple and periorbital area. Some could last up to a day and were associated with nausea and mild vertigo, and some had the features of stabbing headaches. As a child she had suffered from "bilious attacks" with vertigo and nausea, and later developed episodic vertigo associated with a feeling of pressure in her left ear, diagnosed as "Ménière's disease." Her sister suffered from migraine. She did not find betahistine helpful but sumatriptan proved effective in treating the headache attacks. On follow-up four years later, her condition was unchanged but she had found that early use of prochlorperazine and aspirin would usually abort both the headache and vertigo attacks.

CASE 58

A 46-year-old woman had a history of migraine without aura dating back to the age of seven. Ten years prior to consultation, she had begun to experience vertigo attacks independently of the migraine attacks. She also developed tinnitus suggestive of Ménière's syndrome but there was no progressive hearing impairment. She seemed to benefit from betahistine. She was referred when the vertigo attacks began to be followed, usually after some 10 minutes, by her typical migraine headaches on almost every occasion. Neuroimaging and full neuro-otological studies were normal; and these attacks subsequently became infrequent, but she then began to have attacks of typical benign positioning vertigo, precipitated by turning her head to the right. Occasionally, these attacks were also followed by migraine headache. Hallpike test was positive, and she responded to a Semont maneuver that abolished the positioning element, although the other vertigo attacks continued.

Drop attacks: Idiopathic drop attacks are a common neurological challenge. The history is characteristic. The patient, almost invariably a middle-aged woman in otherwise good health, will suddenly find herself on the floor, having fallen without warning or precipitant. The patient can suffer significant trauma, and attacks often recur over a few months. The prognosis, however, is excellent, and the events usually cease spontaneously.

The cause of drop attacks is unknown. They have been attributed to sudden brainstem ischemia, as in "vertebrobasilar insufficiency" (a much overdiagnosed condition), basilar artery spasm, syncope due to cardiac dysrhythmia, autonomic dysfunction, and seizure. However, consciousness is preserved in true drop attacks and the onset is paroxysmal, unlike in all these other conditions.

One group of patients has been identified, in which the mechanism appears to be related to inner ear dysfunction—the *"otolithic crisis of Tumarkin"* (27). It is suggested that Tumarkin falls result from sudden pressure changes across the utricular macule and are a feature of a subset of patients with Ménière's disease. However, while it is certainly true that acute vertigo can cause sudden collapse and prostration, true idiopathic drop attacks are not associated with vertigo. Interestingly, Baloh's group at the

University of California at Los Angeles, have pointed out that patients with Tumarkin falls have a high prevalence of active migraine but normal hearing, unlike typical Ménière's patients (28). Given that the migraine mechanism can cause paroxysmal symptoms, and in the absence of alternative explanations, perhaps idiopathic drop attacks are migraine auras.

Migraine and deafness: We have already mentioned auditory auras, but there is also a suggestion that cochlear dysfunction, the distinctive feature of Ménière's disease, might also be a feature of migrainous vertigo in some cases. This raises the possibility that migrainous vertigo and Ménière's disease could represent a pathophysiological continuum, involving variable brainstem, vestibular, and cochlear dysfunction. It has also been suggested that sudden, unexplained unilateral deafness might result from migraine-associated vasospasm (29). This is considered further in Chapter 4.

Motor auras: Motor auras can exhibit the same sequence of excitatory and inhibitory symptoms as visual and somesthetic auras. *Excitatory* phenomena are rare, but can include involuntary movements such as chorea, dystonia, and akathisia. Indeed, as noted in Chapter 2, Bruyn and Ferrari's observation of chorea in the excitatory phase of migraine aura was early evidence that migraine attacks might originate deep in the basal ganglia or upper brainstem area (30). Dystonic limb "cramps and spasms" can also occur, as can focal seizures, although *migraine-triggered seizure* (IHC-2 1.5.5) is treated as a separate issue (see Chapter 4).

We have encountered a case of what we would interpret as *dystonic aura.*

CASE 59
A 47-year-old woman presented with an eight-year history of stereotyped attacks, occurring monthly. Fatigue and missing a meal seemed provocative. She would experience a prodrome of fatigue, mild drooping of the left eyelid and vague dizziness, followed by progressive dystonia of the left side, with curling of the fingers of the hand and hyperpronation of the left foot, to the extent that the limbs would be functionless. This would be followed by a progressive left-sided headache with severe nausea and vomiting, photo-, and osmophobia. The symptoms would subside over three days, but it might take a week for her to return to normal. Between attacks, she was entirely well.

She had suffered an isolated migraine attack in pregnancy many years earlier, but there was no other migraine history. MRI brain scan was normal. She had tried virtually all antimigraine preparations, responding best to zolmitriptan, although it was only of modest benefit she had not tried an anticonvulsant at the time of consultation.

Hemiplegic migraine: Inhibitory motor aura symptoms occur more often in migraine than positive manifestations, but still much less commonly than sensory symptoms. Feelings of "numbness" in the limbs on one side at the start of an attack are common; and as mentioned previously, patients often interpret these feelings as "weakness," while they are in fact usually sensory. In contrast, true hemiplegic migraine is usually dramatic. The affected limbs are atonic and areflexic during the attack, as in a "cortical stroke," and apraxia may occur during recovery. Naturally, most cases are initially diagnosed as stroke. Stroke from any cause may also be associated with headache, but in hemiplegic migraine, the weakness usually *precedes* headache and has a time course commensurate with aura. Paradoxically, migraine itself can cause stroke (see Chapter 4), but here the hemiparesis or more restricted motor deficit usually *follows* the onset of headache. When hemiplegia due to migraine aura or migrainous infarction occurs without headache, however, the distinction may be impossible to make on clinical grounds alone.

The great majority of instances of hemiplegic migraine are sporadic. We discussed the genetic and pathogenetic aspects of familial hemiplegic migraine (FHM) in detail in Chapter 2, and this interesting condition is considered further in Chapter 4. Here, we will consider only the clinical aspects.

Familial hemiplegic migraine. The IHC-2 diagnostic criteria for FHM (IHC-2 1.2.4) can be summarized as follows:

> At least two attacks of MA, including motor weakness, where at least one first- or second-degree relative has migraine aura, including fully reversible motor weakness, together with at least one of the "typical" forms of aura. Headache begins during the aura or follows aura within 60 minutes.

Of course, it is axiomatic that no other cause for the symptoms can be found after appropriate investigation. Migraine attacks in FHM1 are often associated with unusual symptoms such as disturbances of consciousness, including confusion and coma, fever, ataxia, and CSF pleocytosis. Severe headache is virtually always present. Attacks can sometimes be triggered by mild head trauma, which presumably initiates CSD.

None of the following has been studied genetically, so a diagnosis of FHM can only be presumptive.

CASE 60

A 45-year-old left-handed woman presented with a 10-year history of migraine attacks of variable severity, occurring every four to six weeks. The milder events were typical of MO, comprising a unilateral throbbing temporal headache with blurred vision and vomiting, lasting up to two days. More severe attacks were characterized by a more generalized headache, beginning in the base of the neck, lasting up to a week, with severe vomiting throughout this period. There were often premonitory symptoms of thirst and bloating one to two days prior to attacks, and a subsequent diuresis.

In a number of attacks, she had also developed severe right-sided weakness and aphasia, which would last for one to two days. This would occur about two hours into the event. She described total paralysis and complete inability to communicate. She later said that her younger sister had begun to experience identical hemiplegic attacks, but there was no other known family history.

CASE 61

A 46-year-old woman gave a history of typical migraine with visual aura dating back to her early teens. She had noted that attacks could be precipitated by cheese and chocolate, and later in life she also proved sensitive to red wine and colored liqueurs. Sometimes, she would also experience hemisensory auras with these attacks. Episodes later became catamenial, but were less frequent following hysterectomy.

She was referred following a change in her symptoms over the previous four months. She described recurrent attacks that would begin with a brief visual aura of a colored flash of light, immediately followed by severe pain in and around the right eye, which could become swollen and reddened. Within a few minutes, she would develop complete paralysis of the right arm and leg, which would take about a day to resolve. The headache would last two to three days, and was associated with nausea and vomiting on occasions. Her mother had suffered identical attacks beginning in childhood. A maternal aunt was probably also affected, and the patient's daughter had recently begun to have similar episodes.

Sporadic hemiplegic migraine (SHM). SHM is clinically similar to the common form of FHM, but the major systemic symptoms are usually lacking and, of course, there is no family history of the condition. Although SHM appears to be much more common than FHM, in many instances, hemisensory impairment is probably interpreted as weakness. We have also included some cases of hemiplegia without headache.

CASE 62

A 42-year-old woman, who was six months pregnant, was watching television when she suddenly experienced numbness and weakness of the right arm and leg, and began drooling from the right side of the mouth. Her language function was not affected. After two minutes or so, she developed a severe frontal headache, but there were no other symptoms. She was seen in the Accident and Emergency room about two hours later, at which point the headache was receding, but the weakness persisted. She had a long history of migraine with visual aura, which had become less frequent with the use of pizotifen, and she had had an attack several years previously, comprising left-sided sensorimotor impairment followed by headache and a brief syncope.

On examination there was a mild pyramidal distribution weakness. CT brain scan was normal, and she was discharged the following day. However, a vague feeling of weakness persisted for three months. On review six months after the ictus, she was asymptomatic. MRI brain scan was normal.

CASE 63

A 49-year-old woman, with a long history of leg cramps, developed leg cramp in bed one morning, causing her to jump out of bed. She was immediately aware of a throbbing weakness that ascended up her left side from the foot to the face over some three to five minutes. She felt faint and disoriented, and believed that she was about to die. After ten minutes she recovered completely. There was no headache or nausea. A month later she had an identical attack at a wedding. The weakness down the left side was so profound that she had to sit on the floor. MRI brain scan, MRA, and extracranial ultrasound studies were normal.

A paternal uncle suffered from migraine, and she had a personal history of MA dating from childhood, with attacks once or twice a year. These attacks comprised a prodrome of perception of "time slowing" and repeated yawning, followed by a colored visual aura of "oil on water," photopsia and phonophobia, numbness of the neck and mouth, and dysarthria. A severe "tension-type" headache over the head, like a helmet, would follow, and she would have problems with spatial awareness. After two to three hours, she would have nausea and vomiting, which would usually terminate the attack.

CASE 64

A 51-year-old left-handed man was referred because of symptoms that were clearly episodes of migraine with visual aura. During these attacks he would also often experience numbness in the left arm and hand, and would occasionally develop mild speech impairment. There was a strong family history of migraine with visual aura in his father and brother.

Some 10 years earlier, he had suffered an attack in which, while writing, he became unable to use his left hand, and then developed a dense left hemiplegia and aphasia. There was no associated headache, and he had not experienced any symptoms suggestive of migraine previously. He was extensively investigated but no abnormalities were found, and he recovered fully within 24 hours.

CASE 65

A 37-year-old man was riding in the passenger seat of his wife's car when he suddenly lost consciousness for four minutes. On regaining consciousness, he was paralyzed down the left side, and was developing a severe occipital headache with neck stiffness. His wife rushed him to hospital, but by the time they arrived in the emergency room some 30 minutes later, he had recovered completely. There were no clinical abnormalities, and CT brain scan and CSF examination were normal. A subsequent MRI brain scan was also normal. He had a previous history of migraine with visual auras on a frequent basis, and these continued on follow-up.

CASE 66

A 59-year-old woman was admitted with acute right-sided weakness, coincident with severe headache. She had suffered two earlier attacks of a similar nature. She had a history of migraine with visual aura dating from childhood. The visual auras comprised a chevron pattern beginning in the center of her vision and migrating to the right, leaving a black scotoma. Headache would follow some 30 minutes later, with severe nausea and vomiting. She had experienced a crescendo of such attacks prior to the hemiplegia event, which resolved completely within a day. She had been investigated previously, with negative results. Trials of migraine prophylaxis had been disappointing, but she had found sumatriptan injections to be helpful for the headache phase.

CASE 67

A 47-year-old woman was referred for review with a 14-year history of attacks of sudden weakness of the right arm and leg, lasting from 20 minutes to up to two hours, sometimes followed by severe headaches. In one particularly severe attack, the paralysis was preceded by involuntary movements of the arm, and was followed by loss of consciousness. On some occasions, mild dysphasia and nausea would occur. She had suffered from attacks of migraine with visual aura for years, although the attacks were infrequent. Investigation on several occasions, including ultrasound studies of the extracranial vessels, MRI brain imaging, and MRA had shown no abnormalities.

Sometimes, the motor involvement can be more limited, as illustrated by the following case.

CASE 68

A 76-year-old woman was referred with a three-year history of typical migrainous visual auras without headache. These comprised a non-colored, semilunar scotoma in either the right or left hemifield or a central scintillating scotoma that would resolve over about 20 minutes. Her son and paternal grandmother had quite severe migraine. She recalled that in her 40s, she had experienced frequent stereo-typed attacks beginning with a severe temporal headache, usually on the left but some-times the right, associated with right facial paralysis, but sparing the arm and leg. The facial weakness would persist for four to five days, and the headache for 1 to 10 days, with associated nausea and photophobia. These attacks stopped at the menopause.

DISORDERS OF HIGHER CORTICAL FUNCTIONS

Some of the strangest migraine aura symptoms result from disturbance of higher cortical functions. These include memory disturbances, changes in mood and perception, and alterations in appreciation of time and move-ment. Many of these auras are very rare, but *transient global amnesia* (TGA) is common.

Memory

Alterations of memory function are very common manifestations of migraine. Rarely, this may take the form of déjà vu and jamais vu, as found more often in temporal lobe partial seizures, but amnesia to variable degrees is more often a component of an aura that includes other "typical" aura features.

Amnesia as a Component of "Typical" Auras

CASE 69

A 34-year-old woman began to suffer attacks of visual aura and malaise, followed by weakness of the right hand, lasting between 10 and 30 minutes. During these attacks, she was aware that she was unable to recall recent events. There was no headache, and she recovered fully on each occasion, although she was left with malaise that would last a day or so. She was extensively investigated, including cere-bral angiography, to exclude thromboembolic TIAs, with negative results. These attacks would occur about once or twice a year.

CASE 70

A 31-year-old woman was involved in a road traffic accident, but when interviewed at the scene, it was evident that she had no recollection of events prior to the impact, or of the crash itself. She had not suffered any physical injury. When seen at a local emergency room, she was clearly in the throes of one of her habitual migraine attacks and was complaining of headache and left-sided sensory impairment. There was no medicolegal issue resulting from the accident. She had suffered from migraine with typical aura for many years.

CASE 71

A 24-year-old woman presented with a three-year history of migraine with mild hemisensory aura. The headache was only modest and never disabling, but the attack rate had increased from about twice monthly to almost daily. In addition, she described occasional atypical auras of amnesia and cognitive dysfunction preceding the headache. In the first episode while working in a café, she suddenly became confused. She could not work out denominations of loose change, had difficulty understanding what customers were saying to her, and even had problems putting burgers and hot dogs together in the correct fashion. Instructions to her had to be repeated several times. She was aware of the customary hemisensory disturbance down the right side during this time.

Her most recent attack had been consistent with Transient Global Amnesia (TGA) (see below). She had a premonitory feeling that an attack might be starting and decided to drive home from work. She remembered nothing of the subsequent hour, during which she drove to the wrong town 30 miles away. As her self-awareness returned, she became aware that she was numb down the right side of the body. MRI brain scan showed no significant abnormalities.

CASE 72

A 25-year-old man gave a history of recurrent morning vomiting and attacks of migraine with visual aura extending back over 10 years. The migraine attacks were more likely to occur following sporting activities such as cricket and hockey matches. After one match, he returned home and had a severe migraine attack with almost total loss of vision. He fell asleep for a couple of hours and on waking, he was amnesic. For example, he did not recognize the new shoes he had just bought. The amnesia lasted hours, but there was a fragmentary recovery of the memories of this amnesic period. He had no further amnesic episodes but continued to have attacks of MA.

CASE 73

A 63-year-old man presented with occasional episodes of brief amnesia. On one occasion, he suddenly forgot how to play Bridge, which he had enjoyed for years, and on another, he suddenly found it difficult to remember the names of people and friends. Each amnesic period lasted about 15 minutes, after which his memory function returned to normal, although the memories of the amnesic period never recovered. In the previous six years, he had experienced episodes of throbbing headache behind the right eye, with nausea, and had been admitted to a hospital on one occasion with acute vertigo.

Transient Global Amnesia

The most common form of dysmnesic aura, however, is TGA. Fisher and Adams introduced this term in 1958 to describe a remarkable syndrome characterized by a sudden inability to record or retain new information, usually lasting less than 24 hours, with preservation of consciousness, self-awareness, and higher cognitive functions (31). During attacks, behavior may be reasonably well preserved, and the patient is often able to perform activities such as driving or household tasks, but characteristically there is some confusion, and the affected individual will repeatedly ask questions such as "Where am I?" or "What are we doing?" In effect, the "memory tape recorder" is switched off! Complex tasks or complete journeys may be undertaken satisfactorily during the amnesic period, but there is usually no subsequent recollection of the events that occur during the period of amnesia. A recent study noted that during attacks, patients had marked impairment of both anterograde and retrograde memory, but well-preserved personal and conceptual semantic knowledge. Retrograde memory recovered rapidly and completely, while the extent of recovery of anterograde memory was heterogeneous (32).

Sometimes the amnesia is followed by a headache. This may be migrainous, but more commonly the headache is nonspecific or trivial or there is no headache at all. Although TGA can be very alarming, it is nearly always benign and does not usually recur, although it may do so.

Etiology of TGA: Transient amnesia may have a number of causes, and it is likely that it is a syndrome of heterogeneous origins. Migraine, epilepsy, and focal cerebral ischemia are most commonly implicated, although the phenomenon has also been described in association with a number of structural cerebral lesions. There is also considerable interest in the association between TGA and jugular venous insufficiency, particularly in view of the temporal relationship between onset of attacks and activities that could result in a Valsalva response.

TGA can present at any age, but is most commonly seen in the fifth to seventh decades when risk factors for cerebral ischemia are increasing. However, in the first detailed analysis of the condition in modern times, using case–control and longitudinal studies, John Hodges and Charles Warlow concluded that there was no evidence for a cerebrovascular etiology, at least of the typical thromboembolic (TIA) form, and that the prognosis was much more favorable than for ischemic cerebrovascular events (33). Rare cases of recurrent TGA induced by arm exercise have been reported in patients with the subclavian steal syndrome, suggesting that posterior circulation ischemia might be the cause (34); but interestingly, in one of the patients reported in that study, the attacks were associated with headache and left arm pain, which could have been migrainous.

Transient amnesia can also be a rare manifestation of seizure. Seven percent of patients in Hodges and Warlow's series developed epilepsy, most often of temporal lobe type, and usually within a year of presentation. The authors conceded, however, that these patients probably had complex partial seizures at presentation, incorrectly interpreted as TGA because amnesia had been the most prominent feature. They commented that other series had not reported such a high incidence of epilepsy. Pure amnesic seizures are well recognized in temporal lobe epilepsy, although they apparently never represent the only seizure type in such patients (35). Epilepsy is therefore, an important differential diagnosis, particularly in cases of recurrent TGA.

Another theory, first proposed by Lewis, relates TGA to episodic cerebral venous congestion (36). Although TGA usually occurs spontaneously, there is a well-known association between TGA and various stresses, both physical and emotional, such as exercise, exposure, and shock, which might induce a Valsalva response. For example, an attack was precipitated during an experiment in which a young soldier was immersed in cold water at 35°C (37). Jugular venous incompetence would increase retrograde venous backflow during Valsalva maneuvers, and it was suggested that this could result in venous congestion and consequent venous ischemia in bilateral diencephalic and hippocampal structures involved with memory. Subsequent ultrasound studies by two groups confirmed a significantly higher incidence of increased retrograde jugular venous flow during Valsalva maneuvers in migraineurs compared to controls (38,39).

A number of imaging modalities have been used in an attempt to identify the anatomical substrate of TGA, with conflicting results. In one important recent study, Sedlaczek and colleague from Mannheim, studied 31 consecutive TGA patients by serial MRI diffusion-weighted imaging (DWI) from the day of onset of the attack up to 48 hours later (40). Multiple punctuate lesions were identified in one or other hippocampi (in 15 cases in the left, in 6 in the right, and in 5 in both). These were rarely visible in the early hours after the attack but were observed frequently by 48 hours. All lesions were centered in the pes and fimbria hippocampi and the thalami, regions known to be critical to memory function, consistent with previous SPECT and PET studies that had shown hypoperfusion in these areas in TGA. These studies had also shown that these micro diffusion abnormalities resolved subsequently. The prolonged delay from the onset of TGA to the appearance of these lesions is not consistent with typical thromboembolic ischemia, although nearly all the patients in the Sedlaczek study had significant vascular risk factors. The authors speculated that the lesions were more in keeping with Lewis's venous congestion thesis, but one would have expected that TGA would be more common if that were the case, because jugular venous insufficiency can be demonstrated in about a third of the population (41).

In fact, Hodges and Warlow found that the strongest comorbid association with TGA was with migraine. Jes Olesen had actually proposed this explanation more than 20 years ago (42), and in our view, the evidence that most instances of uncomplicated TGA represent migrainous auras is compelling. However, there are three factors against this hypothesis: the typical age of onset of TGA in middle age and older is not typical of migraine; TGA is more common in men than in women, unlike migraine; and TGA is not usually recurrent, unlike migraine. However, TGA is certainly not confined to the middle-aged and elderly, and other forms of atypical auras are also often nonrecurrent.

Could the delayed DWI lesions be compatible with the migraine mechanism? As noted in Chapter 2, the migraine mechanism does not normally injure the brain but it is associated with white matter lesions on MRI scans, which are thought to be ischemic in origin. In TGA, the area of predilection in the hippocampus lies in the watershed between the upper and lower hippocampal arteries—the hypoxia-susceptible Sommer's sector—and the DWI lesions might result from "misery perfusion" due to the secondary oligemia of CSD. Such stresses could result in enhanced glutamate release (the brain regions involved in memory circuitry are glutamate rich) and locally increased metabolic demands, which might cause focal ischemia, particularly in individuals with age-related small vessel disease.

Another possible etiological link is the observed relationship between migraine and patent foramen ovale (PFO). The concept is that Valsalva manoevres would increase right-to-left shunting if a PFO was present, and this somehow leads to migraine attacks, but again, the relative infrequency of TGA is unexpected under this hypothesis.

When reading the following case histories, the reader might like to reflect on the possible medicolegal implications of TGA, and indeed coital amnesia (see the section on "Coital Amnesia" below), in terms of the definition of "insane automatism!"

CASE 74
A 61-year-old man suffered an isolated episode of amnesia lasting about an hour. He had been working in the garden just prior to the attack. During the event, he otherwise functioned normally and was able to clean his wife's car and conduct a telephone conversation with a relative, who did not notice anything unusual during the conversation. He had a history of MO when young, but had experienced no attacks for years. He had no significant vascular risk factors, save for smoking 10 to 15 cigarettes daily.

CASE 75
A 50-year-old man awoke one morning with a headache and photophobia. He fell asleep in a colleague's car on the way to work. At work, he was unable to remember his computer password, and when told, could not retain the information and had to ask his colleagues again. At home, he could not remember the names of flowers, although he was an avid gardener and would normally have recalled them with ease. Later that day, he developed left facial numbness. For some time afterwards, he had problems with long-term memory, such as recalling important numbers connected with his work. He had a mild recurrence of amnesia a few weeks later but then recovered completely. On inquiry three years later, there had been no further problems. He had no previous personal history of migraine, but his father suffered from recurrent headaches.

CASE 76
A 62-year-old woman was admitted as an emergency as a case of "confusional state," after she had been found standing alone, motionless but holding a dustpan and brush, by her neighbor. The patient said repeatedly, "I don't know what I am doing with these." They had attended a dog-handling class together earlier that day, but the patient had no recollection of the event. By the time she arrived in the hospital, she was complaining of a "thumping" headache, and subsequently

developed nausea and vomiting. Her memory returned to normal within a few hours, and neurological examination and CT brain scan were normal.

She had a history of migraine with visual aura dating back to her 20s. The visual aura phase tended to occur within the headache phase. Nausea and vomiting were almost invariably associated with the attacks.

About a year later, she had another attack of amnesia very similar to the first, but on this occasion, not followed by headache. This attack had been preceded by emotional shock: her dog had been attacked by another, but she was unable to recall any details of the event during the amnesic period or subsequently. She had also opened the front door of her house to a caller, but again had no recollection of the event. She recovered completely in about two hours.

CASE 77

A 27-year-old man suffered an episode of TGA, following a trivial head injury in a rugby match. He did not lose consciousness and completed the game. He seemed normal to his teammates after the match and was able to drive home, but then went to bed in his dirty rugby uniform. The following morning, he had no recollection of any of the previous day's events. A year later, he had another episode. Again, he had been playing rugby, but on this occasion there was no head injury. On his return home, he repeatedly asked his family where he was and what he was doing there. Following this amnesic event, he later suffered repeated migraine headaches in the left frontal area, associated with nausea and photophobia. Some were associated with dysgraphia. There was no previous personal or family history of migraine.

CASE 78

A 41-year-old woman suffered an amnesic attack while giving birth at home. In retrospect, she remembered the midwife arriving, and being given "gas and air," and also remembered saying to her husband that she felt she was "blacking out," but she had no recollection of getting onto the floor for the delivery, the afterbirth, suturing of the episiotomy, having photographs of herself and the baby taken, or giving the baby its first feed. She recovered without further problems. She had a history of occasional headaches with nausea but no family history of headache.

CASE 79

A 65-year-old woman was referred following an attack, witnessed by her general practitioner and husband, during which she suddenly seemed "confused." She made errors on simple tests such as naming the Prime Minister, the year and the date, and she could not remember that her son was living abroad. Her function was otherwise unimpaired. The amnesia lasted about seven hours, after which she was entirely well.

She had suffered two previous attacks of this type about five years earlier, but had not sought medical attention. There was no history of recurrent headaches, but about 20 years earlier, she had awoken with complete blindness of the "left eye" followed by extremely severe headache, nausea, and vomiting. There was no family history of migraine, but her mother and son had each suffered a single epileptic seizure.

CASE 80

A 65-year-old man became amnesic following his morning shower. During this period, he spoke to his wife on the telephone, and while seeming rational, said he could not understand why he was at home and not at work (it was his day off). The episode lasted three hours, and he never recovered the memories of the amnesic period. He suffered a dull headache after the attack. In the previous couple of years, he had experienced mild attacks of migraine with elemental visual auras and severe occipital headache lasting an hour or so.

Three years later, he was referred once more with a further attack of probable TGA. He had been on holiday abroad and was found by the landlady at his accommodation in a slightly bemused state. In retrospect, he had no recollection of events that day over a period of about four hours. He subsequently had a dull headache similar to that he had experienced with the first episode. Investigation revealed no evidence of significant cerebrovascular disease.

CASE 81

A 65-year-old woman was evaluated after three episodes of TGA in the previous year. On each occasion there were prodromal symptoms of malaise and nausea, and sometimes, headache and vomiting. Behavior during attacks was typical of TGA, with anterograde amnesia regarding, for example, her daughter's pregnancy, and inability to recall recent visits to friends. During the attacks, she said and did little. She was visited by her general practitioner during one of the attacks, but had no recollection of the visit. She otherwise recovered completely after each event. She had suffered from MA since childhood. Events could be triggered by foods, starvation, and alcohol, and there was also an extensive family history of such attacks. No abnormalities were found on neuroimaging or vascular screening studies.

CASE 82

A 55-year-old man had been working very hard on a building project for many hours, when he suddenly became amnesic. In retrospect, he remembered calling his wife on the telephone to say he was going to collect some building materials, but then had no recollection of events for the next two hours. During that time, he had driven his van, but he had no idea where he had been or what he had done. Previously, about twice a month, he would experience bilateral pulsatile headaches with nausea lasting about two hours, responsive to paracetamol.

CASE 83

A 74-year-old woman suffered an unprovoked amnesic episode while working in the garden. Her friend witnessed the attack. The patient repeatedly asked "Why am I here?" and "What am I doing?" She was noted to be very pale. Her next recollection was of getting into a car to go to her doctor's office, about an hour later. She had suffered typical migraine attacks in the past, although they had stopped some 15 years ago. She had also suffered two acephalalgic attacks with prostration and unilateral sensory impairment during that period, diagnosed as "possible stroke" or "functional" at the time, but were almost certainly migraine auras.

CASE 84

A 60-year-old woman was referred following a typical attack of TGA. She had returned from work and took a shower. She had no recollection of the next few hours, but she telephoned her husband at some point. He noticed that during conversation, she asked the same questions repeatedly. She recovered fully. She denied a previous history of migraine but had clearly experienced visual auras without headache since her early 30s. These comprised typical scintillating scotomas in the right hemifield, but were infrequent, the last being some five years earlier. Her father had suffered from severe migraine.

Coital Amnesia

The influence of "stress" in the pathogenesis of TGA is probably no better exemplified than by the phenomenon of *coital amnesia*. In this special instance, amnesia with the typical features of TGA is precipitated by sexual intercourse. Most such episodes are isolated, but one of the authors reported a case of recurrent coital amnesia (43). A 64-year-old man was brought to the clinic by his wife, because on five separate occasions over some 20 years, he had temporarily lost his memory after sexual intercourse. At these times, he exhibited behavior typical of TGA, repeatedly asking questions such as "What are we doing?" but he would recognize his wife and was otherwise reasonably preserved, although he appreciated that he was having difficulties. These amnesic periods each lasted about 30 to 60 minutes. He recovered completely on each occasion, but subsequently could recall little of the preliminaries to intercourse. The attacks were not associated with headache but he had a long history of MO and had also experienced attacks of typical coital cephalalgia. He had never experienced TGA under other circumstances. Following the publication of this observation, which was widely reported in the press, a number of people wrote reporting further examples of coital amnesia (see cases below).

Interestingly, coital amnesia has not been reported in women to our knowledge. A cynic might suggest a number of reasons for this, but because migraine as defined by IHC-2 criteria is more common in females than males, this observation is unexplained!

CASE 85
A physician wrote to us describing a male patient who had suffered amnesia following intercourse, with a retrograde amnesia that extended to some 36 hours. With time, this decreased to a 30-minute period immediately following intercourse. Investigations revealed no abnormality, and there were no further events.

CASE 86
A 66-year-old man had been perfectly well until he developed amnesia following sexual intercourse. On that day, he had gone swimming. He came home, made some tea, and then had intercourse with his partner. Afterwards, he carried out a normal telephone conversation with a colleague concerning a forthcoming social event and nothing seemed out of the ordinary. His daughter then called to complain that he had failed to turn up to look after the grandchildren. He had absolutely no recollection of any of these events when asked about them number of hours later, but was aware that some problem had occurred. There was no headache or other symptoms. He had not suffered migraine previously, but had taken aspirin 75 mg daily for years.

CASE 87
A 67-year-old man was referred following two episodes of amnesia, each following sexual intercourse. On the first occasion, following coitus, he got out of bed to go to the bathroom and on his return, he lost his memory completely for about 15 minutes. During that time, he repeatedly asked, "Why am I doing this?" and said "This is not

my shirt" (it was). His wife sensibly suggested that he take some aspirin, but he replied, "I am not on any tablets" (he was). He experienced an identical attack three years later. In the past, he had occasionally experienced severe occipital and vertical headaches lasting 15 to 30 minutes, and his daughter suffered from severe migraine.

CASE 88
A 69-year-old-man was referred following an episode of amnesia associated with sexual intercourse. He remembered that he had woken feeling normal, and had gone downstairs to make a cup of tea. He returned to bed and began to have sex with his partner, but later had no recollection of the act. His next clear memory was of sitting at the top of the stairs, feeling very strange. Over the next few hours, this feeling persisted, and he seemed to have difficulties with memory recall and in assimilating new memories. He then recovered. He was aware that he had experienced a headache at some point in these events but was unable to provide a clear description of the features. He had suffered frequent headaches in the past, usually on waking, which would last an hour or two. There were no other migrainous features however, and no family history of migraine.

One of our correspondents reported a variation on this pattern, which might be termed *"postcoital confusion."*

CASE 89
A 60-year-old-man wrote to say that throughout his adult life, he had suffered a curious decline in his cognitive function the day following sexual intercourse. He referred to it as "an attack of the stupids." He noted a general sense of disorientation, short-term memory problems, poor concentration, and loss of dexterity, for example, when typing. This did not follow every such event, but was sufficiently frequent for him to clearly recognize the association. It was particularly likely to occur after a period of sexual abstinence followed by a particularly vigorous "sexual encounter." He described it as if "the central nervous system had received an overload." He had suffered from migraine since his mid-20s.

Mood Disorders

Alterations in mood are rare as migraine auras, but phenomena such as hyperactivity, pleasure, awe and rapture (as in visions), giggling, hilarity and hysterical behavior, moral indignation, and depression phenomena such as fear, a sense of foreboding, pathological crying, horror, and angor animi have been described.

Disorders of Perception and Planning

Other integrative dysfunctions in migraine may include temporary loss of motor skills and planning, such as how to drive or navigate to a destination, or even how to do very simple household tasks (*scotoma of action*). *Astereoagnosia* may occur, in which the nature of an object held in the hand cannot be perceived, despite normal primary sensory function. Curious disturbances of time perception have also been reported. Hughlings Jackson described the phenomenon of *"doubling of consciousness"* in which the altered state runs in parallel with normal consciousness.

CASE 90
A 39-year-old woman presented following an attack four days previously, in which she had suddenly felt drooping of her right eyelid, followed by an illusion in which she believed the film she was watching on television was moving too fast. Later that evening, she experienced a nonspecific right-sided headache radiating into the neck. The following day she had right arm pain (presumably migrainous), which progressed to include a feeling of weakness with dragging of the right leg, face pain, and difficulty swallowing. By the time she was evaluated, the symptoms had resolved, and there were no abnormal findings on examination. She had a history of MO, invariably with right-sided headache, dating back to childhood.

CASE 91
A 56-year-old-woman was driving passengers in a mini-bus at the Airport. While reversing her vehicle, her vision "evaporated," and she suddenly felt while "reversing backwards at 100 mph." She jammed her foot on the brake so hard that she sprained it. No one in the bus noticed but she was so alarmed by this event that her doctor signed her off work for six weeks! She was then well until a year later when, while watching television, she developed a visual aura "like interference," followed by bilateral white central scotomas that persisted for several days. She had a further event of this type a few days later, followed by syncope. She had suffered severe migraine with visual auras as a young woman. On follow-up two years later, she had reported that she had no further illusions, or, indeed, any more migraine attacks.

CASE 92
A 32-year-old man, referred for other medical issues, mentioned a six-month history of recurrent paroxysmal symptoms. These included episodes of sudden speech arrest or expressive dysphasia lasting seconds, sudden attacks of inability to masticate properly, again lasting seconds, and sudden "blinding headaches" with nausea and photophobia lasting only a few minutes. He also mentioned that for many years, he had periodically felt that suddenly "things were going faster than they should." For example, people seemed to be speaking unusually quickly or moving very fast. This would last for a few seconds to a minute and occurred about twice a year. He had never sought medical opinion previously about these feelings because he felt he would not be taken seriously.

CASE 93
A 33-year-old man, again referred for other clinical issues, mentioned in passing that from time to time "things suddenly seem to be going incredibly fast—people speaking, movement and so on," and this was of concern to him, because it occurred without warning or explanation. He had never mentioned this to a doctor before. There was however, no personal or family history of migraine.

CASE 94
A 43-year-old man presented with a one-year history of visual disturbances that would occur exclusively when he was driving, particularly on long journeys on roads where there were interrupted white lane lines on the road. He would suddenly feel that he was in fact stationary, but the environment was moving in relation to him. This feeling would persist for anywhere from 10 minutes to an hour, during which he would feel unsteady and "off balance," even though he was sitting. He had a history of MA, with weekly attacks of "splitting" frontal and periorbital headache, sometimes associated with elemental visual auras. There was, however, no family history of migraine.

The "menagerie of migraine" continues to surprise us with its repertoire. The phenomena we have described are benign and reversible, but sometimes frightening, and certainly inconvenient. In the next chapter, we will consider some situations where migraine really gets nasty!

Dreams and Nightmares

As we discussed in Chapter 2, there is an interesting relationship between sleep and primary headache syndromes. For example, it is well established that sleep disturbance or deprivation can provoke migraine attacks, migraine and cluster headache often start during sleep, and hypnic headache occurs exclusively from sleep.

Dreaming occurs in all stages of sleep. Dreams are reported by 80% of persons who are awakened during REM sleep and sleep onset (NREM stages 1 and 2), and by 40% of persons who are awakened from a deep sleep (NREM stages 3 and 4). However, the content of dreams seems to depend on the sleep stage in which they occur. Dreams experienced during REM sleep tend to be bizarre and detailed. Most frightening dreams and nightmares occur during REM sleep, whereas dreams experienced in deep sleep are less well formed and the dreams of stages 1 and 2 are simpler and shorter than the dreams of REM sleep (44). The ability to recall dreams may reflect the "distance" of the dream from the awake thought processes, and the best recall seems to occur during sleep stages, with electroencephalographic patterns that are most like those in the waking state.

There is some evidence that dreams and nightmares occur more commonly among migraineurs. This was first noted by Caro Lippman who, as noted above, was particularly interested in the psychic aspects of migraine (45). Some migraineurs will experience a significant headache if woken during a dream (46,47) and "lucid dreams," in which imagery is particularly vivid and readily recalled when the subject awakes, seem to be more common among migraineurs (48,49). While the function of dreams is debated, these observations raise the real possibility that dreams are yet another manifestation of the migraine mechanism. Could 'dreams' be a form of migraine aura?

REFERENCES

1. Headache classification subcommittee of the International Headache Society. The International Classification of Headache Disorders. 2nd ed. Cephalalgia 2004; 24 (suppl 1):1–160. Oxford, UK: Blackwell Publishing, 2004.
2. Kelman L. The aura: a tertiary case study of 952 migraine patients. Cephalalgia 2004; 24:728–734.
3. Alvarez WC. The migrainous scotoma as studied in 618 cases. Am J Ophthalmol 1960; 49:489–504.
4. Cohen S, Blau JN. Lifelong migraine aura without headache: change of pattern with upper respiratory tract infection. J R Soc Med 2003; 96:504–505.

5. Bucholz DW, Reich SG. The menagerie of migraine. Semin Neurol 1996; 16: 83–93.
6. Hadjikhanani N, Sanchez del Rio M, Wu O, et al. Mechanisms of migraine aura revealed by functional MRI in the human cortex. Proc Natl Acad Sci 2001; 98:4687–4692.
7. Richards W. The fortification illusions of migraine. Sci Am 1971; 224:88–96.
8. Panayiotopoulos CP. Visual phenomena and headache in occipital epilepsy: a review, a systematic study and differentiation from migraine. Epileptic Disord 1999; 1:205–216.
9. Atkinson RA, Appenzeller O. Deer woman. Headache 1978; 37:229–232.
10. Wilkinson M, Robinson D. Migraine art. Cephalalgia 1985; 3:151–157.
11. Fuller GN, Gale MV. Migraine aura as artistic inspiration. Br Med J 1988; 297:1670–1672.
12. Podoll K, Ayles D. Inspired by migraine: Sarah Raphael's "Strip!" paintings. J R Soc Med 2002; 95:417–419.
13. Caplan LR. Top of the basilar syndrome. Neurology (Minneapolis) 1980; 30:72–79.
14. McKee AC, Levine DN, Kowall NW, Richardson EP. Peduncular hallucinosis associated with isolated infarction of the substantia nigra pars reticulata. Ann Neurol 1990; 27:500–504.
15. Lippman CW. Hallucinations in migraine. Am J Psychiatry 1951; 107:856–858.
16. Lipmann CW. Certain hallucinations peculiar to migraine. J Nerv Ment Dis 1952; 116:346–351.
17. Lipmann CW. Hallucinations of physical duality in migraine. J Nerv Ment Dis 1953; 117:345–350.
18. Todd J. The syndrome of Alice in Wonderland. Can Med Assoc J 1955; 73: 701–704.
19. Goodacre SH. The illnesses of Lewis Carroll. Practitioner 1972; 209:230–239.
20. Kew J, Wright A, Halligan PW. Somesthetic aura: the experience of "Alice in Wonderland". Lancet 1998; 351:1934.
21. Leon-Sotomayor LA. Cardiac migraine. Report of twelve cases. Angiology 1974; 25:161–171.
22. Guiloff RJ, Fruns M. Limb pain in migraine and cluster headache. J Neurol Neurosurg Psychiatry 1988; 51:1022–1031.
23. Isler H. Historical background. In: Olesen J, Tfelt-Hansen P, Welch KMA, eds. The Headaches. New York: Raven Press, 1993:1–8.
24. Brandt T. A chameleon among the episodic vertigo syndromes: migrainous vertigo' or 'vestibular migraine'. Cephalalgia 2004; 24:81–82.
25. Neuhauser H, Lempert T. Vertigo and dizziness related to migraine: a diagnostic challenge. Cephalalgia 2004; 24:83–91.
26. Von Brevern M, Zeise D, Neuhauser H, Clarke AH, Lempert T. Acute migrainous vertigo: clinical and oculographic findings. Brain 2005; 128:365–374.
27. Tumarkin A. On Ménière's disease. Proc R Soc Med 1961; 54:907–912.
28. Ishiyama G, Ishiyama A, Baloh RW. Drop attacks and vertigo secondary to a non-Ménière otological cause. Arch Neurol 2003; 60:71–75.
29. Lee H, Lopez I, Ishiyama A, Baloh RW. Can migraine damage the inner ear? Arch Neurol 2000; 57:1631–1634.

30. Bruyn GW, Ferrari MD. Chorea and migraine: "Hemicrania choreatica"? Cephalalgia 1984; 4:119–124.

31. Fisher CM, Adams RD. Transient global amnesia. Trans Am Neurol Assoc 1958; 83:143–146.

32. Guillery-Girard B, Desgranges B, Urban C, Piolino P, DE la Sayette V, Eustache F. The dynamic time course of memory recovery in transient global amnesia. J Neurol Neurosurg Psychiatry 2004; 75:1532–1540.

33. Hodges JR, Warlow CP. The aetiology of transient global amnesia. Brain 1990; 113:639–657.

34. Blasco MR, Arjona A, Jiminez C, Escamillla C. Global transient amnesia and subclavian steal syndrome. Lancet 1996; 347:1636.

35. Palmini AL, Gloor P, Jones-Gotman M. Pure amnestic seizures in temporal lobe epilepsy. Brain 1992; 115:749–769.

36. Lewis SL. Aetiology of transient global amnesia. Lancet 1998; 352:387–399.

37. Castellani JW, Young AJ, Sawaka MN, Backus VL, Canete JJ. Amnesia during cold water immersion: a case report. Wilderness Environ Med 1998; 9:153–155.

38. Sander D, Winbeck K, Etgen T, Knapp R, Klingelhofer J, Conrad B. Disturbance of venous flow patterns in patients with transient global amnesia. Lancet 2000; 356:1982–1984.

39. Akkawi NM, Agosti C, Rozzini L, Anzola GP, Padovani A. Transient global amnesia and venous flow patterns. Lancet 2001; 357:639.

40. Sedlaczek O, Hirsch JG, Grips E, et al. Detection of delayed focal MR changes in the lateral hippocampus in transient global amnesia. Neurology 2004; 62:2165–2170.

41. Tong DC, Grossman M. What causes transient global amnesia? New insights from DWI. Neurology 2004; 62:2154–2155.

42. Olesen J, Jorgensen MB. Leao's spreading depression in the hippocampus explains transient global amnesia. A hypothesis. Acta Neurol Scand 1986; 73:219–220.

43. Lane RJM. Recurrent coital amnesia. J Neurol Neurosurg Psychiatry 1997; 63:260.

44. Pagel JF. Nightmares and disorders of dreaming. American Family Physician 2000; 61:2037–2044.

45. Lippman CW. Recurrent dreams in migraine: an aid to diagnosis. Journal of Nervous and Mental Diseases 1954; 120:273–276.

46. Levitan H. Dreams which culminate in migraine headaches. Psychotherapeutics and Psychosomatics 1984; 41:161–166.

47. Heather-Greener GQ, Comstock D, Joyce R. An investigation of the manifest dream content associated with migraine headaches: a study of the dreams that precede nocturnal migraines. Psychotherapeutics and Psychosomatics 1996; 65:216–221.

48. Irwin HJ. Migraine, out-of-body experiences and lucid dreams. Lucidity Letter 1983; 2:2–4.

49. Irwin HJ. Lucidity dreams and migraine: a second investigation. Lucidity Letter 1986; 5:1–2.

4

Complications

INTRODUCTION

In Chapter 2, we discussed the migraine mechanism and concluded that its underlying processes were pathophysiological rather than due to a "disease." Thus, migraine is a function of the normal human brain, and it is our contention that nearly all of us will experience some manifestation of the condition during our lives.

Despite the tumult of potentially toxic neurochemical events that occur during migraine, it is nearly always benign—as Thomas Willis observed with regard to the frequent and disabling attacks that afflicted his patient Anne, Countess of Conway (see p. 18).

> Having pitched its tents near the confines of the brain, had so long besieged its regal tower, yet it had not taken it.

Nevertheless, the migraine mechanism can sometimes cause complications that can be serious. These complications and the possible reasons for the failure of the intrinsic mechanisms that normally protect the brain from injury by the migraine mechanism are the subject of this chapter.

The International Headache Classification Version 2 (IHC-2) denotes the following as "complications of migraine":

- Chronic migraine
- Status migrainosus
- Persistent aura without infarction
- Migrainous infarction
- Migraine-triggered seizures

We take the view that "chronic migraine" and "status migrainosus" simply represent protracted manifestations of the migraine mechanism rather than true complications, and we will discuss these conditions in Chapter 5. On the other hand, we do consider *migrainous syncope* and *migraine coma* to be additional true complications.

PERSISTENT AURA WITHOUT INFARCTION

Migraine auras generally last around 20 minutes, and the rubric of the IHC-2 definition of aura (see Chapter 3, p. 92) allows a duration of up to one hour. It is well recognized, however, that aura symptoms may continue for much longer and, indeed, may (although rarely) last months or even years.

Persistent aura without infarction appears to be uncommon, and of course, the diagnosis rests entirely on the patient's account. It is defined under IHC-2 (1.5.3) as:

> Aura symptoms that persist for more than two weeks without radiographic evidence of infarction. The aura should be typical of those that have occurred in previous attacks, the only difference being the duration.

Persistent Visual Aura

Haas described two patients with persistent visual aura (1). One reported an elemental colored hemifield hallucination accompanied by ipsilateral parasthesia and clumsiness that lasted five weeks. The second patient gave a seven-month history of concentric grey circles, either bilaterally or in the left hemifield. Luda described a patient who reported a year's history of teichopsia in the right hemifield (2). In a more recent study by Liu and colleagues (3), 10 patients with persistent positive visual aura lasting months to years were examined. The aura symptoms were entirely elemental (such as TV static, snow, lines of ants, dots, and rain), but were bilateral, with full field involvement. Electroencephalograms (EEGs) and magnetic resonance imaging (MRI) brain scans showed no clinically relevant abnormalities. We have not encountered cases of persistent visual aura with features of this type, although several of our patients with presumed retinal migraine (see Chapter 5, p. 213) had persistent subjective visual impairment in the affected eye. However, the following two cases seemed to have features of a persistent *hemianopic* aura.

CASE 95: PERSISTENT HEMIANOPIC VISUAL AURA IN ACEPHALALGIC MIGRAINE

A 29-year-old woman was referred after she had suddenly developed a bright white scotoma in the left visual hemifield while driving her car some 10 weeks previously. The scotoma had persisted ever since, but there was no headache, visual or other neurological symptoms. Ophthalmological examination had revealed no abnormality, and she could detect objects in the scotomatous area on charting, but said that the area just seemed bright and blurred. She had first experienced a similar visual aura some five years before referral, but it had resolved in about 20 minutes to be followed by typical migrainous headache with nausea and vomiting. She had then experienced migraine attacks once or twice a year. Both parents had severe migraine. On review 12 years later, the scotoma persisted unchanged, and her migraine attacks had become more frequent over the years. Neuroimaging was normal.

CASE 96: PERSISTENT VISUAL AURA
A 37-year-old man began to experience occasional visual disturbances in which he thought his right pupil seemed bigger than the left. He would also notice a shimmering or flickering hallucination in the right upper temporal field that was also present with the eyes closed and worsened on looking at a white background. Neurological and ophthalmological examinations and MRI brain scans were normal. This visual aura was still present on review six months later.

Persistent Somesthetic Aura

To date, persistent aura without infarction has been largely confined to reports of visual aura, although one of Haas's cases had additional symptoms, as noted above. However, we have occasionally seen patients with what appeared to be persistent somesthetic, hemiparetic, and dysphasic auras.

CASE 97: PERSISTENT SENSORY AURA WITH SOMESTHETIC METAMORPHOPSIA
A 35-year-old woman was admitted with a suspected stroke. She had been sitting in her garden when she suddenly experienced visual distortion in the left hemifield, as though a photograph had been ripped down the middle. She then developed a muzzy head, and her left arm, face, and tongue went numb. The sensory disturbance was maximal after 90 minutes. Over this period, she felt like ''a very small person in a very large room.'' Neuroimaging and other appropriate investigations were normal. Her left face recovered over three days, but the tongue and left arm took six weeks. Repeat MRI scan two months later showed no abnormalities. The day before this attack, she had suffered an extremely severe headache, having not previously suffered significant headaches.

CASE 98: EXTENSIVE AURA PHENOMENOLOGY INCLUDING FEATURES OF BASILAR TYPE MIGRAINE WITH DEVELOPING PERSISTENT HEMISENSORY AURA
A 46-year-old woman presented with a year's history of sudden feelings of faintness, followed by bilateral arm dysfunction during which her arms would become mildly cyanosed. Her hands would then go white and tingly, and she would recover after about a minute or two. During these spells, she would be fully aware, but found it hard to speak. About three months later, she began to have more extensive attacks of sudden numbness and weakness of the left face, arm, and leg, lasting seconds, during which she was unable to move or talk. Recovery from these symptoms was associated with light-headedness and left-sided paresthesia. She presented to an emergency room following a particularly severe attack in which she dropped the telephone she was holding. By the time she was examined, she had recovered completely, and computed tomography (CT) brain scan and extracranial ultrasound were normal.

She had a 20-year history of migraine with both visual and hemisensory aura, with severe nausea and vomiting, but no family history of migraine.

Over the next few years, she also began to suffer presyncopal and syncopal episodes, some of which were associated with left hemiparesis and apparent speech arrest. There was no associated headache with these episodes, which would occur every 7 to 10 days. She was re-referred after one episode in which the left-sided weakness failed to resolve. Examination two weeks after the onset of this attack revealed mild pyramidal weakness in the left arm without subjective or objective sensory impairment. An MRI brain scan, including diffusion-weighted imaging, showed no abnormality, and magnetic resonance angiography (MRA) was also normal. On review 14 months later, she continued to feel weakness in the left arm and left-sided numbness, and had developed persistent allodynia over the left side of the body and head, together with marked sensitivity to sensory stimuli such as bright light and noise. Following a protracted period of irritating loud noise at work caused by a photocopier, she suddenly experienced left leg weakness followed by severe nausea and vertigo, and lost her vision for about an hour. As it returned, she experienced a kaleidoscope of colored visual flashes and sparks over a three-hour period before recovering completely.

CASE 99: PERSISTENT HEMISENSORY AURA AND DYSPHASIA

A 38-year-old woman suddenly felt weak on her right side while walking down the stairs at home. She tried to call her husband, but she had become aphasic. Within minutes she was hemiplegic and fell to the ground but did not lose consciousness. She remained in this state for approximately four hours and later developed a severe throbbing right-sided headache with nausea and photophobia that lasted several more hours. The aphasia had largely resolved after some 10 hours, but the right hemiparesis persisted.

She had a history of migraine with visual aura comprising bright scotomas or shattering of the image, and at one time had been getting weekly attacks until she was put on pizotifen. Between attacks she typically experienced visual discomfort when looking at striped or checked patterns. There was no family history of migraine. CT brain scan on admission was normal, as was a subsequent MRI scan and EEG.

On review four months later, she continued to experience sensory problems down the right side together with vague confusion and nominal problems. Neuropsychometric examination five months after the attack revealed difficulties with word finding and selection, syntax, problem solving, and high-level language function. She had to give up the course of study she had been pursuing. She had a similar attack a month after the assessment, but this resolved within two hours. She has been left with mild persisting functional deficit, but a recent MRI brain scan again failed to show abnormality. She has continued to experience her typical migraine attacks, despite trials of treatment with beta-blockers.

CASE 100: PERSISTENT HEMISENSORY OR HEMIPARETIC AURA

A 37-year-old woman began to have disabling migraine without aura attacks following the birth of her first child some six years before referral. The attacks comprised severe vertex headache followed some two hours later by nausea and vomiting. Attacks would typically last two or three days but were infrequent, occurring only every few months and stopped following treatment with regular slow-release propranolol. Following the birth of her second child two years later, she suffered an acute attack of right-sided numbness and weakness. This persisted for a day. There was no headache. She was followed up by a neurologist but declined investigation at that stage. She then experienced a flurry of her habitual migraine attacks despite the propranolol, and a further episode of the right-sided sensorimotor symptoms, again without headache. These headaches continued despite a number of other prophylactics.

About a year later, she had a recurrence of the right-sided sensorimotor symptoms, but on this occasion, they were progressive and later associated with increasing malaise, nausea, vomiting, and marked photophobia, but again without headache.

She was admitted and investigated, but no laboratory or neuroimaging abnormalities were found.

The right-sided sensorimotor symptoms persisted for some two months until another neurologist started treatment with topiramate. Since then, she has had only occasional attacks of her customary migraine without aura, which respond well to sumatriptan.

The basis of persistent aura is not known, but it would be reasonable to assume that in such cases, the effects of spreading depression are somehow unusually protracted or even permanent. It will be recalled that routine neuroimaging in migraine with aura rarely discloses abnormalities relevant to the neurological symptoms, although in cases of familial hemiplegic migraine (FHM), protracted hemiplegia can be associated with striking focal abnormalities in the affected hemisphere, indicating cytotoxic cerebral edema secondary to neuronal dysfunction (see p. 154). Recently, the first single photon emission computed tomography (SPECT) and perfusion MRI study of a patient with persistent visual aura was reported. The patient had experienced migraine with visual aura for many years, but at the time of the study, the aura had persisted for over one month. While there were no clinical abnormalities, and routine visual evoked potentials, EEG, brain CT, and standard sequence MRI were normal, both SPECT and brain perfusion MRI showed hypoperfusion reflecting secondary oligemia in areas corresponding to the visual symptoms. The aura did eventually remit, and a repeat study seven months later was normal (4).

MIGRAINOUS INFARCTION

An association between ischemic stroke and migraine has long been recognized. As noted in Chapter 1, the Swiss physician Wepfer first described migrainous infarction in the seventeenth century. In 1881, Fére published a review of Charcot's teachings on the subject and noted that occasionally, the transient symptoms of aura could become prolonged and even permanent (5). This was believed to be the result of constriction and thrombosis of vessels secondary to migrainous vasospasm (*Charcot-Fére syndrome*) (6). This relationship has since been the subject of much research, debate, and speculation. A large number of retrospective and more recent prospective studies have been published examining the relative risk of ischemic stroke in migraine sufferers compared to "non-migraine" control populations at different ages. However, it is difficult to draw confident conclusions from many of the earlier studies because knowledge of the causes of cerebral infarction was more limited.

Is Migraine a Risk Factor for Stroke?

Migraine and stroke could be associated in several ways:

- An ischemic stroke might occur in a migraine sufferer but not in association with a migraine attack.

- Stroke might be attributed to migraine erroneously. Stroke symptoms sometimes include features of "migraine," such as "vascular headache," nausea, and vomiting.
- An ischemic infarct might result directly from a migraine attack—a true *migrainous infarction.*

The current International Headache Society classification defines a migrainous infarction (IHC-2 1.5.4) as follows:

> One or more migraine aura symptoms associated with a relevant ischaemic lesion demonstrated by neuroimaging. Previous attacks fulfil criteria for migraine with aura and the index attack is typical of previous attacks, but one or more aura symptoms last more than 60 minutes. Neuroimaging demonstrates ischaemic infarction in a relevant area, which cannot be attributed to another disorder.

This definition implies that migrainous infarction is dependent on aura. As we will show, this is not true. While some authorities would accept a diagnosis of migrainous infarction only if it evolved sequentially from a typical migrainous aura, in keeping with the International Headache Society (IHS) definition, many studies have not drawn a distinction between stroke occurring during migraine attacks with aura and without aura.

Epidemiology

Migrainous infarction is generally believed to be a rather rare occurrence, but its true incidence is unclear because it is essentially a diagnosis of exclusion. The number of investigations available to identify "rare" causes of stroke, which are particularly important in "young" stroke patients—the group in which migrainous infarction is most common—has increased significantly over recent years. These investigations might now include an extensive search for coagulopathies and antiphospholipid antibodies, genetic screening for mitochondrial cytopathy and *notch 3* mutations (for CADASIL— *cerebral autosomal dominant arteriopathy with subcortical infarcts and leuco-encephalopathy*, which can present with migraine, strokes, and stroke-like events) (7), magnetic resonance imaging and angiography (MRI, MRA), and CT angiography to look for abnormalities of intra- and extracranial blood vessels, particularly vessel dissection. Cardiac sources of embolism are of particular practical importance, and investigation would also typically include transthoracic echocardiography; and if negative, transoesophageal echocardiography (TOE) to look for structural abnormalities. There is particular interest at present in the possible relationship between migraine and patent foramen ovale (PFO, see below). Contrast echocardiography and transcranial Doppler (TCD) studies following intravenous injection of air-agitated saline ("bubble study") have increased the detection rate for intracardiac right-to-left shunts. Ambulatory electrocardiogram (ECG) monitoring for occult dysrhythmias would also be considered. Interestingly, the "prolapsing mitral valve," much vaunted in the past as a cause of stroke, is no longer considered important (8).

These new insights have reduced the apparent incidence of strokes attributable to migrainous infarction. For example, in a retrospective study from the Mayo Clinic based on records from the mid-1970s, migrainous infarction was thought to account for 25% of ischemic strokes in patients of up to 50 years of age (9), while a series of more recent studies puts the incidence between 10% and 15% in this age group (10).

There is now a general consensus that migrainous infarction is most often encountered in young women and that migraine is an independent risk factor for stroke in this group. Smoking and the use of oral contraceptives increase the risk of stroke still further.

In 1993, Marie-Germaine Bousser's group in France published a prospective, case-controlled, hospital-based study that examined whether migraine (as defined by IHC-1 criteria) was a risk factor for stroke. In the first study, 212 stroke cases were compared with 212 controls, matched for age, sex, and history of hypertension. The prevalence of migraine in the whole control population was 16%, and in women under 45, it was 30%. The prevalence of migraine among the stroke patients did not differ from the controls overall, but was four times greater in all women with stroke, under age 45, and 10 times greater among women under 45 if they smoked (11). In fact, the association was strongest for *migrainous aura without headache*, which can be easily confused with a transient ischemic attack (TIA).

This association was explored further in a second study by this group, published in 1995 (12). Seventy-two women under age 45 with ischemic stroke were compared with 173 random controls among patients visiting hospitals for non-neurological problems. Ischemic stroke was, again, strongly associated with migraine, with a threefold increased risk for migraine without aura and a sixfold increase for migraine with aura. The risk of stroke among young female migraineurs was increased about 10 times if they were heavy smokers (at least 20 cigarettes/day) and 14 times if they were using oral contraceptives. The following year, an Italian prospective, case-controlled, hospital-based study was published, comparing the incidence of either stroke or TIAs in 308 patients aged 15 to 44 years with 591 age- and sex-matched controls (two controls per patient, one being a patient admitted for non-neurological reasons and the other selected from "non-travelling railway system personnel"!). Migraine was about twice as common in the stroke and TIA group overall, but was three to four times greater, and indeed the only defined risk factor, in women less than 35 years of age (13).

A recent European collaborative study, organized through the World Health Organization, compared the type and frequency of migraine in 86 cases of ischemic stroke in women aged 20 to 44 with age-matched controls. The adjusted risk was more than four times higher with migraine of more than 12 years duration, and eight times higher for migraine with aura, independent of oral contraceptive (OCP) use (14). A prospective primary-care study of patients based on 3873 cases in the Lausanne Stroke Register identified 130 cases with first ever ischemic stroke and "active migraine" (at least two attacks in the previous two months). Sixty-six patients (74% women) were under the age of 45 and comprised 15.8% of all strokes in this age group. Nine of these (13.7%) had migrainous infarcts (ischemic stroke developing during a typical attack of migraine with aura), *but 15 (22.7%) suffered ischemic stroke during a migraine attack without aura*, in the absence of any other defined cause (15).

Peter Goadsby and colleagues at the National Hospital Queen Square, have provided a helpful summary of the relative risks of stroke in young female migraineurs, based on published evidence (Table 1). The intrinsic risk associated with migraine in this group is similar to that posed by smoking and oral contraceptives, but the risk rises dramatically when these risks act in concert (16).

In conclusion, the available evidence suggests:

- Migrainous infarction accounts for about 10% to 15% of "young strokes";
- Migraine is a significant independent risk factor for ischemic stroke, especially in young women;

Table 1   Stroke Risks for Female Migraineurs Under 45 Years of Age Compared to Age-Matched Female Non-Migraineurs, Based on Published Case-Controlled Studies

	Odds ratios (confidence intervals)	
	Females with migraine	Females without migraine
Stroke risk	4.3 (1.2–16.3)	
	3.5 (1.8–6.4)	
	3.7 (1.5–9) <35 yr	
	1.9 (1.1–3.3) 15–44 yr	
	3.54 (1.3–9.61)	
With aura	6.2 (2.1–18)	
	3.81 (1.26–11.5)	
Without aura	3.0 (1.5–5.8)	
	2.97 (0.66–13.5)	
Smoking	10.2 (3.5–29.9)	3.0 (1.0–9.0)
	7.39 (2.14–25.5)	0.82 (0.36–1.89)
OCPs	13.9 (5.5–35.1)	3.5 (1.5–8.3)
	16.9 (2.72–106)	2.76 (1.01–7.55)
OCPs + smoking	34.4 (3.27–361)	

Abbreviation: OCPs, oral contraceptive pills.
Source: From Boes CJ, Matharu MS, Goadsby PJ. Migraine and stroke. Stroke Review 2002; 6:1–4.

- The basic risk of stroke is three to four times greater in females under the age of 45 with "active migraine" than in the non-migraine young female population, and is probably greater still in migraine with aura.
- The risk of migrainous infarction may increase with the duration of migraine history and attack frequency.
- The relative risk is age dependent, becoming insignificant in comparison with other stroke risk factors by age 40 to 50.
- The stroke risk due to migraine rises dramatically with smoking and the use of oral contraceptives, and in combination may be 30 times greater than in non-migraine controls.

Cases of migrainous infarction: Clearly, a diagnosis of migrainous infarction can only be presumptive through exclusion of other known causes of infarction. In all the following cases, alternative causes of stroke were excluded by the standard techniques available at the time. These included coagulopathy screening, extracranial ultrasound studies, Holter monitoring, and transthoracic echocardiography. TOE and other studies were performed where described. None of the patients had other significant risk factors for stroke, but the patients were not studied using contrast echocardiography or TCD techniques for detecting PFO. The data is summarized in Table 2. Follow-up information was not available for some of the patients (indicated in the table as "not recorded").

In general, the patients were relatively young, and infarction occurred most often in the posterior circulation territory, in keeping with previous observations. Most patients had experienced recurrent headaches prior to ictus, but not necessarily "typical" migraine attacks, and in some, the stroke had been heralded by a crescendo of migrainous symptoms over a short period. Oddly, there was a family history of migraine in only a minority of cases. Most continued to have recurrent headaches on follow-up, but none suffered further cerebrovascular symptoms. As noted by others, the prognosis for migrainous infarction seems to be excellent.

CASE 101

A man aged 40 was jogging when he suddenly developed scintillating scotoma followed by severe headache, nausea, and vomiting. The headache persisted until the following day; when on his way home from work, it suddenly worsened and he developed a right hemiplegia and aphasia. CT brain scan showed an infarct in the left posterior frontal cortex. He had experienced recurrent unilateral headaches from childhood, and his sister was similarly affected. No other risk factors were identified, and he made a complete recovery.

On review 13 years later, he had reported that he had no further migraine attacks, although he suffered occasional "stress headaches."

CASE 102

A 40-year-old General Practitioner suddenly developed teichopsia with disorientation and light-headedness. His teichopsia evolved into a left homonymous

Table 2 Authors' Cases of Presumed Migrainous Cerebral Infarction

Case no.	Age, sex	Personal history of migraine?	Family history of migraine?	Infarct territory	Subsequent migraine?
101	40, M	Yes, from childhood	Yes. Sister	MCA posterior frontal lobe	No, but "stress headaches"
102	40, M	Caffeine headaches	Yes. Mother	PCA occipital pole	Yes
103	21, F	No	Yes. Multiple	PCA posterior thalamus and occipital lobe	Not recorded
104	44, F	Yes, but only 6 wks	Not recorded	MCA posterior frontal lobe	Yes, but responded to pizotifen
105	48, M	1 yr visual auras	Not recorded	PCA occipital lobe	Yes
106	57, M	Yes, 2–3 yrs	No	MCA parietal lobe	Yes
107	54, F	No, but 3 mo occipital headaches	No	Basilar pons	Yes
108	39, M	Yes, 2 yrs	No	Basilar medulla	Yes
109	37, F	Yes, yrs	No	PCA occipital lobe, cerebellum	Yes
110	33, M	Possible	No	PCA occipital lobe	Not recorded
111	33, F	Yes, 10 yrs	No	PCA posterior thalamus and occipital lobe	Not recorded
112	28, F	Possible	Yes. Mother	PCA posterior thalamus and occipital lobe	No, but taking propranolol
113	19, F	Possible	No	PCA deep parietal lobe and occipital lobe	Not recorded
114	33, F	Yes, 20 yrs	No	Diffuse brain stem and both cerebellar lobes	Yes
115	38, F	Yes, 20 yrs	No	MCA parietal	Yes, refractory to treatment

Abbreviations: MCA, middle cerebral artery; PCA, posterior cerebral artery.

macular-splitting hemianopia over some two minutes. CT showed a right occipital pole infarct. No other risk factors were identified, but he had experienced recurrent headaches after drinking coffee in the past, and his mother had migraine. On follow-up over a 10-year period, he suffered no further vascular events, although he continued to experience occasional migrainous headaches.

CASE 103
A 21-year-old woman developed, over three days, a typical throbbing migrainous headache over the right temple, followed by light-headedness, nausea, and vomiting. On the fourth day, she developed left-sided weakness and sensory symptoms. CT showed a right parietal infarct, and MRI revealed in addition, a right posterior thalamic lesion with mass effect and also a right occipital lesion, both lesions being in the posterior cerebral artery territory. Repeat MRI one month later showed marked resolution (Fig. 1). TOE and MRA were normal. Three months later, MRI showed only mild gliotic scarring.

Several other family members had apparently suffered migrainous infarctions but were not available for evaluation.

CASE 104
A 44-year-old woman began to experience increasingly severe and frequent migraine attacks over a six-week period, not having suffered from migraine previously. One day, she suddenly developed left-sided weakness and dysarthria. CT showed no abnormality, and she recovered with the exception of persistent mild dysarthria. Repeat CT three months later, however, revealed an infarct in the posterior aspect of the right frontal lobe. Nine months later, she began to experience severe

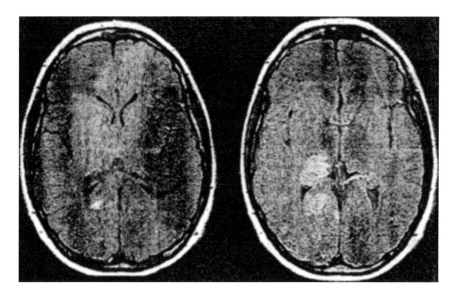

Figure 1 Case 103. Magnetic resonance imaging brain scans. T2-weighted fluid-attenuated inversion recovery images (FLAIR), showing high signal compatible with infarction in right medial occipital lobe and posterior thalamus (*right panel*), with marked resolution three months later (*left panel*).

migraine attacks with syncope. These episodes settled with pizotifen, and she had only one further moderate attack the next year.

CASE 105

A 48-year-old man began to experience episodes of visual aura, comprising brightly colored scotomata in the left hemifield lasting only 20 to 30 seconds. These recurred over about a year. There was no associated headache. On one occasion, a typical scotoma was followed by a right hemisensory loss and hemianopia. CT showed a left occipital infarct. He made a full recovery, but subsequently developed typical migraine with visual auras.

CASE 106

A 57-year-old man had a two- to three-year history of migraine with visual aura (blurring). He developed a right-sided headache over one to two days, with incoordination of the left arm and difficulty with spatial judgment on the left side. On examination, he had slight clumsiness of the left arm. CT showed a right parietal lobe white matter infarct. He improved gradually but on review, continued to experience migraine with aura several times a year.

Three years later, he was investigated for chest pain. ECG was equivocal for ischemic heart disease, but seven years later he suffered an inferior myocardial infarction.

CASE 107

A 54-year-old woman had a three-month history of right occipital headaches, lasting several hours every other day. These were nonspecific, and there were no other features. She suddenly experienced a particularly bad attack, and was admitted. CT and other baseline tests were negative. She was discharged after five days. The very next day, she developed a right hemiplegia. CT was again normal, but MRI two weeks later demonstrated a left pontine infarct. She continued to have recurrent occipital headaches, now more typical of migraine and associated with nausea and vomiting. There were no further stroke-like events, however, and no new lesions were seen on several subsequent MRI scans. She had no previous or family history of migraine.

CASE 108

A 39-year-old man presented with a two-year history of hemicranial headache, with nausea and vomiting. One year earlier, he had experienced an attack of left facial and arm weakness and numbness, evolving over six hours, but without headache. On examination, he had subjective left-sided sensory impairment. MRI revealed an infarct in the right medulla. There was no family history of migraine. On follow-up, he continued to experience frequent right-sided headaches with nausea and was treated successfully with propranolol, and an aspirin and metoclopramide combination.

CASE 109

A 37-year-old lady with a previous history of recurrent episodes of migraine without aura developed a nonspecific headache, which she tried to "sleep off." However, it was still present when she awoke and indeed became progressively worse. She developed nausea, vomiting, sweating, and shaking. In addition, she began to experience visual disturbances that she found hard to describe, numbness of the tongue, and numbness and clumsiness of the left arm. She was admitted to an emergency room. Although she complained of problems with her visual fields, no investigations were performed. She was discharged. She was still experiencing difficulties in standing or walking. She spent the next two days in bed before recovering, but consulted her optician who found a right-sided upper quadrantinopia. She smoked 15 cigarettes daily and had been on OCPs for six months.

MRI brain scan revealed an infarct in the left occipital lobe and superior cerebellum, but MRA was normal. When last reviewed 10 months later, she had subsequently suffered more typical migrainous headaches with visual aura of flashing lights, and the right upper quadrantanopia persisted.

CASE 110

A 33-year-old man suddenly experienced a severe right occipital headache, which evolved over three days. He noticed immediate loss of vision in the left hemifield, which reduced subsequently to an upper quadrantic field defect. CT showed an infarct in the right occipital lobe. Cerebral angiogram was normal. He had previously experienced occasional headaches over the left eye, lasting about two hours, but no other migrainous symptoms. There was no family history of headache.

CASE 111

A 33-year-old woman suffered a stroke 10 years prior to presentation, without any previous personal or family history of note. This had started with a severe pain over the left supraorbital and frontal area and was followed by tingling and heaviness of the left arm, leg and perioral area. The pain gradually subsided, and she became aware of the loss of vision to the left. On examination shortly afterwards, she had an incongruous hemianopia to the left and a mild left-sided ataxic hemiparesis with sensory impairment. CT brain scan revealed infarction of the right occipital and posterior temporal region, encroaching into the brain stem. Cerebral angiogram demonstrated a right posterior cerebral artery occlusion, without evidence of dissection in the vertebral or carotid arteries.

Subsequently, she began to experience occasional migraine headaches without aura, but was referred with severe migraine preceded by a right-sided visual auras, consisting variably of wavy lines, tunnel vision, or a shimmering, moving triangle. MRI demonstrated only the old right occipital and thalamic infarct.

CASE 112

A 28-year-old woman was admitted when nine weeks pregnant, with protracted nausea and vomiting. She recovered without further problems. One month later, she developed a severe, throbbing left frontal headache, followed by right hemiparesis and a macular-splitting right homonymous hemianopia. She eventually recovered except for the field defect. CT was normal on admission, and investigations including TOE were normal or negative. One year later, she presented with recurrent attacks of spontaneous coma (see p. 189) lasting 10 to 15 minutes, followed by severe headache, nausea, and vomiting. MRI showed an old left occipital and thalamic infarct. Her mother had suffered from severe migraine. On review two years later, she had had no further migrainous events while taking propranolol.

CASE 113

A 19-year-old woman developed progressive malaise followed by increasing headache, and then a brief period of loss of consciousness. On recovery, she had severe visual blurring, visual hallucinations, nausea, and severe headache. CT showed a hemorrhagic infarct in the left trigonal area. Cerebral angiogram was normal. Over the next 18 months she suffered a number of epileptic seizures, but then recovered fully. Twelve years later, she experienced an attack very similar to the first event, except that she did not lose consciousness. The headache persisted for three days. MRI now showed the previous lesion in the left trigonal area and a new left occipital infarct. There was no cavernoma, and EEG changes were nonspecific. There was no family history of migraine.

CASE 114
A 33-year-old woman with a typical history of very infrequent migraine without aura attacks dating back to her teens, awoke with a severe generalized headache. On opening her eyes, she was also immediately aware of "involuntary movements" of her arms, which continued for about a minute during which she was fully conscious. She then experienced severe nausea and tenesmus. By this point, the headache had become right sided. On attempting to walk to the bathroom, she noted that she felt weak down the left side. She then vomited and returned to bed to sleep, but was restless. The weakness persisted. She feared she may have suffered a stroke, and an ambulance was summoned. On admission, she was found to have mild pyramidal weakness down the left side but no other signs. CT brain scan and cerebrospinal fluid (CSF) examination on admission were normal, but a subsequent MRI brain scan showed diffuse infarction in the posterior circulation territory (Fig. 2). Both vertebral arteries and the basilar artery were patent on MRA, and MR venogram showed no venous sinus defects. Extracranial ultrasound, bubble TOE, and coagulopathy screen were negative. She eventually recovered without significant clinical deficit. Her vascular risk factors included the use of OCP and smoking, but there was no family history of migraine.

CASE 115
A 38-year-old woman had suffered weekly attacks of migraine with visual aura lasting several days, for over 20 years. She then had a two-year period of acephalalgic attacks, with visual auras only, occurring every two days. The auras included hallucinations of movement, as if peering into a swimming pool, followed by teichopsia in either visual hemifield. After one aura, she developed left hemisensory impairment and then left hemiplegia, which resolved in 30 minutes. She subsequently had several further hemiplegic attacks preceded by visual aura, on either side. On examination, she seemed to have mild upper motor neuron signs on the left. MRI showed a right parietal infarct and small infarcts in the right internal capsule. Chest X-ray (CXR) showed multiple pulmonary arteriovenous malformations, but she had no cerebral vascular malformations or other stigmata of hereditary telangiectasia, nor a family history of this condition. The attacks settled with pizotifen and propranolol.

Migrainous deafness. Curiously, although migrainous infarcts are largely confined to the posterior circulation, migrainous infarction seems to be uncommon in association with basilar-type migraine (see p. 209). However, it is possible that microinfarction of the auditory nerve secondary to *migrainous vasospasm* might account for some instances of otherwise unexplained isolated unilateral deafness. We noted in Chapter 3 that aura can rarely include auditory symptoms (see p. 111), and instances of acute deafness have been reported in relation to migraine attacks (17,18). The internal auditory artery (IAA), a branch of the anterior inferior cerebellar artery (AICA), supplies the labyrinth. The anterior vestibular branch of the IAA supplies the

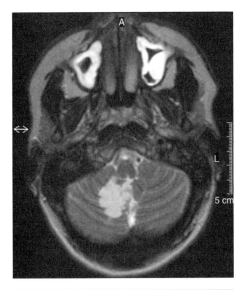

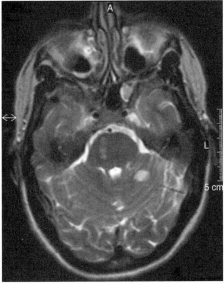

Figure 2 Case 114. T2-weighted magnetic resonance imaging showing infarction of the right cerebellar hemisphere (*upper panel*), superior aspect of the left cerebellar hemisphere, and diffuse brain stem infarction (*lower panel*).

anterior and lateral semicircular canals and the utricle, and has a poorer collateral supply than other branches of this vessel, which supply the cochlea. This may be why vertigo, and not deafness, is the most common symptom of ischemic stroke in this territory.

Cases of possible migrainous deafness

CASE 116: POSSIBLE MIGRAINOUS DEAFNESS

A 49-year-old woman presented with sudden numbness of the left side of the tongue, which spread to the lips, face, and then the whole of the right side of the body over about 20 minutes. There was no motor or speech dysfunction and no headache. The symptoms resolved over a few days, save for a faint feeling of tingling in the tips of the radial three fingers of the right hand, and the lips. MRI brain scan and MR angiogram were normal.

Two years earlier, she had suddenly developed complete right-sided deafness. There were no other symptoms, vestibular function was unaffected, and the audiogram of the left ear was normal. MR angiogram showed a normal, patent vertebrobasilar system, and no other cause for the deafness could be found. She had suffered recurrent nonspecific headaches with some nausea for years, but there was no family history of migraine, stroke, or deafness, and her only risk factor for vascular disease was a modest smoking history.

CASE 117: POSSIBLE MIGRAINOUS DEAFNESS AND
INCIDENTAL MENINGIOMA

A 40-year-old woman awoke with a headache, and found she was deaf in the right ear. There were no other symptoms. She was examined at a local hospital. Audiogram revealed an almost complete sensorineural deafness across all frequencies. MRI brain scan was completely normal. There was no recovery of her hearing. She then began to suffer recurrent and progressively severe headaches. These were typically triggered by loud noises, had a pulsatile quality, and were located chiefly in the occipitonuchal area, which would become markedly tender during the attacks. There was no photophobia or nausea, but she would be severely phonophobic. There was no previous personal or family history of migraine.

These occasional episodic headaches continued, but four years later, she presented with an altogether different headache syndrome, a slowly progressive, constant left retro-orbital pain, without any other symptoms. There were no signs on examination, but MRI brain scan now showed a left parasaggital meningioma. This head pain resolved completely following excision of the tumor, but she later had a further episode of hearing impairment during one of her habitual migraine headaches, this time on the left side—which was alarming but fortunately without permanent sequelae on this occasion.

The following case might be construed as a particularly severe example of migrainous deafness.

CASE 118: UNILATERAL DEAFNESS DUE TO MIGRAINOUS AICA
TERRITORY INFARCTION

A 48-year-old man was straining at stool when he suddenly experienced acute whistling tinnitus and then total deafness in the left ear. Within a few seconds, he became severely vertiginous and nauseous, and vomited. He fell to the left when trying to stand, and the left side of his face felt numb. An ambulance was summoned, and he was taken to an emergency room. By the time he arrived there, about half an hour later, he had developed a severe left-sided headache. On examination, he had nystagmus to the right in the primary position and marked gaze-evoked nystagmus to the left. He also had mild left-sided facial weakness. He had ataxia of the left arm and leg, and an equivocal left plantar response. MRI brain scan confirmed infarction

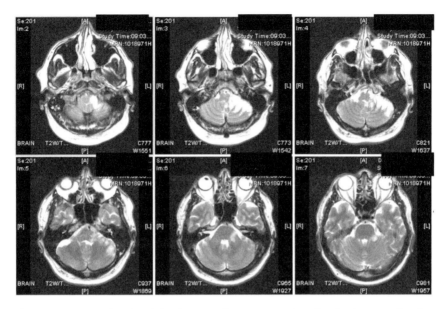

Figure 3 Case 118. T2-weighted magnetic resonance imaging brain scan showing infarction in the distribution of the left anterior inferior cerebellar artery. The neurological symptoms included left-sided sensorineural deafness and vertigo, due to occlusion of the internal auditory artery, and were followed by typical migrainous headache.

in the distribution of the left anterior inferior cerebellar artery (Fig. 3). He underwent extensive screening for stroke risk factors, with negative results, with the exception of a PFO without atrial septal aneurysm, with a large right-to-left shunt demonstrated on bubble TOE. The shunt was occluded without complication using a septal repair implant via a femoral vein approach.

He had a history of disabling migraine without aura attacks, usually lasting at least two days, dating back to his teens.

"Cluster headache" and stroke. We have also encountered a patient who suffered a posterior circulation stroke at a very young age and who went on to experience headaches with characteristics more typical of cluster headache than migraine, beginning within a few months of the stroke.

CASE 119: STROKE FOLLOWED BY CHRONIC CLUSTER HEADACHE

A 37-year-old man, who had never previously suffered headaches or neurological symptoms, awoke one morning with a nondescript generalized headache. This lasted all day, and he became aware of a visual field abnormality to the right. He went to the local emergency room, and a CT brain scan demonstrated an infarct in the left occipital lobe. He smoked 15 cigarettes per day and had mild hypertension. There was no family history of headache or vascular disease. Investigations failed to disclose a source of emboli, and he was treated with ramipril, aspirin, clopidogrel, and atorvastatin.

About five months later, he began to experience stereotyped nocturnal headaches several times a week, waking him from sleep at around 1 or 2 A.M. These consisted of very severe pain in the right nasal and periorbital area, spreading to the right temporoparietal area and jaw, associated with epiphora but no other trigeminal autonomic symptoms. The attacks would last about 45 minutes, during which he would be restless. He also noted that his scalp would feel tender, and he had some photophobia, but there was no nausea or vomiting. MRI and MRA were normal apart from the mature left occipital infarct. Individual attacks responded to oral zolmatriptan within 15 minutes, and the frequency reduced with verapamil sustained release 120 mg at night. Eventually, he began to have occasional diurnal attacks of this type. The characteristics of these daytime attacks gradually changed. They became more prolonged and were associated with nausea, and he would prefer to lie still, suggesting a more "migrainous" phenotype.

Pathogenesis of Migrainous Infarction

Migraine is, therefore, clearly a risk factor for ischemic stroke, but does migraine *cause* stroke? In Chapter 2, we explored the current knowledge of the migraine mechanism, and noted that cerebral blood flow changes, and in particular oligemia associated with spreading depression, are evident in at least some migraine attacks. Following the thesis of Fére and Charcot, it would seem reasonable to believe that occasionally, the impairment of blood flow during an attack might become critical, leading to infarction. However, as discussed, there is actually rather little evidence to support this hypothesis. Cerebral oligemia associated with migraine is not normally sufficiently severe to cause ischemia.

Does Spreading Depression Injure the Brain?

Another possibility is that spreading depression could lead to microvascular changes that, injure the brain. If so, it might be anticipated that recurrent attacks of prolonged hemiplegic aura in hemiplegic migraine would be particularly likely to result in abnormalities on neuroimaging.

A series of recent studies have addressed this issue. In one report (19), a 13-year-old boy with FHM, who had suffered repeated hemiplegia attacks, was scanned serially. During the attack, the MRI showed cerebral edema, dilatation of cerebral vessels, and decreased water diffusion contralateral to the hemiparesis, not respecting vascular territories, in keeping with the primary neurogenic and secondary vascular pathogenic mechanisms outlined in Chapter 2 (Fig. 4). However, there was complete resolution of the imaging abnormalities as the clinical signs resolved. This observation is the more remarkable because there were significant changes on diffusion-weighted imaging during the symptomatic period, generally taken to reflect cytotoxic edema due to parenchymal damage. In another study of a woman who developed hemiplegic migraine during pregnancy (20), there was no evidence of ischemia on diffusion-weighted MR imaging, despite the presence of vasospasm on cerebral angiography. Hypoperfusion (presumably related to spreading oligemia) was seen diffusely, while depression of cortical electrical activity on EEG was seen for several days over the affected hemisphere. In another case (21), a patient with FHM experienced a right-sided hemiparesis and aphasia lasting 10 days. Slowing of cortical rhythms over the left hemisphere on the magnetoencephalogram normalized as the symptoms improved. Positron emission tomography (PET) six days after onset demonstrated glucose hypometabolism in the left frontobasal cortex, caudate, and thalamus, although in this case no abnormalities were seen on MRI (including perfusion- and diffusion-weighted images). In the 21-year-old patient with a hemiplegic attack lasting over three weeks, studied via serial imaging by Oberndorfer and colleagues (22), the affected cortex showed normal diffusion-weighted imaging (DWI) throughout, while perfusion-weighted imaging and SPECT revealed hypoperfusion (secondary to the neural processes of migraine aura), which gradually resolved as the patient recovered.

Thus, despite the marked and protracted cerebral hypoperfusion found in such cases, no permanent damage seems to occur. Indeed, to our knowledge, there is no reported instance of ischemic infarction occurring during the course of an attack in a patient with familial or sporadic hemiplegic migraine, although permanent deficit and even fatality has been reported in this condition due to the profound hemisphere swelling that can occur (23,24).

Similarly, persistent aura does not seem to cause structural damage to the brain. We noted above the eventual complete resolution of the abnormalities on cerebral perfusion MRI in the patient with persistent visual aura reported by Relja et al. (4), and the 10 patients with persistent positive visual aura lasting months to years studied by Liu et al. were found to have essentially normal routine MRI brain scans (3). In addition, a voxel-based morphometric study showed no difference in global gray or white matter volumes, comparing migraine patients with aura to those without aura, or with controls, nor were there global or regional macroscopic structural differences comparing migraineurs with controls (25).

On the present evidence we would therefore conclude that the migraine mechanism per se does not normally injure the brain. Some other factor or factors must therefore be operative in those instances in which ischemic damage does occur.

Neuroimaging in Migraine

Paradoxically, in direct contrast to the above conclusion, active migraineurs are more likely to demonstrate "white matter lesions" (WML) on MRI brain scans than control subjects. Because of its relatively benign outcome, there was little opportunity to study the pathogenesis of migrainous infarction before the advent of scanning. The few pathological and arteriographic studies that were conducted in rare fatal cases generally found the cerebral vessels to be normal (26). Instances of vasospasm (27) and occlusion of intracranial vessels (28) were recorded on rare occasions. In a more recent study of a case of what was described as "fatal migraine" (29), now more

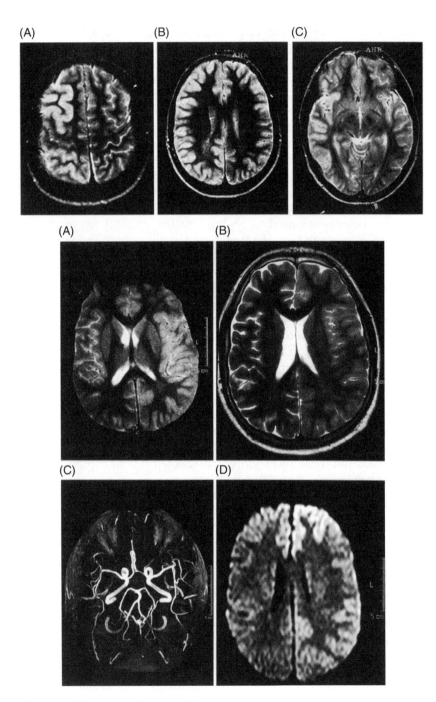

Figure 4 (*Caption on facing page*)

correctly diagnosed as "malignant stroke secondary to migraine," a 58-year-old woman with a history of migraine with aura developed a typical attack comprising visual blurring, photophobia, and flexor spasms in the left hand, followed by right-sided hemicrania. Within hours, she developed a progressive left hemiplegia with paralysis of conjugate gaze to the left. CT showed a large right-sided temporoparietal infarction, which caused coning and death. At autopsy, the extracranial vessels were essentially normal and the intracranial vessels were free of atheroma. The right middle cerebral artery contained fresh thrombus, but the histological findings indicated that the infarct antedated the development of the thrombus by several days. The authors concluded that the infarction had been the consequence of migrainous vasospasm—the pathogenesis suggested by Fére and Charcot. In support of this concept, a report from the Houston Headache Clinic cited the case of a 47-year-old woman with migraine with aura (MA), who presented with status migrainosus that progressed to cortical blindness and quadriparesis due to bilateral hemispheric infarction. Profound and extensive intracranial vasospasm was shown on cerebral angiography, and no other pathologies or risk factors for stroke were evident (30).

In 1976, Hungerford et al. reported an unexpectedly high incidence of abnormalities on CT brain scans in severe migraineurs (31). The same year, Cala and Mastaglia reported CT abnormalities in 37 of 46 patients referred because of increasing frequency or severity of migraine (32). Some of their findings, such as "a mild degree of edema in the white matter" in 21 of the cases, might be considered rather subjective, but areas of occipital infarction were found in four cases with permanent visual field defects, together with unexpected temporal lobe infarctions in two others.

A series of studies dating from the late 1980s also revealed a high frequency of MRI scan abnormalities in migraineurs. In an uncontrolled study (33), Soges et al. found that 11 of 24 cases (46%) had well-defined high signal lesions on T2-weighted images, mainly in the periventricular white matter, while additional cortical lesions compatible with infarcts were found in four patients with "complicated" migraine (i.e., with focal symptomatology). In a subsequent controlled study (34), 36 of 91 migraineurs (39.6%)

Figure 4 (*Figure on facing page*) Magnetic resonance imaging in familial hemiplegic migraine. *Top panel* (**A–C**). On admission with left hemiplegia T_2-weighted images showed extensive gyral enhancement throughout the right fronto-parietal and temporo-occipital regions. *Bottom panel* (**A–D**). On re-admission 21 months later, with right hemiparesis and aphasia, T_2-weighted images now showed similar enhancement in the left insular and parieto-occipital cortex (**A** and **B**), (**C**) Time of flight MR angiogram showing slightly dilated left proximal middle cerebral artery. (**D**) Diffusion-weighted image (DWI) showing high signal throughout to left fronto-parietal cortex. *Source*: From Butteriss DJ, Ramesh V, Birchall D. Serial MRI in a case of familial hemiplegic migraine. Neuroradiology 2003; 45:300–303.

were found to have WML on T2- and proton density–weighted images, and among cases under 40 years of age without vascular risk factors, the incidence was 29.4%, nearly three times higher than that of the controls (11.2%) (Fig. 5).

Subsequent studies gave broadly similar results; WML were found two to three times more often in migraineurs than in controls, although the overall observed frequency varied from about 10% to 40% (35,36). Interestingly, one study found that the frequency of these lesions varied with the type of headache (35). Of 38 cases, the incidence was 18% in migraine without aura, 53% in cases with typical aura, and 38% in basilar migraine. However,

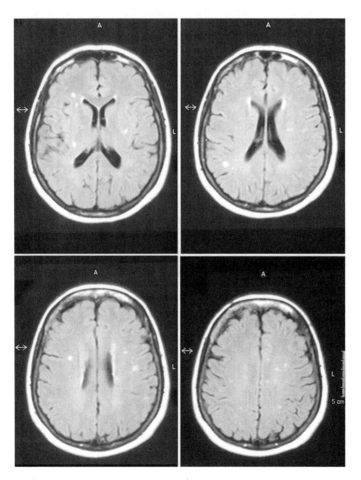

Figure 5 Scattered white matter lesions at all levels in the hemispheres. Believed to be ischemic in origin, these lesions are significantly more common in migraineurs than in individuals without active migraine. *Source*: From Butteriss DJ, Ramesh V, Birchall D. Serial MRI in a case of familial hemiplegic migraine. Neuroradiology 2003; 45:300–303.

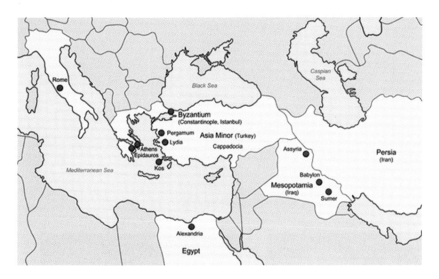

Figure 1.2 The Ancient World of Eurasia. (*See p. 3*)

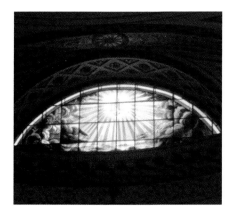

Figure 1.6 Stained glass window in the Chapel of All Saints. (*See p. 9*)

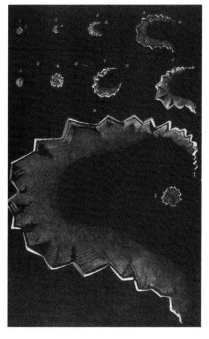

Figure 1.7 Dr. Hubert Airy's sinistral teichopsia. (*See p. 12*)

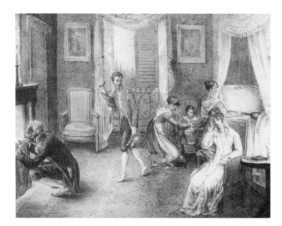

Figure 1.10 The Countess of Conway. (*See p. 17*)

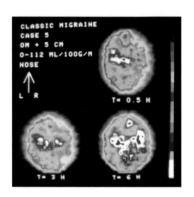

Figure 1.17 Study of regional cortical blood flow during spontaneous migraine. (*See p. 33*)

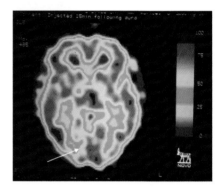

Figure 1.18 HMPAO. (*See p. 34*)

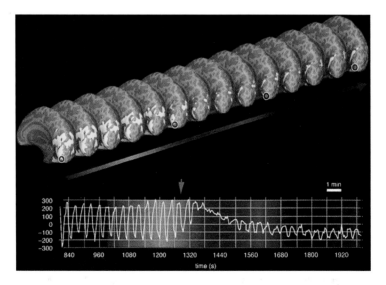

Figure 2.3 Neural activity underlying visual aura. (*See p. 54*)

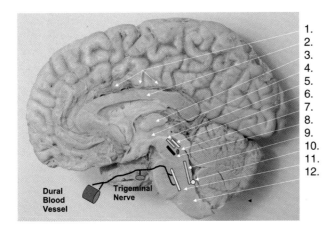

Figure 2.4 Sagittal section of the human brain. (*See p. 58*)

1.
2.
3.
4.
5.
6.
7.
8.
9.
10.
11.
12.

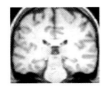

Dural Blood Vessel

Trigeminal Nerve

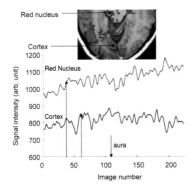

Figure 2.7 Neuroimaging of brainstem in migraine. (*See p. 64*)

Red nucleus

Cortex

Red Nucleus

Cortex

aura

Signal intensity (arb. unit)

1200
1100
1000
900
800
700
600

0   50   100   150   200

Image number

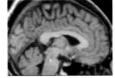

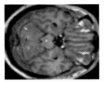

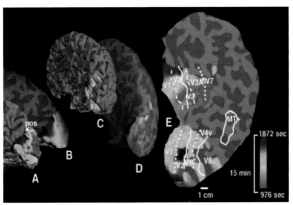

pos

A   B   C   D   E

V1 V2 V3A V7
V3

MT

V4v

V1

V2 V3 V8

1872 sec

15 min

976 sec

1 cm

Figure 3.2 Site and time of onset of fMRI signal changes during visual aura. (*See p. 98*)

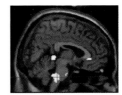

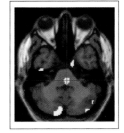

Figure 2.8 PET studies in GTN-triggered migraine. (*See p. 69*)

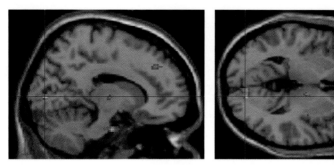

Figure 2.9 PET in cluster. (*See p. 70*)

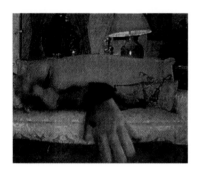

Figure 3.4 Macrosomatognosia. (*See p. 109*)

(E)

(F)

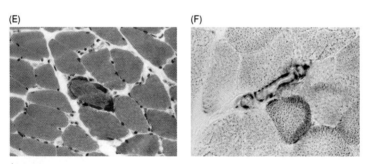

Figure 5.10 (E and F). (*See p. 254*)

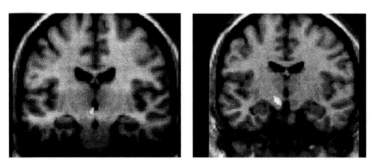

Figure 6.2 Activation of the posterior hypothalamus in a patient during a spontaneous attack. (*See p. 270*)

in another study, although WML were found much more commonly in patients with "primary headache" compared to controls (33.3% vs. 7.4%), they occurred with about equal frequency in patients with "tension headache" (34.3%) and "migraine" (32.1%) (37).

It is difficult to reconcile the earlier observations based on CT scan findings with the MRI data. Indeed, a comparative study of 74 patients with migraine with aura revealed typical WML in 26% of patients, but CT detected none of these lesions (38).

In a recent cross-sectional study of Dutch adults aged 30 to 60 (39), MRI scans of 161 patients with migraine with aura were compared with that of 134 migraine without aura cases and 140 controls, with regard to evidence of silent infarction and periventricular and deep WML. None had a history of cerebrovascular events. Overall, the prevalence of infarcts was similar in the migraineurs and controls (8.1% vs. 5%), but the prevalence was significantly higher in the posterior circulation territory in migraineurs, particularly in aura cases and in those with frequent attacks (OR 15.8; CI 1.8–140). Deep WML were about twice as common in female migraineurs than in men or controls, while the prevalence of periventricular WML did not differ in the three groups.

A meta-analysis of seven informative studies confirmed that WML were almost four times as likely to be present in patients with active migraine than controls, and this risk was independent of any coexisting risk factors for cerebrovascular disease (40). In contrast, however, a study of cerebral WML in patients with CADASIL, comparing those who had suffered attacks of migraine with aura and those who had not, found no difference in the frequency of lesions in the two groups (41).

The nature of WML is not yet clear. Recent evidence suggests that they might not be microinfarcts but result from extravasation of plasma proteins across arteriolar walls leading to perivascular neuronal and glial cell damage (42). Is it possible then that the migraine mechanism might be a factor in the local breakdown of the blood–brain barrier, leading to these "lesions"?

We would, therefore, conclude as follows:

- Migraine is not just a risk factor for stroke. The migraine mechanism itself can also sometimes precipitate ischemia and cerebral infarction.
- Migraine accounts for some of the deep WML encountered during routine MRI imaging, particularly in the posterior circulation territory. These may be ischemic but might also result from the effects of periodic breakdown of the blood–brain barrier, possibly caused by neurogenic inflammation.
- The great majority of migrainous cerebral infarctions occur in the posterior circulation. This would accord with the location of the migraine mechanism in the brain stem and occipital cortex, as described in Chapter 2.

- However, the processes underlying migraine aura, including spreading oligemia, probably cannot *in isolation* account for migrainous infarction under normal circumstances. Additional factors acting in concert with the migraine mechanism seem to be necessary for infarction to occur.

Comorbidity Factors and Migrainous Infarction

As discussed in Chapter 2 (see p. 56), a number of neuroprotective mechanisms are normally mobilized to counteract the potentially toxic effects of the neurochemical and microvascular changes that occur in the brain during a migraine attack. But it is certainly possible that these might sometimes be overwhelmed. For example, in Chapter 2, we noted that Moskowitz had shown that upregulation of matrix metalloproteinases, in his model of the trigeminovascular system, caused leakage of the blood–brain barrier, allowing potassium, nitric oxide, adenosine, and other products released by cortical spreading depression to reach and sensitize the dural perivascular afferents. We also noted that in similar experimental studies, high K^+ and blockade of nitric oxide synthase could abolish the hyperperfusion phase associated with the initial depolarization in spreading depression (SD), resulting in more severe hypoperfusion and cortical infarction (43). The WML seen on MRI might be due to such processes, perhaps in concert with factors such as platelet dysfunction (see Chapter 1, and see also "Symptomatic Migraine" in Chapter 5), coagulopathies, or microembolism from structural cardiac abnormalities, as we will discuss shortly.

It would be anticipated that the presence of additional known risk factors for stroke might increase the likelihood of a migraine attack causing cerebral infarction. The impact of oral contraceptives and smoking has already been discussed. By analogy, hormone replacement therapy (HRT) might also be a risk factor, as the following case illustrates.

CASE 120: HORMONE REPLACEMENT THERAPY

A 42-year-old woman developed severe migraine with aura shortly after receiving an HRT implant following hysterectomy and bilateral salpingo-oophorectomy for endometriosis and fibroids. Initially, the aura comprised phosphenes and scintillations, but subsequently, she began to have hemianopic attacks, affecting the right side exclusively. She then began to suffer crescendo episodes, culminating in status migrainosus (see p. 206).

The attacks were associated with severe nausea, vomiting, photophobia, and prostration. She had no previous history of migraine, but her father was a migraineur. The implant was removed and substituted first with an oral HRT preparation and subsequently transcutaneous HRT patches, but the severe migraine attacks continued. Her gynaecologist insisted that the estrogen replacement therapy be continued, but changed to a low-dose preparation. The attacks reduced in frequency to one every month or so. She then began to experience episodes of syncope and chest and arm pain. Extensive cardiological investigation proved negative. It was concluded that the episodes were probably due to migrainous pseudoangina (see Chapter 3).

The attacks of migraine with aura continued with similar frequency. She was referred once more some six years later, following the development of episodes of right-sided paresthesia and visual blurring. MRI brain scan revealed a mature infarct in the left inferior occipital pole. Screening for coagulation disorders (thrombin time, anti–thrombin III, protein S, lupus anticoagulant, Factor V Leiden, prothrombin gene mutations, Factor VIII, fasting homocysteine, and anticardiolipin antibodies) was entirely negative. She eventually stopped the HRT and following this, the migraine attacks decreased dramatically in frequency and severity.

In our experience, the most common additional factor predisposing to migrainous infarction is platelet dysfunction, but platelet diseases seem to increase the risk of migraine attacks in general and are, therefore, discussed in the section on Symptomatic Migraine in Chapter 5 (see p. 240). Otherwise, coagulopathies and microvascular diseases can be occasional *agents provocateurs.*

CASE 121: OCP AND PROTHROMBIN GENE MUTATION

An 18-year-old girl was admitted as an emergency following the rapid onset of dysphasia, right hemiparesis, and hemisensory impairment, together with a dull headache. Examination revealed a very mild right hemiparesis, particularly affecting the leg. CT brain scan on the day of admission showed no abnormality, but a subsequent study two days later showed some signal attenuation and swelling in the left hemisphere, particularly in the basal ganglia region. A subsequent MRI scan (Fig. 6, *top panel*) showed a watershed infarct in that region, together with high signal within the left middle cerebral artery, consistent with reduced flow.

She had a previous history of abdominal migraine as a child, and the previous month, she had suffered an attack of dysphasia and visual blurring lasting some 15 minutes, without headache. She was taking the OCP, and her mother had suffered deep vein thrombosis and pulmonary embolism while taking the OCP. While in the hospital she had two further episodes of headache with right-sided sensorimotor disturbance. Extracranial ultrasound, transthoracic echocardiography, and TOE showed no abnormality, and a basic thrombophilia screen was normal. She was treated with aspirin, clopidogrel, and pizotifen.

Following discharge, she continued to experience attacks comprising left frontal headache followed 20 to 30 minutes later by "deadness" in the right leg with footdrop, and a sense of heaviness and numbness in the right arm lasting several hours, relieved by sleep. During these episodes, she was unable to speak. Nausea and photophobia would also occur in some of these attacks. She also found that when exercising, she would sometimes experience sudden weakness of her right arm and particularly the right leg. Three months after her first admission, she had a more severe attack with dysphasia, and was readmitted and treated with intravenous heparin.

Further thrombophilia screening revealed that she was heterozygous for the prothrombin gene mutation (G20210A) and had raised fibrinogen levels and borderline increased homocysteine of 15.6 (normal range 5–15). (This prothrombin gene mutation is present in about 2% of the population and results in a two- to three-fold increased risk of venous thrombosis, similar to the OCP).

Lactate responses to exercise were normal, and screening for mitochondrial DNA mutations was negative. Magnetic resonance angiogram (MRA) (Fig. 6, *bottom panel*) and subsequently formal angiography, demonstrated complete occlusion of the right middle cerebral artery. She was treated with warfarin to an International normalized ratio (INR) of around 3, together with folic acid, but the attacks continued. Warfarin

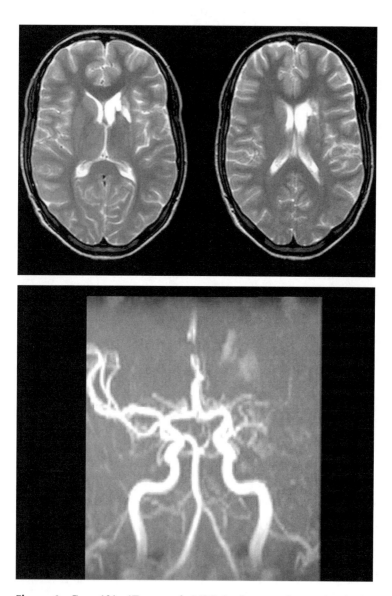

Figure 6 Case 121. (*Top panel*) MRI brain scan shows signal abnormality in the head of the left caudate nucleus and basal ganglia in the distribution of the lenticulostriate branches of the left middle cerebral artery. (*Bottom panel*) Magnetic resonance angiogram showing occlusion of the left middle cerebral artery from its origin.

was eventually stopped without deterioration. On review 18 months after presentation, the episodes of paresis had become less frequent, but she continued to have migrainous headaches. The hyperhomocysteinemia was corrected with folate supplements.

She later had an uneventful pregnancy, using subcutaneous heparin to try to prevent further thrombotic events. However, she subsequently started to have recurrence of the episodes of right-sided weakness, again chiefly affecting the leg. She was referred for further neurovascular studies, which demonstrated a low-perfusion state in the left hemisphere on Xenon scanning, reversed by acetazolamide, consistent with focal hypoperfusion. This was treated with a bypass from the carotid to the distal middle cerebral artery and the attacks of right leg weakness ceased.

Clearly, this was a most unusual case. It is possible that the middle cerebral artery occlusion was unrelated to the migraine mechanism, although this pathology has been reported previously on at least two occasions in connection with migrainous infarction (44,45).

With regard to the issue of coagulopathies, a recent meta-analysis by Pankaj Sharma and colleagues of all informative published studies of genetic factors in stroke showed a significant association with factor V Leiden Arg 506Gln (OR 1.33, 95% CI 1.12–1.58), methylene-tetrahydrofolate reductase C677T (OR 1.24, 95% CI 1.08–1.42), prothrombin gene G20210A (OR 1.44, 95% CI 1.11–1.86), and insertion or deletion mutations in angiotensin-converting enzyme (OR 1.21, 95% CI 1.08–1.35) (46).

CASE 122: MIGRAINOUS INFARCTION WITH DIABETIC SMALL VESSEL DISEASE, THEN MIGRAINE-TRIGGERED SEIZURES

A 46-year-old woman with insulin-dependent diabetes complicated by retinopathy, polyneuropathy, and severe obesity, and with degenerative arthropathy, hypertension, and asthma, developed a severe occipital headache that woke her from sleep. There was no nausea, vomiting, or other symptoms. The headache was short-lived, and she went back to sleep, but the next day the headache was still present and she felt numb and weak down the left side. She had a 20-year history of migraine without aura, which was infrequent, occurring only two or three times per year. The episodes were, however, incapacitating. On one previous occasion, she had experienced a brief period of numbness in the left arm during an attack.

She was seen at a local hospital and considered to have suffered a migraine attack. The headache resolved, but she was left with persistent mild weakness on the left side. She returned to hospital. On examination, she now had a left-sided macular-sparing hemianopia and a mild pyramidal distribution weakness. CT brain scan confirmed infarction in the right parieto-occipital region (Fig. 7, *top panel*). MRI also revealed extensive white matter abnormality compatible with ischemic small vessel disease (Fig. 7, *bottom panel*), but extracranial ultrasound studies and MRA were normal. A previous CT study undertaken eight years earlier following the migraine attack associated with the left arm numbness had been normal.

About a year after the stroke, she experienced a unilateral headache followed rapidly by numbness affecting the right side of the tongue, which then persisted to a degree for several weeks. At this time, she would often develop a severe headache while swimming, usually followed by involuntary head movements lasting about a minute. Walking home from the pool one day, she had a drop attack with feelings of disorientation. She was readmitted briefly for observation, but she recovered without further problems.

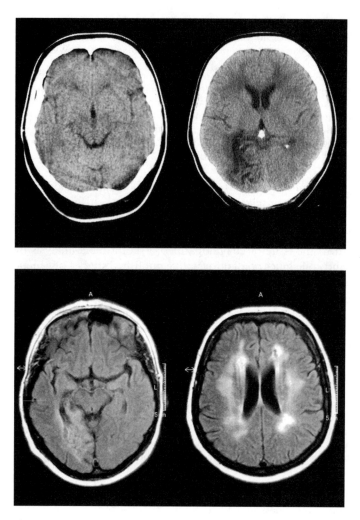

Figure 7 Case 122. (*Top panel*) CT brain scans. The image on the right shows an infarct in the right parieto-occipital region. The CT image on the left was taken eight years previously and is normal. (*Bottom panel*) Magnetic resonance imaging scans showing the infarct (*left panel*) and extensive white matter ischemic disease, presumably secondary to diabetes.

Four months later, she had a further episode of involuntary head movement, during which she felt her head was being repeatedly thrust backwards. This was then followed by a "movie shutter" visual hallucination in which images oscillated between black and white very rapidly for two minutes. She felt strange and weak but recovered fully in the emergency room after about two hours. All these symptoms resolved, but it was felt that she might have epilepsy and was started on sodium valproate. A few days after starting treatment, she had a generalized epileptic seizure, again preceded by the involuntary "head thrusting." Several months later, she had an attack of status epilepticus. This began with a progressive right-sided parietal and vertical headache similar to the previous headaches following swimming. She became increasingly nauseous, and after two hours suffered a series of generalized seizures without recovery between events, requiring hospital admission. She recovered rapidly and without further deficit.

CASE 123: MOYAMOYA DISEASE AND MIGRAINOUS INFARCTION

A 32-year-old left-handed man with a history of migraine with aura dating from early childhood, presented with a persistent left-sided hemianopia and symptoms of right parieto-occipital dysfunction, including marked dressing apraxia, which developed during the course of a more than usually severe migraine attack. His habitual migraine episodes had begun in childhood. These comprised a visual aura of 'lines in front of the eyes' lasting up to an hour, followed by an occipital headache spreading forwards, with nausea and photophobia. The attacks would last several hours but were not frequent.

At the age of 7 he had an attack that was associated with sudden onset of right arm and leg weakness that evolved during the headache phase, and then persisted. Investigation elsewhere revealed "a left cerebral infarction" and angiographic features of moyamoya disease. At age 14, he had an attack at school in which he lost his vision completely for an hour, but there was no permanent deficit. In adult life, the attacks had become much less frequent. MRI brain scan and MR angiogram (Fig. 8) confirmed moyamoya, with a new infarction in the right parieto-occipital area in addition to the older infarct in the left frontal lobe. Coagulation screen and TOE were normal, and no other source of emboli was found.

His father had suffered a stroke in his 50s, and there was a strong family history of migraine on his mother's side of the family. The same year the patient was admitted, one of his younger brothers, aged 30, was also admitted having suffered two events comprising headache with nausea together with left-sided hemisensory symptoms and dysphasia. His MRI, MRA, and CSF examination were normal, and the attacks were interpreted as due to migraine with aura.

Migraine, Stroke, and Structural Cardiac Abnormalities

Migraine and stroke have both been linked to a number of structural cardiac abnormalities, including prolapsing mitral valve (47), atrial myxoma (48), and most recently, patent foramen ovale (PFO) (49). Such lesions might serve as niduses for platelet aggregation and avenues for microemboli to pass directly into the cerebral circulation from the heart, and either precipitate a migraine attack or cause TIA or stroke.

In 1988, Lechat et al. from Paris (49) reported that PFO, detected by contrast echocardiography, was four times more common among 60 stroke patients under age 55 than in 100 controls. The incidence was 54% in 26 stroke cases in whom no other cause of stroke could be identified. It was suggested that stroke resulted from paradoxical embolism from clinically silent venous thrombosis. This is compelling, but mindful of the now largely discredited relationship between prolapsing mitral valve and stroke; there are also problems with the association between PFO and stroke.

- Like prolapsing mitral valve, PFO is found in a substantial proportion (perhaps 30%) of the normal population.

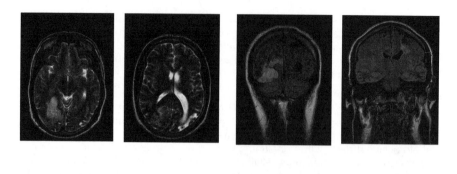

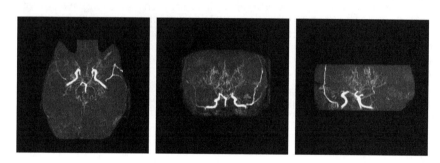

Figure 8 Case 123. Recurrent migrainous infarction in a patient with migraine with aura and known moyamoya disease. Presented with left hemianopia and dressing apraxia that developed during a particularly severe attack of his habitual migraine syndrome. He had suffered a right hemiplegia as a child under similar circumstances. (*Top panels*): Magnetic resonance imaging brain scan showed extensive infarction in the right posterior temporoparietal region, in keeping with his acute presentation, and an extensive patchy infarction in the left hemisphere, including the frontal and posterior parietal regions, relating to the childhood stroke. (*Lower panels*): The MR angiogram revealed the typical features of moyamoya (Japanese = "*puff of smoke*") disease, with severe attenuation or absence of components of the circle of Willis and characteristic proliferation of collateral microvessels, particularly in the basal ganglia regions. The cause of moyamoya is unknown.

- The association between PFO and stroke seems to be largely confined to young people. Stroke, in general, occurs primarily in the elderly; so why is the association lost, given that PFO would presumably persist throughout life?
- A systematic review found a wide range of detection rates in case-controlled studies of PFO in cryptogenic stroke (50), suggesting problems with case definition and criteria for detection of PFO.
- As the Lausanne group first noted (51), a source of venous embolism is found in only about 5% of cases of stroke associated with PFO, and the risk of recurrence is low, at around 2% per year.

PFO may be relevant to stroke pathogenesis only if a significant right-to-left shunt can be demonstrated by contrast TOE or TCD during Valsalva manoeuvre. The presence of an atrial septal aneurysm increases the stroke risk further. It is also possible that emboli might arise from the canal of the PFO, or septal aneurysm if present, or arise from atrial dysrhythmias.

Surprisingly, a study in 1998 reported that, using contrast TCD, the incidence of PFO in patients with migraine with aura (44%) was similar to that of a comparison group of young strokes (35%) and significantly higher than in normal subjects (16%) (52). This relationship between migraine with aura and cardiac right-to-left shunts was then studied in a UK series, reported by Peter Wilmshurst and colleagues from Shrewsbury (53). Of 37 patients who had undergone a PFO closure procedure for various clinical indications (prevention of decompression sickness, stroke prevention, or for hemodynamic reasons), 57% of the operated patients had a history of active migraine prior to the procedure (which at first glance seems surprisingly high), but on follow-up, about half experienced no further migraine attacks, and most of the others reported a significant reduction in the frequency. Subsequently, Sztajzel et al. from Geneva examined the prevalence of PFO and migraine in 74 consecutive patients presenting with "stroke of unknown origin" (54). Overall, PFO was demonstrated in 57% of their cases, and in 36% of patients with migraine with aura, compared to 13% in those with migraine without aura. About half the stroke cases in which PFO was considered causative had migraine with aura, compared to only 16% in cases where the PFO was considered unrelated. Half the patients treated by closure of the PFO or with anticoagulants experienced complete resolution of migraine with aura attacks.

Several groups have embraced this concept vigorously and report remarkable success in the treatment of PFO by percutaneous transcatheter procedures (55,56). One group also reported that among 17 migraineurs (eight with aura, and nine without) with PFO detected by TCD, followed up six months after the procedure, five became free of attacks, 10 were much improved, and two were unchanged. Aura also stopped in six of the eight migraine with aura patients (57). However, the outcome is not always so favorable, and in one case report, infrequent episodes of migraine with aura were transformed into daily attacks for six months, following closure of a PFO (58).

These observations are striking, and it would seem that intracardiac right-to-left shunts somehow predispose to migraine attacks, and in particular attacks of migraine with aura, presumably because humoral factors reach the brain by escaping the pulmonary filter. Despite the observations of the Lausanne group, it seems most likely that this humoral factor is paradoxical platelet emboli. It has indeed been shown that certain prothrombotic conditions, notably factor V Leiden and prothrombin G20210A mutations (as in Case 121 above), are significantly associated with cryptogenic stroke in patients with PFO (59). In addition, the Valsalva maneuver, which increases shunting, has been linked to transient global amnesia (TGA), which is probably a migraine aura in most cases (see p. 125).

Interestingly, PFO was found in four of five patients in a single family with CADASIL (in which patients may have migraine attacks, see Chapter 2, p. 81), and the authors suggested that mutations in the *notch 3* gene might result in abnormal development of the endocardial cushion (60). Further evidence of genetic influences comes from a more recent study by Peter Wilmshurst's group. They looked at the prevalence of intracardiac shunts (PFO and atrial septal defects) and history of migraine with aura among relatives of 71 subjects with such defects. They found that the inheritance of shunts was consistent with autosomal dominant inheritance. In addition, when the subject had migraine with aura and an atrial shunt, over 71% of first-degree relatives with a significant right-to-left shunt also had migraine with aura, compared to 21% without a shunt. They concluded that inheritance of a shunt was linked to migraine with aura in some families (61).

We have encountered a patient with a history that suggested that an intracardiac shunt might have been the source of migrainous infarction— but none could be demonstrated!

CASE 124: MIGRAINE AND FOCAL SYMPTOMS PRECIPITATED BY VALSALVA MANEUVER

A 53-year-old man was admitted because of acute right-sided weakness and sensory impairment, which had been precipitated by a sneezing fit. He was a heavy smoker and mildly hypertensive, and had a previous history of migraine with typical visual, hemisensory, and dysphasic auras from the age of 12, although he had been free of attacks for several years prior to presentation. The acute sensorimotor symptoms had evolved much more quickly than his typical auras but had been followed by the familiar migraine headache with nausea, lasting about two hours. MRI brain scan demonstrated an infarct in the left lentiform nucleus and anterior limb of the internal capsule. MR angiogram did not demonstrate dissection. He recovered completely. Subsequently, he began to experience his habitual migraine attacks once more.

Some two years later, he again experienced a right-sided weakness and sensory disturbance precipitated by a sneezing attack, on this occasion associated with dysphasia and followed by a migrainous headache. However, repeat MRI scan showed no new lesions. TOE with bubble study failed to demonstrate a PFO.

On the other hand, the following case illustrates, very nicely, the possible connection between PFO and the migraine mechanism, and in particular, cortical spreading depression.

CASE 125: VISUAL AURA WITHOUT HEADACHE IN A PATIENT WITH PFO, DISCOVERED DURING INVESTIGATION FOLLOWING "THE BENDS"

A 41-year-old man had suffered an episode of "the bends" while diving some eight months previously, and was referred because of persisting sensory symptoms in the left leg. He was an experienced diver and had performed hundreds of dives previously without problem. The dive had been to a depth of 43 m. He had followed the approved decompression program during the ascent, but at 3 m, he had suddenly experienced back pain, mainly on the left side. This became progressively worse over the next 20 minutes on reaching the surface, and he then developed severe rotatory vertigo. The back pain gradually resolved but was replaced by a curious numb sensation from the left loin down the lateral aspect of the left leg. He was diagnosed as having spinal and vestibular bends and was treated in a hyperbaric oxygen chamber.

Vestibular function testing was performed four months later because of on-going vertigo, and demonstrated a right-sided peripheral abnormality. However, the symptom had largely resolved by the time he was evaluated in the neurology clinic. On examination, he exhibited mild hyper-reflexia down the left side with some ill-sustained ankle clonus, and slight sensory impairment over the left thigh. MRI of the brain and spinal cord was normal, however.

He denied any history of headache, but on direct questioning, he confessed to experiencing stereotyped episodes dating back to childhood, in which he would suddenly develop a kaleidoscopic scotoma sufficient to impair his ability to read. There was no headache, but several members of his family had suffered recurrent headaches. Transthoracic and baseline TOE showed no abnormality, but a bubble study during TOE showed a PFO during Valsalva maneuver. Expert opinion was that the patient's neurological symptoms were due to paradoxical gas embolism and that the habitual visual symptoms were migraine auras due to the same mechanism.

Individuals who demonstrate a right-to-left atrial shunt only during provocation, such as Valsalva, can often perform very many dives before developing neurological symptoms due to bends, while individuals with a demonstrable shunt at rest are far more vulnerable and usually develop symptoms after only a few dives.

While the relationship between structural cardiac disease and migraine is difficult to understand, the prospect of a surgical solution to intractable migraine (and therefore possibly other intractable primary headaches) is tantalizing and clearly requires more careful and detailed investigation. At the time of writing, the preliminary findings of the first randomized, placebo-controlled clinical trial of transcatheter closure of PFO in selected migraine patients have just been reported and are discussed at the conclusion of Chapter 7.

As mentioned, migraine has also been linked to other cardiac abnormalities, such as atrial myxoma (47,48,61,62), and can be precipitated by cerebral angiography. This raises the possibility that the migraine mechanism might be triggered by some factor originating in the vasculature. One possibility is that intracardiac abnormalities in general might give rise to platelet microemboli. As noted in Chapter 2, another possibility is that release of endothelin-1, the most potent of all vasoconstrictors, from vessel walls might be involved. Endothelin-1 levels are increased in blood at the start of a migraine attack (63), and, experimentally, endothelin-1 is a potent trigger of spreading depression (64).

We encountered a possible example of structural cardiac abnormality causing an exacerbation of migraine.

CASE 126: MIGRAINE AND AORTIC VALVE REPLACEMENT

A woman of 80 years of age presented with frequent and troublesome attacks of migraine with visual aura. Attacks comprised typical "zigzag" visual obscurations lasting about 30 minutes, followed by a severe headache for three to four hours. These had begun when she was in her 50s but had become much more frequent following the insertion of a prosthetic aortic valve for aortic stenosis at the age of 73. She did not receive anticoagulation or antiplatelet drugs. Her cardiac function on ECG and echocardiography was otherwise normal. She failed to respond to beta-blockers but the frequency of migraine attacks dropped dramatically with the use of aspirin 75 mg daily. When she stopped taking the aspirin, as a trial, the migraine attacks returned with a vengeance, but stopped once more when aspirin was restarted.

Migrainous TIAs

If migraine can cause stroke, it would not be surprising if it could also cause transient, reversible "stroke-like" events: *migrainous TIAs*. The difficulty is in distinguishing such events from migrainous auras, and indeed, it may not be possible to do so with confidence. Thromboembolic TIA symptoms would result from focal cerebral ischemia, while auras (probably) do not. If headache is associated with the symptoms, the clinical distinction is more straightforward; auras usually precede headache, while the symptoms of migrainous TIAs are coincident with or follow the headache phase. However, this is not invariably true, as we discussed in Chapter 2. Another possible distinguishing feature is that auras usually include "positive" symptomatology, such as tingling paresthesiae, while ischemic lesions largely cause negative symptoms, such as numbness and weakness.

It is well recognized that migrainous auras can occur in the absence of headache. We believe that many of the cases of recurrent "funny turns" that present at emergency rooms and neurology clinics, for which no cause can be established even after extensive investigation, are probably caused by migraine. As discussed in Chapter 3, migraine auras can include a wide variety of symptoms, including unilateral weakness and sensory impairment, dysphasia, and recurrent dizziness and vertigo. Such symptoms are frequently misdiagnosed as thromboembolic TIAs or "ministrokes" and have been referred to variously in the literature, as "acephalgic migraine attacks," "migrainous equivalents," or "migrainous accompaniments" (*migraine accompanée*).

C. Miller Fisher of the Mayo Clinic, who was the first to clearly define the clinical characteristics and pathogenesis of thromboembolic TIAs (65), was also the first to identify patients with similar symptoms of probable migrainous origin among patients in the "stroke age group" (over 45 years). In an abstract published in 1979, he described "Transient Migrainous Accompaniments (TMAs) of late onset"—recurrent episodes mimicking

Table 3 Miller Fisher's Late-Life Migrainous Accompaniments

Visual (excluding scintillating scotoma)
  Blindness
  Homonymous hemianopia
  Blurred vision, difficulty focusing
Visual + paresthesia
Visual + speech disturbance (dysarthria or aphasia)
Visual + parasthesia + speech
Visual + brain stem symptoms
No visual symptoms but any of the other symptoms mentioned above

---

thromboembolic TIAs but with normal cerebral angiograms and no other source of emboli as defined by the techniques of the time (66). While migrainous visual auras without headache had been recognized for centuries, Miller Fisher identified 60 analogous cases in which parasthesia, aphasia, dysarthria, paresis, diplopia, etc. evolved *slowly*, in a manner similar to that of classical visual aura, as distinct from the more rapid development of negative symptoms in thromboembolic TIAs, or the even more rapid march over seconds of focal sensory or motor seizures.

By 1986, this experience had extended to 205 cases and comprised several categories of symptoms (Table 3) (67). In all these patients, the probability that the symptoms were migrainous was supported by:

- Occurrence in patients with a previous or current personal history of migrainous visual aura in addition to the presenting symptom.
- Serial progression from one symptom to another in individual attacks (not a feature of thromboembolic events).
- Recurrence of stereotypic symptoms, often in "flurries" of repeated events over a short period.
- A generally benign course.
- Lack of evidence of an alternative explanation for the symptom.

Headache was associated with these auras in only about half of the cases, and two-thirds had a previous history of recurrent headaches.

In contrast to the general prevalence of migraine, these "TIAs" were more common in men (60%) than women (40%), and the duration of the symptoms seemed to vary much more widely than in the earlier study (66), lasting anywhere from seconds to several days, blurring the distinction between auras, ischemic TIAs, and focal seizures (Table 4).

Visual Symptoms

Miller Fisher excluded cases of typical scintillating scotoma from his series (because this is virtually diagnostic of migraine) and also transient monocular blindness (which could be amaurosis fugax due to thromboembolism), but

Table 4 Duration of Migrainous Episodes in
205 Cases of Late-Life Migrainous Accompaniments

1 min or less	4%
1–5 mins	25%
6–15 mins	20%
16–30 mins	18%
30 min–1 hr	4%
1–4 hrs	11%
5–24 hrs	10%
24–72 hrs	3%
Less than 72 hrs	3%

Source: Adapted from Fisher CM. Late-life migraine accompaniments—further experience. Stroke 1986; 17:1033–1042.

included examples of homonymous hemianopia, total blindness (bilateral homonymous hemianopia), and bilateral superior or inferior altitudinal quadrantanopia. He also included "visual blurring" (e.g., heat haze effects) and examples of visual metamorphopsia, which he described graphically as "a phantasmagoria of visual effects almost beyond description."

Sensory Symptoms

These included positive phenomena such as tingling, and pins and needles, and negative symptoms of "numbness," which could occur in isolation. Speech disorder could include any type of dysphasia, as well as dysarthria in brainstem attacks.

Motor Symptoms

Weakness or paralysis was not then widely regarded as a typical manifestation of migraine, except in FHM and "alternating migrainous hemiplegia of childhood," but Miller Fisher provided a number of examples in both young and older patients. Very often, the paralysis was described as profound, and could be bilateral.

Brainstem Symptoms

These could include diplopia, a feeling of "misalignment of the eyeballs," dizziness, tinnitus, and oscillopsia.

We have encountered several examples of this type of case, some of which have proved extraordinarily resistant to treatment.

CASE 127: MIGRAINOUS HEMIPARESIS

A 53-year-old man developed an acute attack of weakness and sensory impairment of the left arm and leg, without headache. This resolved over some nine days. MRI brain scan showed evidence of "small vessel ischemic disease" but no clear infarction, and extracranial ultrasound was normal. He was treated with aspirin. He subsequently began to have typical migraine without aura attacks. Two years after the first event, he had a further left-sided event, affecting the arm only, which resolved within an hour. There was no headache. He subsequently left the area and was lost to follow-up.

CASE 128: MIGRAINOUS HEMIANESTHESIA

A 76-year-old man was referred after he had suddenly developed paresthesia in the left arm while writing. This feeling then spread to his left leg over a few minutes. He felt muzzy headed, but there was no headache. The symptoms resolved in about 20 minutes. He had an identical episode in church two weeks later, and the next day a more severe attack with left facial numbness and dysarthria. On this occasion, the symptoms took 30 minutes to resolve and he felt muzzy headed for the rest of the day.

He had a history of transient unexplained neurological symptoms dating back some 30 years. On the first occasion, he had been running for a bus when he began to develop the same left-sided paresthesia, which resolved after about 10 minutes. He underwent extensive investigation, including cerebral angiography, with negative results. He had also been investigated following a similar attack six years before referral, including MRI brain scan, with negative results. He had been advised to take aspirin 75 mg daily and was taking this at the time of the most recent events.

CASE 129: COMPLEX MIGRAINOUS AURAS PRESENTING AS "TIAS"

A 42-year-old woman suddenly developed blindness in the left eye, followed in sequence by left hemianopia, left hemisensory impairment, and then weakness beginning in the left hand and ascending slowly up the arm, sparing the face and leg. The symptoms resolved over 20 minutes. There was no headache and no personal or family history of migraine. She had an increasing number of such attacks over the next few days, refractory to aspirin 300 mg daily. She was admitted urgently for anticoagulation, with heparin and then warfarin. However, screening for thromboembolism, including MRI brain scan, extracranial ultrasound and TOE, was negative. The attacks stopped, but one month later she was readmitted with a severe recurrence of left-sided weakness, again without headache, despite an INR of greater than 2. Repeat MRI brain scan and MRA were normal. The warfarin dose was increased, and she had no further attacks for six months, after which the drug was stopped. Soon afterwards, she had another attack of left-sided weakness without headache. All the investigations were repeated, again with negative results. No further treatment was instituted, and she was then asymptomatic for two years.

She then began to have attacks of classical migraine with visual aura, some of which were followed by left-sided sensory disturbance and weakness of the left arm, reminiscent of her earlier attacks. Occasionally, the sensory symptoms included an illusion of enlargement of the limb, and sometimes of the face and tongue (somesthetic metamorphopsia, see p. 107). In one dramatic attack, while driving her car, she suddenly felt that both her arms were swollen and detached from her body, and the car felt as if it were tipping over. She then experienced a mild tetraparesis lasting 15 to 20 minutes, and then recovered completely. There was no associated headache with any of these events.

CASE 130: MIGRAINOUS HEMIPLEGIC TIAs

A 52-year-old left-handed man suddenly developed weakness and numbness of the left face and arm, and mild slurring of speech. This resolved after some 10 minutes, but he was investigated at a local hospital. Clotting studies, CT brain scan, and extracranial ultrasound were normal. He was a smoker and had suffered a mild myocardial infarction five years earlier. He was treated with aspirin. About 18 months later, he had a sudden attack of total left arm paralysis, sparing the face and leg, lasting seconds, with complete recovery. He was fully investigated again, including MRI brain scan and MRA, with negative results, and was then asymptomatic for over a year. He then had further attacks of transient left arm paralysis, and also unassociated episodes of severe frontal headache lasting 10 minutes at a time. These attacks recurred over the next two years at frequent intervals, with complete recovery on each occasion. On some occasions, the headache was preceded by a "cracked glass" visual aura in the left hemifield.

About five years after first presentation, he suddenly experienced a black scotoma in the right eye on two occasions. An ophthalmologist identified retinal artery vasospasm during one of these attacks. Six months later, he had a similar attack in the left eye, followed by sensory disturbance down the right side, with recovery over two minutes. He had further episodes of the original left-sided symptoms over the next year. An MRI brain scan now revealed a mature infarct in the left occipital lobe. A week later, he suddenly developed a dense right hemiplegia due to a middle cerebral artery thrombosis. He made only a poor recovery from this, but was anticoagulated (INR > 2). Despite this, he continued to experience the transient left-sided attacks as before. A further extensive screening, including a full coagulation study, MR angiograms of the aortic arch and cerebral vessels, and a further TOE were all normal.

He continues to experience the left-sided sensorimotor attacks but they tend to last longer, 10 minutes to an hour, and may be followed by right-sided headaches without other migrainous characteristics in about 20% of instances.

CASE 131

A 58-year-old woman was referred following admission for a period of acute unsteadiness and malaise, followed by nonspecific headache. She had a long and complex background history of neurological symptoms of unclear origin.

At school, she had experienced migraine without aura. Some 30 years before referred, she had suffered episodes of deep vein thrombosis in two successive pregnancies. The second pregnancy was complicated by pre-eclampsia, and she developed a postpartum nephrotic syndrome. Thereafter, she had brittle hypertension. Her migraine attacks returned, but she had no associated neurological symptoms until 18 years prior to referral, when she had an episode of sudden "deadness" of the right leg. This lasted 20 minutes, but she then developed acute vertigo and a left-sided hemiparesis. She underwent extensive investigation. We do not know the results, but the hemiparesis took two years to resolve. She subsequently began to experience further transient stroke-like events affecting either leg, each preceded by a curious prodrome of faintness and nausea. None was convincingly associated with headache. She was repeatedly investigated by neuroimaging and coagulopathy screening, with negative results, and the events continued despite treatment with dipyramidole and aspirin. MRI brain scan two years prior to admission showed only numerous foci of hyperintensities throughout the white matter, as seen in some cases of migraine (see "Neuroimaging in migraine," above), and a repeat MRI study showed no significant change.

Lactate responses to exercise, and genetic screens for mitochondrial cytopathy and CADASIL were negative.

CASE 132

While attending a function, a 71 year old man found himself "rooted to the spot." He was able to move his arms, and there was no alteration of consciousness. He was eventually able to walk again with difficulty, but had to climb stairs using the banisters. The right leg felt particularly weak. He recovered completely after 20 minutes, and there was no headache. Four days later, he had an attack of paresthesia beginning in the right arm and spreading to the face, which lasted about four minutes. He had half a dozen similar episodes that day and the next, each lasting 5 to 10 minutes. He was referred to the local emergency room where "TIAs" were diagnosed. He had no significant vascular risk factors, and screening tests including CT brain scan and extracranial ultrasound studies were normal. He was treated with aspirin, clopidogrel, and ramipril, but the attacks continued at the same frequency.

He had no previous personal or family history of migraine. It was noted that his sensory symptoms, were entirely "positive"; there was no associated numbness or weakness. Subsequently, EEG, MRI brain scan, and MR angiogram (MRA) were entirely normal. He was anticoagulated to an INR of 2.2 with warfarin, but this did not influence the attacks. It was thought that the attacks might, therefore, represent late-life migrainous accompaniments, and he was treated with topiramate. Six months later, he reported that he had had no further attacks.

In a 1987 article Richard Peatfield (68), drew attention to the reported high frequency of unilateral headache in cases of thromboembolic TIA, while conversely, focal neurological symptoms of presumed migrainous origin were not associated with headache in about 50% of cases. He speculated that focal deficit and headache in TIA might result from platelet aggregation in the microcirculation. While the mechanism of headache in thromboembolic TIAs is unclear, the headache and focal symptoms seem to occur on the same side of the head, suggesting a local disturbance. He reasoned that small emboli might trigger spreading depression, resulting in migraine aura with headache in a migraine-susceptible individual; or in more rapid-onset focal symptoms without headache that would then be diagnosed as a typical thromboembolic TIA. Larger aggregates might result in infarction with or without headache. The diagnosis would thus vary with the clinical picture, but the "thromboembolic" and "migrainous" TIA events would have a common pathogenesis.

Some support for this concept comes from an earlier study of 22 patients with TIAs of unknown origin (i.e., no evidence of atherosclerotic, vascular, or cardiac disease, and no coagulopathy or previous history of migraine). The only abnormalities found, which might have explained the TIAs, were increased platelet aggregation and adhesiveness in vitro. The TIAs remitted with antiplatelet drugs but recurred when these were discontinued (69). However, as discussed elsewhere in this book, there is diversity of opinion concerning the relevance of in vitro platelet function studies in migraine.

Migrainous Microangiopathy?

In conclusion, it seems timely to propose a view regarding the relationship between migraine, ischemic infarction, and migrainous "TIAs." It is evident that migraine is a risk factor for cerebral ischemia, and that a significant proportion of events diagnosed as "TIAs" are likely to have a basis in the migraine mechanism in the absence of evident vascular risk factors or source of emboli, particularly in patients under 50 years of age. Because there is no good evidence that the neuronal processes of spreading depression and associated oligemia cause cerebral ischemia under normal circumstances, additional factors must be considered. First, it is possible, on the basis of experimental studies, that the intrinsic neuroprotective mechanisms invoked by the migraine mechanism might be overwhelmed, leading to parenchymal damage. Second, vascular injury might result in the release of endothelin-1, causing vasospasm.

More likely, however, is a link between migraine and cerebral ischemia through the behavior of platelets, either as a result of local aggregation in the cerebral microcirculation or by direct or paradoxical embolism via the heart. As discussed in several contexts elsewhere in this book, platelet function in migraineurs is abnormal, showing particular tendency to increased aggregation. The high prevalence of PFO among migraineurs, and the reported reduction in the frequency and severity of attacks of migraine with aura, and aura alone, following closure of shunts, is striking. The increased tendency of platelets to aggregate to form platelet emboli in the cerebral microcirculation might explain the high prevalence of WML on MRI scans in migraine patients (although the basis of these WML is debated—see above). Similar asymptomatic lesions occur in divers subject to decompression sickness, where PFO is found up to four times as often than in normal controls (70). The relatively high prevalence of PFO in the normal population might also explain the frequency of these MRI scan abnormalities in normal asymptomatic subjects.

It might thus be argued that such factors acting in concert could affect the cerebral microcirculation sufficiently to produce infarction. These considerations will no doubt lead to greater scrutiny of migraine patients for evidence of PFO and platelet abnormalities in the future, and to more careful controlled trials of antiplatelet drugs in migraine.

MIGRAINE AND BLACKOUTS

Blackouts and "funny turns" are among the most common symptoms that confront neurologists. The usual diagnostic issue is whether the patient's symptoms are due to syncope or near syncope, or seizure, or vertigo. The migraine mechanism can cause all of these, but, curiously, migraine does not even appear as part of the differential diagnosis for such symptoms in some major texts.

Migrainous Syncope

Syncope is a common clinical problem and may be dangerous and disabling. Population-based studies suggest that syncope affects some 3.5% of the general population, three times more than epilepsy. However, unlike epilepsy, syncope attracts remarkably little attention. It also accounts for about 3%

of admissions to accident and emergency departments and up to 6% of hospital admissions annually (71). Some 40% of cases of syncope remain undiagnosed, and 30% of patients experience recurrent episodes (72).

Pathogenesis of Syncope

Syncope or near syncope is associated with a halving of the cerebral blood flow, although such a fall will not necessarily cause symptoms. When we adopt the upright posture, there is a pooling of some 300 to 800 mL of blood in the vessels of the lower extremities. Responses from mechanoreceptors in the vessel walls result in increased sympathetic and reduced parasympathetic output from the brainstem. The physiological response is thus tachycardia and vasoconstriction, resulting in an increase in blood pressure (73).

Syncope is most likely to occur in otherwise normal individuals when standing motionless in warm environments (which promotes vasodilatation), following meals (diversion of blood to the splanchnic vessels), or when dehydrated. The mechanism in these circumstances seems likely to reflect excessive venous pooling or reduced intravascular volume. Syncope can also follow emotional and other "stresses," and can be triggered by reflexes associated with micturition and defecation. This might be related to the marked release of catecholamines, that has been found to occur just prior to the onset of syncope. Such stimuli might be expected to generate an even greater normal physiological response, but in some individuals, the opposite occurs.

The term "*vasovagal syncope*" was introduced by Thomas Lewis to describe this paradoxical response of vasodilatation and bradycardia. It is not known why this abnormal response occurs. A current suggestion is that some form of cerebral rather than a cardiogenic reflex is likely, and the phenomenon is now generally referred to as "*neurocardiogenic syncope*" (73). The tilt table test, wherein individuals are maintained motionless at an angle of 60° to 80° for up to 30 minutes, can precipitate syncope in susceptible individuals. Subsequent provocation with infusions of a variety of adrenergic, cholinergic, and vasodilator drugs can enhance the paradoxical reflex and increase sensitivity. In fact, a variety of abnormal responses can be observed. These include

- Vasovagal syncope—as described, a sudden drop in blood pressure associated with bradycardia.
- POTS (*postural orthostatic tachycardia syndrome*)—hypotension with tachycardia.
- Cerebral syncope, in which a normal cardiovascular response is associated with *cerebral vasoconstriction*, as observed by TCD studies.

In addition, the test can identify cases of postural hypotension due to for example dysautonomia, as found in a variety of neurodegenerative diseases.

Syncope in Migraine Attacks

In earlier epidemiological studies, episodes of impairment of consciousness were reported in about 10% and 20% of migraineurs in various series, mainly in the young (74–76). Syncope accounted for most instances while seizures were uncommon, occurring in perhaps 1% to 2% of cases. A recent survey of 16,809 admissions to three hospitals in Florence, Italy, during 1998 found that 775 admissions (4.46%) were due to syncope. Of these, about half were vasovagal attacks and half were associated with a variety of diseases, including orthostatic hypotension, heart block, gastrointestinal hemorrhage, "chronic cerebral disease," aortic dissection—and also migraine (77). A study of 108 children aged 2 to 19 years, referred with a diagnosis of idiopathic syncope, found that 75% of cases were vasovagal and the remainder were due to other causes, with 11% being considered migrainous (78).

Pathogenesis of migrainous syncope: No systematic study of migrainous syncope *per se* has been undertaken to our knowledge, and its mechanisms are not clear. However, as we noted previously (see p. 48). Sicuteri et al. found a marked hypersensitivity to bromocriptine in patients with presumptive migraine syncope. The drug caused marked hypotension, which was reversed by domperidone, suggesting dopamine receptor hypersensitivity (79). This observation has been supported by subsequent observations (80,81). As discussed in Chapter 2, there are indeed features of dopaminergic activation in migraine attacks in both prodromal symptomatology and nociception, and there is evidence of increased sensitivity of both peripheral and central dopamine receptors during attacks (81).

We have encountered numerous instances of syncope and near syncopal "funny turns" that do not appear to have been clearly provoked in circumstances normally associated with vasovagal, posturally induced or cardiogenic syncope. In many such instances, which affect young people particularly, we have noted a previous or recent history of migraine. We have also documented instances in which migraine attacks seem to have lead directly to syncope. Each of the following cases of presumptive migrainous syncope fulfilled at least three of the following four criteria:

- Attacks were unprovoked.
- Blackout was preceded by or associated with symptoms compatible with migraine aura on at least some occasions.
- Syncope was associated with headache having migraine characteristics.
- There was a personal or family history of migraine.
- There was no alternative explanation following investigation.

CASE 133: SYNCOPAL ATTACKS WITH VISUAL MIGRAINE AURA
A 31-year-old woman was referred because of "blackouts" dating back some 16 years. They would occur weekly for several weeks, separated by months of freedom

from attacks. Without provocation or warning, she would develop progressive bilateral tunnel vision, with scintillations in the central scotoma, associated with a numb, cold, clammy feeling in the head. Attacks only occurred while standing and could be aborted by lying or sitting, but in about 20% of instances, she would lose consciousness for a minute. In those instances, she would awake with a severe generalized pulsatile headache, without nausea or vomiting. The visual symptoms would resolve, and she would recover after a short sleep. On one occasion, she lost consciousness for 30 minutes. In addition, she had frequently experienced attacks of idiopathic stabbing headache, and there was a strong family history of migraine.

CASE 134: SYNCOPE, FOLLOWED BY MIGRAINE HEADACHE AND FAMILY HISTORY OF MIGRAINE

A 20-year-old woman was referred with a recent history of unprovoked blackouts on six or more occasions. There were no premonitory symptoms, and she would be unconscious for five or six minutes. On waking, she would experience a severe, pounding headache. She would feel groggy and disorientated. For some months, she had also been troubled by very frequent unilateral pounding headaches, often accompanied by nausea and vomiting, and her mother suffered from migraine.

CASE 135: CHILDHOOD SYNCOPAL ATTACKS, FOLLOWED BY ADULT MA

A 30-year-old woman was referred for evaluation of frequent episodic sensory symptoms. From the age of nine years, she had suffered repeated stereotyped attacks comprising sudden visual blurring and polyopia in the left hemifield followed by hemisensory paresthesia on either side, usually the left, and then loss of consciousness lasting seconds to minutes. She was extensively investigated in her teens, but no abnormalities could be found to explain the attacks. In her 20s, the sensory disturbances were followed by typical migraine headache, usually left sided, rather than syncope.

CASE 136: SYNCOPAL ATTACK WITH MIGRAINE ON RECOVERY AND PREVIOUS PERSONAL AND FAMILY HISTORY OF MIGRAINE

A 43-year-old woman developed a nonspecific headache, which persisted throughout the day. She felt exhausted on return from work. On climbing the stairs, she began to experience vague chest pain followed by dizziness and malaise, and felt she might faint. She knelt down over the toilet, but passed out. Her husband found her very pale, barely breathing, and she had been incontinent of urine. She was unconscious for a few minutes, and on recovery, her vision seemed yellow. She was slightly aggressive and then developed nausea and vomiting. She went to bed. At about 4 A.M., she awoke to find she could not see properly. She remained unwell for 72 hours, and her memory seemed impaired for some two weeks, after which she recovered completely.

She had a previous history of typical migraine with visual aura, and both her parents were migraine sufferers.

CASE 137: PRESYNCOPAL MIGRAINOUS SYMPTOMS IN A PATIENT WITH MA

A 61-year-old woman began to experience recurrent stereotyped attacks about once a week, in which she would suddenly feel ill and tremulous, and then develop a vague headache. She would then become pale, flushed, and clammy for a number of minutes. Subsequently, she would feel very sleepy and would lie down and go to sleep for a period, awaking refreshed. These episodes would last around 15 minutes.

She had a previous history of migraine with visual aura, and also acephalalgic attacks. She had suffered from "vertigo" for years and had probably had abdominal migraine as a child. There was a strong family history of migraine.

On enquiry four years later, she reported that these attacks had continued for about six months but had then stopped, and her migraine had become less frequent.

CASE 138: MIGRAINOUS SYNCOPE

A 45-year-old lady was referred with a year's history of recurrent blackouts, which would occur without warning or precipitant. She would suddenly fall to the ground, and lie unconscious and immobile for 10 to 15 minutes. On regaining consciousness, she would usually feel thirsty and confused. In about 20% of events, recovery would be associated with a severe thumping headache, which would last for one to two hours, together with an odd taste in the mouth. She also experienced similar headaches without loss of consciousness, from time to time. Her mother had also suffered from attacks of headache and blackout.

CASE 139

A 14-year-old girl was referred for investigation of "funny turns." The first had occurred at age 4 when she fainted briefly, and over the next few years, she had several more syncopal attacks. At age 11, she suffered two episodes in one day. After showering, her jaw began shaking, and the shaking then spread to the rest of the body. Consciousness was unaffected, but she felt vaguely numb. Later that day, she had a recurrence, associated with involuntary elevation of the right arm. EEG was normal.

Her mother had experienced similar attacks in childhood and adolescence and had recently been diagnosed as having migraine, and her younger sister was being evaluated for similar problems. The sister's EEG also proved to be normal.

A year after first evaluation, the patient had another event. On this occasion, however, the symptoms were typical of migraine with visual aura. On recent review, she had continued to experience occasional migraine with aura attacks, sometimes accompanied by typical syncopal events with secondary anoxic seizures. Further EEGs, including a sleep study, were entirely normal.

CASE 140: SYNCOPE FOLLOWING ONSET OF MIGRAINE HEADACHE, SOMETIMES WITH BASILAR TYPE MIGRAINE AURA

A 15-year-old girl presented with attacks comprising sudden onset of throbbing frontal headache, mainly over the eyes, with visual blurring. After about two minutes, she would feel light headed and would then lose consciousness. She would be unconscious for about three minutes and then awake with a severe headache and nausea. In an attack witnessed by her mother, she was noted to be deathly pale and lying completely still. In another attack, numbness of the mouth, tongue, and both arms preceded the loss of consciousness. A paternal cousin suffered severe migraine attacks.

On follow-up 12 years later, the patient indicated that the syncopal attacks had stopped, but that she continued to get attacks of migraine without aura.

CASE 141: MIGRAINOUS SYNCOPE

A 48-year-old woman woke in the night with a severe throbbing headache in the right frontal region. This worsened over the next two days. She suddenly noticed darkening of her vision, felt faint, and then lost consciousness for two minutes. On recovery, she was drowsy, slightly dysarthric, and a little confused for a few minutes, but she recovered completely. She did not seek medical attention because she had been investigated for a similar event a year earlier. On that occasion, she suddenly developed a severe occipital headache and lost consciousness rapidly. She was found on the bathroom floor, pale and peripherally cyanosed, with shallow breathing. She underwent urgent CT brain scan and lumbar puncture, which were entirely normal, and was told she had suffered a thunderclap headache. She had a long history of migraine with aura that seemed to have been triggered by taking an oral contraceptive. The attacks had stopped when this was discontinued. Her sister also had migraine.

CASE 142: MIGRAINE WITH AURA AND SYNCOPE

A 37-year-old woman presented with infrequent but stereotyped attacks. These were heralded by the onset of tunnel vision and altered awareness and giddiness. One episode, witnessed by her husband, was associated with subsequent loss of consciousness. She slumped forwards in her seat, looking very pale, and lay completely still for some two minutes. Attacks were followed by headache with some nausea. Her mother suffered from migraine, and her brother had blackouts and had been advised to "avoid caffeine."

On follow-up eight years later, she was still experiencing attacks of dizziness, nausea, and faintness, now lasting much longer, although her headaches were less of a problem.

CASE 143: MIGRAINOUS SYNCOPE INDUCED BY CHEESE

A 27-year-old man had a history of six blackouts over nine years. All had occurred after eating raw but not cooked cheese and had been identical in nature. On each occasion, having eaten cheese the previous evening, he had awoken the following morning with a severe pulsatile headache. Within half an hour of getting out of bed, he would feel progressively faint, nauseous, sweaty, and tachycardic, and would slump to the floor for about 30 seconds. On recovery, he would remain unwell, and the headache would persist for the rest of the day. He had not experienced such symptoms under any other circumstance, and he was on no other medication. There was no personal or family history of headache.

CASE 144: HISTORY OF PRESYNCOPE AND LATER MIGRAINOUS SYNCOPE

A 36-year-old man was referred for evaluation of a 14-year history of "funny turns." These were felt to be near-syncopal symptoms, and investigations were negative. He also had a history of independent episodic headaches. He was not followed subsequently but continued to have these events.

Six years later, he was admitted as an emergency following an episode that had begun while he was lying in bed in the early hours. He became dizzy and sweaty, and increasingly pale. He then lost consciousness with his eyes rolled up in his head for a couple of minutes. On recovery, he had a dull generalized headache, similar to headache episodes in the past. Investigations were normal or negative.

CASE 145: MIGRAINOUS SYNCOPE—RESPONSE TO PROPRANOLOL

A 32-year-old man had been driving his lorry when he began to experience severe nausea followed by a "blinding headache." He came to a halt and then lost consciousness for a minute or two. He self-referred to a local hospital. CT brain scan was normal, and he was discharged, although he felt unwell for a few days after this. He had an identical attack a week later and was admitted for investigations, which again proved normal. He had a long history of migraine with typical visual auras but no family history of headache. The headache attacks subsequently reduced in frequency with propranolol prophylaxis, but he had two further syncopal attacks, both without headache, in the following few weeks.

CASE 146: SYNCOPE WITH MIGRAINOUS FEATURES AND FAMILY HISTORY OF MIGRAINE
A 44-year-old woman presented with stereotyped attacks heralded by light-headedness. After about 20 minutes, she would become very pale and lose consciousness, lying motionless on the ground for about 10 minutes. On recovery, she would experience a severe, pounding headache in the frontal and bitemporal regions, with nausea and photophobia, and would have to "sleep it off." On waking after a short period, she recovered completely on each occasion. She had no personal history of migraine, but a nephew had severe attacks.

Migraine and Epilepsy

The relationship between migraine and epilepsy has intrigued neurologists for more than a century (82). Some consider the presence of both disorders in an individual as no more than chance, given that they are both common. Others have suggested that one can lead to the other, and even that they might have a common pathogenesis.

Sieveking combined his early interest in headache with work in epilepsy and, in 1858, was the first to clearly define a relationship between the two conditions (83). He described and documented many such cases, referring to the syndrome as *cephalalgia epileptiformis*. Of course, we cannot be sure that some of these cases did not have underlying structural pathology but the association conformed well with Liveing's later nerve-storm hypothesis (1873) and Gowers' views, as expressed in his work "Border-land of Epilepsy" (1907) (see Chapter 1, p. 23).

Not surprisingly, there is a significant incidence of underlying structural abnormalities in patients presenting with both migraine and epilepsy, particularly with focal epilepsy. In addition, migraine and seizures can both be manifestations of mitochondrial cytopathies, particularly MELAS (*mitochondrial encephalomyopathy with lactic acidosis and stroke-like episodes*) (84,85). Clearly, such disorders must be excluded by appropriate investigations in all cases presenting with this syndrome before considering a diagnosis of migraine-related seizures.

There are several compelling similarities between migraine and epilepsy. First, headaches with migrainous features are common following epileptic seizures (86). In one recent outpatient survey of 110 epilepsy patients (87), 43% reported seizure-associated headaches. The vast majority were postictal, but one patient had exclusively preictal headache and three other cases had both pre- and postictal headaches, suggesting possible migraine-triggered seizures. One-third of the headaches in these patients conformed to IHC criteria for migraine headache, but there was no relationship between headache localization and epilepsy features.

Second, EEG abnormalities, sometimes including spike and wave patterns typical of epilepsy, have been recorded in patients during migraine attacks (82). Finally, anticonvulsants are increasingly favored as migraine prophylactics (see Chapter 7).

There is some evidence that although there is a significant incidence of active migraine among patients with epilepsy and vice versa, there may be subtle distinguishing features in these different patient groups. In a recent study, 61 patients with comorbid migraine and epilepsy were compared to 280 patients with epilepsy alone and 248 patients with migraine alone (88). As expected, there were more females in the comorbidity and migraine groups than the epilepsy group, but the epilepsy diagnoses did not differ between the comorbid and epilepsy groups. However, the prevalence of migraine with aura was significantly higher in the comorbidity group than in the migraine group, and the patients with both migraine and epilepsy tended to have more severe migraine attacks.

Certain forms of epilepsy and migraine have been shown to be due to neuronal channelopathies. FHM in particular may be associated with seizures, including status epilepticus (89). As noted, a prolonged hemiplegia in FHM may be associated with striking MRI scan abnormalities indicating reduced cerebral blood flow secondary to protracted spreading depression (see p. 154), and similar reversible abnormalities have recently been reported in a patient with recurrent *migralepsy*, who showed MRI brain scan abnormalities consistent with the neurological deficits (90).

The ICH-2 classification defines migraine-triggered seizure, or migralepsy, as

> A seizure fulfilling diagnostic criteria for one type of epileptic attack occurring during, or within 1 hour after, a migraine aura.

Andermann (91) defined three non-symptomatic "migraine epilepsy" syndromes:

- *Epilepsy occurring during migraine aura.* This was the largest group among the patients studied. It was suggested that such patients had a low threshold for seizure, with attacks triggered by the aura process. Many showed response to migraine prophylactics or anticonvulsants.
- *Patients who developed an independent seizure disorder.* A smaller group initially had migraine-triggered seizures but went on to develop temporal and occipital seizures independent of the migraine aura.
- *Benign occipital epilepsy with intercalated migraine.*

The following cases are examples of these groups. In all cases, detailed imaging and other appropriate investigations were normal or negative, except where specified.

Cases of Migraine-Triggered Seizures

CASE 147: SEIZURES PRECIPITATED BY MIGRAINE AURA

A 29-year-old woman was evaluated after an isolated grand mal seizure. Eight years earlier, she had begun to experience frequent acephalalgic migraine attacks, comprising visual auras. She would suddenly see white patches in the visual fields, usually followed by typical teichopsia and would feel "muzzy headed" as the aura resolved. However, since childhood, she had also experienced recurrent "feelings of indecision." When faced with choices (such as which way to turn when driving), she would feel suddenly completely unsure but would make a choice, which was "invariably wrong." This feeling would pass in seconds.

She had been on a train some months prior to referral when she experienced this aura, after which she lost consciousness briefly. The grand mal seizure that prompted her admission had been preceded by a similar aura.

CASE 148: SEIZURE PRECIPITATED BY MIGRAINOUS SYNCOPE PROVOKED BY CHOCOLATE

A 19-year-old woman was walking when she suddenly felt dizzy and faint. She eventually had to sit down, whereupon she fell to the ground and suffered a tonic-clonic seizure. Afterwards she had a "screaming sound" in the back of her head and seemed a little confused. She resumed walking, but the symptoms recurred. She attended an emergency room. On arrival, she experienced blurred vision and then developed a progressive unilateral and occipital headache, and diarrhea. Detailed investigations were unremarkable. She subsequently began to suffer occasional migraine headaches. She had had "bilious attacks" as a child and recalled eating a large amount of chocolate cake just before the presenting attack.

CASE 149: SEIZURE PRECIPITATED BY MIGRAINE PROVOKED BY LIGHT

A 55-year-old man presented following three migraine attacks, each of which had triggered a grand mal seizure. He had suffered from migraine with visual aura about once every two years for many years. Bright lights and orange juice could trigger attacks. His father was also a sufferer. He acknowledged that he had been under more stress recently and had been drinking two bottles of wine daily. The familiar visual blurring of his migraine aura heralded the first epileptic attack. This lasted about four minutes, but he had no subsequent memory of events until he was coming to, surrounded by paramedics. There was no distinct headache. His wife had witnessed the seizure, and he had bitten his tongue. About four months later, he had another attack, identical in character and yet another within the month, possibly provoked by bright lights.

On follow-up six months later, no further attacks had occurred. He had stopped drinking whisky, coffee, and orange juice.

CASE 150: MIGRAINE-TRIGGERED SEIZURES

A 32-year-old man was referred following a seizure preceded by headache. He had developed epilepsy at around seven years of age. Every attack began with a severe, throbbing, frontal headache with nausea, photophobia, and phonophobia.

After 10 to 15 minutes, he would have a typical generalized tonic-clonic seizure. On recovery, he would vomit. The headache usually continued for an hour or so, and he would then recover completely. He suffered two such attacks per week; and in addition, he experienced headaches of a similar type without seizures. He was treated with valproate and eventually became attack-free by age 18. He had continued treatment until some two years prior to referral, and the recent attack seemed to have been precipitated by stopping the anticonvulsant. This attack was identical to those earlier in his life. MRI brain scan and EEG showed no significant abnormalities.

CASE 151: MIGRAINE-TRIGGERED SEIZURE

A 19-year-old girl was referred following a witnessed grand mal seizure. She had a long history of migraine with visual aura. She had been working hard on her homework when she began to experience her habitual aura, followed by migraine headache. This was still present when she went to bed. She had a grand mal seizure in her sleep. The next day, she was aware of problems with photophobia and visual blurring. She was given sodium valproate for a short while but did not continue the medication. She was subsequently treated with atenolol, and this significantly reduced the frequency of her migraines. However, a year later, she suffered a further seizure while awake, preceded by an elemental visual aura of "flashing lights." Her EEG was normal. She was treated thereafter with carbamazepine. On follow-up 12 years later, she had had no further problems with either migraine or seizures.

CASE 152: MIGRAINE-TRIGGERED SEIZURE

A 21-year-old woman was referred following two possible nocturnal seizures. She had a history of migraine with teichopsic aura dating back to her teens. One day, having been exercising hard and eating inadequately, she experienced a fuzzy but vividly bright visual aura and became strange and distant, according to her companions. She had no memory of this. She had to lie down. Her consciousness was clouded, and she was not easily roused. After about half an hour, she vomited and then recovered sufficiently to resume her activities. Six months later, while drifting off to sleep one night, she experienced a visual aura and then suddenly fell asleep. On waking the next day, she had generalised muscle pain and had bitten her tongue. She had an identical episode four months later. She had a strong family history of migraine.

Cases of Migraine Evolving into Epilepsy

CASE 153: MIGRAINE-TRIGGERED EPILEPSY EVOLVING INTO
SEIZURE DISORDER WITH EPILEPTIC AMNESIA ATTACKS

A 17-year-old girl presented with a six-year history of infrequent migraine headaches preceded by elemental visual auras. One day, she had a witnessed grand mal seizure after a visual aura had started while she was watching a visual display unit screen. The seizure was followed by a typical migraine headache. She had a further seizure preceded by similar migrainous symptoms some weeks later. Her CT brain scan was normal, but her EEG showed diffuse epileptic activity. She was started on sodium valproate. Her seizures and migraine headaches stopped completely for some years, but she later developed attacks of epileptic TGA, lasting up to 10 minutes, followed by migraine headache with nausea and photophobia. These attacks also stopped eventually, and she was then asymptomatic until three years later, when the amnesic attacks recurred.

CASE 154: MIGRAINOUS SYNCOPE EVOLVING INTO MIGRAINE-TRIGGERED SEIZURES AND NOCTURNAL EPILEPSY

A 16-year-old boy was referred with recurrent episodes of loss of consciousness dating back some seven years. These seemed to be typically syncopal but occurred without provocation. His father had suffered similar events in childhood. For some three years, he had also experienced nocturnal pounding headaches associated with nausea that would wake him from sleep, and also occasional episodes of visual aura, comprising an expanding, multicolored scotoma in the left hemifield, followed by mild headache. He was referred when one of these migraine with aura attacks was followed by loss of consciousness associated with jactitation and postictal drowsiness. EEG was normal except for episodic sharp waves during overbreathing. This attack was interpreted as a migrainous syncope with secondary hypoxic seizure.

He was referred once more three years later following the onset of nocturnal seizures. He had continued to experience the migraine with aura attacks and had sometimes been unconscious for up to half an hour. The new events were heralded by a pounding headache, forcing him to retire to bed where he would have a fit in his sleep of such severity that he would bite his tongue and develop cyanosis and petechial hemorrhages around the eyes and over the forearms. EEG was normal. On follow-up six years later, he recorded that the migraine headaches had eventually stopped, but he had continued to have visual auras and nocturnal seizures.

CASE 155: FOCAL EPILEPSY AND MIGRAINE

A 31-year-old woman presented with a 12-year history of occasional, untreated generalized nocturnal seizures, associated with very severe migraine headaches. The migraine attacks were not associated with aura and were unilateral, occurring in the left temporal or right occipital region. On such occasions, she would lie down to "sleep it off," and the seizures would occur while she was asleep. She also experienced the migraine headaches without subsequent seizures. Her mother had suffered identical attacks.

Neuroimaging and EEG, both when awake and asleep, were normal, and baseline studies for mitochondrial disorder were negative. She was treated with pizotifen, which reduced the frequency of attacks, and valproate was added to reduce seizures. After a year, the headaches had resolved significantly, but she continued to get nocturnal seizures once monthly.

She was re-referred four years later, following an attack during which she suddenly developed uncontrollable shaking of the left leg and numbness of the left arm. This continued for some 30 minutes, after which the limbs were weak for some days. Her headaches returned after this event. MRI brain scan was normal.

Benign Occipital Epilepsy with Intercalated Migraine

CASE 156

A 10-year-old girl presented with typical migraine with visual auras, nausea, vomiting, and acroparesthesia. The attacks lasted a few hours. There was a history of migraine in her father and a maternal uncle. The attacks stopped completely after a year but were succeeded by nocturnal grand mal epilepsy. During these episodes, she would jactitate with such violence that she would be projected from her bed onto the floor, where she would exhibit a typical tonic-clonic generalized convulsion, lasting several minutes. She would not wake fully after these events but simply resumed sleeping. She would be amnesic for the events the following day but said she had had "dreams." CT brain scan was normal, but her EEG showed continuous occipital epileptic discharges compatible with the diagnosis of benign occipital epilepsy with intercalated migraine. The attacks remitted completely with sodium valproate.

Migralepsy: Finally, one occasionally encounters patients who seem to suffer attacks of migraine and epilepsy both independently and in conjunction. The term "migralepsy" seems particularly appropriate to such instances.

CASE 157: MIGRALEPSY

A five-year-old girl was referred following four stereotyped attacks. Three had occurred on a single day and the fourth about six months later. Each began with a headache and stomach ache followed by clouding of consciousness, with automatisms such as repetitive tugging at her shirt and the eyes rolling from side-to-side. Each event lasted about four minutes, and she was noticeably flushed at the end of the attacks. CT brain scan was normal, but EEG showed spike–wave paroxysms arising in the right temporal region. She initially showed a good response to valproate but developed some behavioral abnormalities that seemed to settle when she was switched to lamotrigine. Some four years later, she presented with recurrent nonspecific headaches and dizziness, which seemed to respond to pizotifen. Repeat EEG was normal. Having been seizure free for more than five years, anticonvulsant cover was withdrawn.

About seven years later, she began to have recurrent attacks of dizziness, nausea, and visual blurring, with possible mild clouding of consciousness lasting only a minute or two. Quite often, throbbing occipital headache with nausea, which could last all day, preceded these symptoms. In retrospect, she now felt these symptoms had also been present in the childhood attacks. Her mother had suffered recurrent migraine attacks as a young woman.

EEG now showed irregular, sharp theta discharges with occasional spikes during hyperventilation and photic stimulation (Fig. 9), but these responses did not outlast the photic stimulus (and were, therefore, not indicative of photosensitive epilepsy).

CASE 158: MIGRALEPSY

A 37-year-old lady presented with a history of "funny turns" dating back to her early teens. She was investigated with scans and EEG, but no firm conclusions were drawn. These episodes eventually stopped for many years but later recurred.

Each episode comprised sudden clouding of consciousness lasting seconds, in which she would be aware but unable to talk or move. Observers noted that she was extremely pale and would stare blankly. As she recovered, she would experience a severe frontal headache, with nausea and sometimes vomiting but without photo- or phonophobia. In addition, she also suffered headaches two or three times a week that were unassociated with alteration in consciousness but which were otherwise very similar to the headaches following the episodes of impaired consciousness.

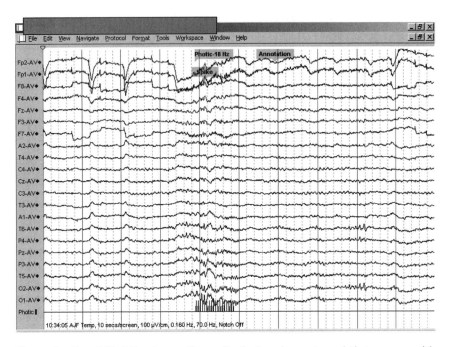

Figure 9 Case 157. Migralepsy. Generalized, sharply contoured theta waves with some spiking prominent in the occipital region.

MRI brain scan showed no abnormality, but her EEG showed some nonspecific abnormalities. She was treated with pizotifen, which seemed to reduce the frequency of both the "funny turns" and headaches.

Two years later, she suddenly began to experience the "funny turns" again on a frequent basis and was then admitted following a typical nocturnal tonic-clonic seizure. In the ward, she had a further seizure, followed by headache and vomiting. At this point, she was started on lamotrigine and the pizotifen was stopped. On review three months later, she had had no further seizures, but the migrainous headaches had returned and were frequent and disabling. They reduced considerably in frequency once more after the pizotifen was reinstituted.

Can Migraine Induce Epilepsy?

The pathogenesis and manifestations of the common forms of migraine and epilepsy are clearly different; although, as discussed, some forms of both are neuronal channelopathies.

It is instructive to contrast these pathophysiologies. Epilepsy results fundamentally from electrical instability of neuronal membranes in the cortex, with rapid spread of depolarization. Partial seizures (epileptic auras) progress quickly, for example, from hand to face to leg over a matter of seconds. By contrast, migraine is a "neurochemical" event triggered in the brain

Table 5 Relative Frequencies of Auras in Migraine and Epilepsy in Relation to Cortical Origin

Auras	Migraine	Epilepsy	Cortical origin
Visual	++++	+	Posterior
Somesthetic	+++	+	
Aphasic	++	++	
Olfactory		+++	
Motor	+/−	+++	
Epigastric	+/−	++++	Anterior

stem, cortex, or both, and the timeframe of events is orders of magnitude slower. In addition, epilepsy has a predisposition for the "front of the brain," while the migraine mechanism chiefly involves posterior structures, as evidenced by the frequency of the aura types in the two conditions (Table 5). Paradoxically, injury to posterior neural structures seems prone to induce seizures. Occlusion of the posterior cerebral artery during posterior fossa surgery can result in "temporal lobe" epilepsy. Olivier et al. demonstrated an occipitotemporal pathway, which, it was suggested, might be involved in secondary epileptogenesis in migraine (92).

MIGRAINE COMA

It has been recognized for many years that migraine can be associated with altered states of consciousness and even coma. This is particularly so in cases of migraine of basilar type and in children with certain forms of FHM, in which coma can follow trivial head injury. Nevertheless, migraine coma is rare in practice. Early surveys identified a significant number of episodes of posttraumatic coma that were difficult to explain, and which may have included instances of migraine coma (93). A later series of sporadic cases of migraine associated with impaired consciousness was reported from Australia (94).

Coma in FHM

We have discussed FHM in connection with migraine pathogenesis (Chapter 2), migraine auras (Chapter 3), and in this chapter with regard to consideration of possible brain injury by the migraine mechanism. Studies of patients with FHM have also noted that coma is a common manifestation of the disorder. Fitzsimons and Wolfenden observed that hemiplegic migraine was a cause of recurrent coma associated with life-threatening cerebral hemisphere edema, fever and CSF pleocytosis mimicking viral meningoencephalitis. Moreover, attacks could be precipitated or exacerbated by cerebral angiography (95). Corbin et al. described a child with recurrent migraine coma with very similar systemic symptoms, but generalized motor dysfunction rather than hemiplegia. One episode of coma in this patient was precipitated by mild head injury. It was not possible to determine the family history in this case (96).

Surveying the situation with regard to FHM patients with mutations in *CACNA1* (see p. 79), Ducros et al. found that about one-third of attacks were associated with coma (97). Recently the mutation S218L was found to be specifically associated with delayed cerebral edema and coma after minor head injury (98). This mutation results in a severely reduced threshold for opening of the neuronal voltage-gated calcium channel, and produces remarkably prolonged depolarization. This would predicate protracted cortical spreading depression (CSD) effects and the development of brain swelling through hyperperfusion and cytotoxic edema. Indeed, attacks may sometimes cause irreversible brain damage or even death, as noted above. Interestingly, episodes of reversible encephalopathy and coma with very similar general features to those of coma in FHM have also been reported in cases of CADASIL in which, it will be recalled, the culpable *notch 3* gene lies in the vicinity of the *CACNA1A* gene (99).

Syncope and Coma in Basilar-Type Migraine

Migraine of basilar type will be discussed in Chapter 5, but a brief summary is pertinent here because attacks can cause loss of consciousness. This syndrome was first characterized by Bickerstaff in 1961 (100) and is now defined under IHC-2 (1.2.6) as a form of migraine with aura, in which the aura includes symptoms suggestive of brain stem dysfunction. These can include decreased level of consciousness. Originally, the term "basilar artery migraine" or "basilar migraine" was used, but many patients have symptoms that are intermingled with symptoms of "typical" aura, indicating cortical involvement. For example, Bickerstaff described the syndrome in its complete form as causing

> Vivid teichopsia, with impairment or loss of vision in the whole of both fields, dysarthria, vertigo, tinnitus, unsteadiness of gait, and paraesthesiae in the periphery of both hands, both feet, and around both sides of the mouth and the tongue .... succeeded after 10–45 minutes by throbbing headache, usually occipital and accompanied by vomiting.

Eight of Bickerstaff's 32 cases had a history of impaired consciousness during attacks. This was described as a trance-like or dream state during the aura phase, following which patients might fall into a "sleep," lasting a few minutes to half an hour from which they were difficult to rouse. Bickerstaff believed that the impaired consciousness resulted from ischemia of the reticular activating system.

Migraine of basilar type, is mostly seen in young adults. Patients with FHM also have basilar-type migraine symptoms in 60% of attacks; so, strictly speaking, migraine of basilar type should only be diagnosed when no clear motor signs are present—although this is debatable.

There are relatively few case reports of basilar migraine with coma (101,102). The patients described did not have features of hemiplegia, pyrexia, or CSF abnormalities typical of coma in FHM, and neurophysiological studies such as EEG and auditory-evoked potentials were abnormal and pointed to brain stem dysfunction. Interestingly, in one series of four cases, one patient awoke spontaneously with intense bulimia, and coma was reversed in the other three patients by intravenous flumazenil, suggesting gabaergic dysfunction in the reticular activating system as the basis of pathogenesis of the coma (103).

We have encountered occasional cases of brief loss of consciousness in migraine of basilar type, and one case that might be considered an example of migraine coma.

CASE 159: SYNCOPE IN MIGRAINE OF BASILAR TYPE

A 67-year-old man was referred because of recurrent blackouts. These had begun some six years earlier. On the first occasion, he lost consciousness without warning for a minute or so while working in the garden. He was found to be sweaty, pale, and shaking, and took some 48 hours to recover fully. He continued to have paroxysmal symptoms in the succeeding weeks, comprising a curious sensory disturbance from the chest to the head with faintness but no loss of consciousness. Subsequent attacks began with sudden pain in the left side of the head followed by brief loss of consciousness, after which he would notice numbness of the left side of the face and narrowing of the left palpebral fissure. He would typically wish to sleep after such events. Between events, he was perfectly well. Over the years, he had several MRI brain scans, MR angiograms (MRA) and EEGs, which showed no significant abnormalities.

CASE 160: MIGRAINE COMA

A 44-year-old man developed a generalized headache one evening, associated with an overwhelming desire to sleep. He slept that night, but his wife found him almost impossible to rouse throughout the next day. A day later, he had recovered somewhat but he could only stagger about, and his speech was very slurred. He was admitted to another hospital, where CT and subsequent MRI brain scans were normal. He eventually recovered completely but had no memory of these events.

Subsequently, he suffered repeated migrainous headaches lasting up to a week at a time, sometimes waking him at night. For many years previously, he had suffered recurrent vertigo of such severity that he had been discharged from military service on medical grounds. He had undergone extensive neuro-otological investigation with negative results and had not developed tinnitus or deafness.

Subsequent investigation, including trimodality-evoked potentials, CSF examination, and plasma lactate and ammonia levels, was normal. He was treated with atenolol and the migraine attacks became much less frequent, but he continued to have further episodes of coma and then severe obtundation, developing out of sleep in a similar fashion to the first attack. On some occasions, attacks were accompanied by a severe, throbbing headache.

In conclusions, in addition to producing a plethora of transient, fully reversible neurological symptoms, the migraine mechanism can, on occassions produce severe and sometimes permanent cerebral injury. Generally, severe sequelae are unpredictable and not necessarily related to the "severity" of the attack, but additional comorbidities, such as vascular disease or platelet abnormalities, may play a part in determining such consequences.

REFERENCES

1. Haas DC. Prolonged migraine aura status. Ann Neurol 1982; 11:197–199.
2. Luda E, Bo E, Sicuro L, et al. Sustained visual aura: a totally new variation of migraine. Headache 1999; 31:582–583.
3. Liu GT, Schatz NJ, Galetta SL, Volpe NJ, Skobieranda F, Kosmorsky DO. Persistent positive visual phenomena in migraine. Neurology 1995; 45: 664–668.
4. Relja G, Granato A, Ukmar M, Ferretti G, Antonello RM, Zorzona M. Persistent aura without infarction: description of the first case studied with both brain SPECT and perfusion MRI. Cephalalgia 2005; 25:56–59.
5. Fére C. Contribution à l'étude de al migraine ophthalmique. Revue de Médecin Paris 1881; 1:625–649.
6. Ramadan NM. Migrainous infarction: the Charcot-Fére syndrome. Cephalalgia 1993; 13:249–252.
7. Lesnik Oberstein SA, van den Boom R, Middelkoop HA, et al. Incipient CADASIL. Arch Neurol 2003; 60:707–712.
8. Ricci S. Embolism from the heart in the young patient; a short review. Neurol Sci 2003; 24(suppl 1):S13–S4.
9. Broderick JP, Swanson JW. Migraine-related strokes. Arch Neurol 1987; 44:868–871.
10. Milhaud D, Bogousslavsky J, van Melle G, Liot P. Ischemic stroke and active migraine. Neurology 2001; 57:1805–1811.
11. Tzourio C, Iglésias S, Hubert J-B, et al. Migraine and risk of ischemic stroke: a case controlled study. Br Med J 1993; 307:289–292.
12. Tzourio C, Tehindrazanarivelo A, Iglésias S, et al. Case-control study of migraine and risk of ischaemic stroke in young women. Br Med J 1995; 310:830–833.
13. Carolei A, Marini C, de Matteis G. de Matteis G and the Italian National Research Council Study Group on Stroke in the Young. Lancet 1996; 347:1503–1506.
14. Donaghy M, Chang CL. Poulter N and the European Collaborators of The World Health Organization Collaborative Study of Cardiovascular Disease and Steroid Hormone Contraception. J Neurol Neurosurg Psychiat 2002; 73:747–750.
15. Chang CL, Donaghy M. Poulter N and The World Health Organization Collaborative Study of Cardiovascular Disease and Steroid Hormone Contraception. Migraine and stroke in young women: case control study. Br Med J 1999; 318:13–18.

16. Boes CJ, Matharu MS, Goadsby PJ. Migraine and stroke. Stroke Review 2002; 6:1–4.

17. Lee H, Lopez I, Ishiyama A, Baloh RW. Can migraine damage the inner ear? Arch Neurol 2000; 57:1631–1634.

18. Piovesan EJ, Kowacs PA, Werneck LC, Siow C. Oscillucusis and sudden deafness in a migraine patient. Arq Neuropsiquiatr 2003; 61:848–850.

19. Butteriss DJ, Ramesh V, Birchall D. Serial MRI in a case of familial hemiplegic migraine. Neuroradiology 2003; 45:300–303.

20. Gonzalez-Alegre P, Tippin I. Prolonged cortical electrical depression and diffuse vasospasm without ischaemia in a case of severe hemiplegic migraine during pregnancy. Headache 2003; 43:72–75.

21. Gutschalk A, Kollmar R, Mohr A, et al. Multimodal functional imaging of prolonged neurological deficits in a patient suffering from familial hemiplegic migraine. Neurosci Lett 2002; 332:115–118.

22. Oberndorfer S, Wober C, Nasel C, et al. Familial hemiplegic migraine: follow-up findings of diffusion-weighted magnetic resonance imaging (MRI), perfusion-MRI and [99mTc] HMPAO-SPECT in a patient with prolonged hemiplegic migraine. Cephalalgia 2004; 24:533–539.

23. Hayashi R, Tachikawa H, Watanabe R, Honda M, Katsumata Y. Familial hemiplegic migraine with irreversible brain damage. Intern Med 1998; 37:166–168.

24. Kors EE, Terwindt GM, Vermeulen FL, et al. Delayed cerebral edema and fatal coma after minor head trauma; role of the CACNA1A calcium channel subunit gene and relationship with familial hemiplegic migraine. Ann Neurol 2001; 49:753–760.

25. Matharu MS, Good CD, May A, Bahra A, Goadsby PJ. No change in the structure of the brain in migraine: a voxel-based morphometric study. Eur J Neurol 2003; 10:53–57.

26. Guest IA, Woolf AL. Fatal infarction of brain in migraine. Br Med J 1964; 1:225–226.

27. Dukes HT, Vieth R. Cerebral arteriography during migraine prodrome and headache. Neurology (Minneapolis) 1964; 14:636–640.

28. Connor RCR. Complicated migraine: a study of permanent neurological and visual defects caused by migraine. Lancet 1962; 2:1072–1075.

29. Selby G, Fryer JA. Fatal migraine. Clin Exp Neurol 1984; 20:85–92.

30. Sanin LC, Mathew NT. Severe diffuse intracranial vasospasm as a cause of extensive migrainous cerebral infarction. Cephalalgia 1993;13:289–292.

31. Hungerford GD, du Boulay GH, Zilkha KJ. Computerised axial tomography in patients with severe migraine: a preliminary report. J Neurol Neurosurg Psychiat 1976; 39:990–994.

32. Cala LA, Mastaglia FL. Computerised axial tomography findings in a group of patients with migrainous headaches. Proc Aust Neurol Assoc 1976; 13:35–41.

33. Soges LJ, Cacayorin ED, Petro GR, Ramachandran TS. Migraine: evaluation by MR. Am J Neuroradiol 1988; 9:425–429.

34. Igarashi H, Sakai F, Kan S, Okada J, Tazaki Y. Magnetic resonance imaging of the brain in patients with migraine. Cephalalgia 1991; 11:69–74.

35. Fazekas F, Koch M, Schmidt R, et al. The prevalence of cerebral damage varies with migraine type: an MRI study. Headache 1992; 32:287–291.

36. Robbins L, Friedman H. MRI in migraineurs. Headache 1992; 32:507–508.
37. De Benedittis G, Lorenzetti A, Sina C, Bernasconi V. Magnetic resonance imaging in migraine and tension-type headache. Headache 1995; 35:264–268.
38. Kuhn NJ, Shekar PC. A comparative study of magnetic resonance imaging and computomography in the evaluation of migraine. Comput Med Imaging Graph 1990; 14:149–152.
39. Kruit MC, Van Buchem MA, Hofman PA, et al. Migraine as a risk factor for subclinical brain lesions. J Am Med Assoc 2004; 291:427–434.
40. Swartz RH, Kern RZ. Migraine is associated with magnetic resonance imaging white matter abnormalities: a meta-analysis. Arch Neurol 2004; 61: 1366–1368.
41. Vahedi K, Chabriat H, Levy C, Joutel A, Tournier-Lasserve E, Bousser MG. Migraine with aura and brain magnetic resonance imaging abnormalities in patients with CADASIL. Arch Neurol 2004; 61:1237–1240.
42. Wardlaw JM. What causes lacunar stroke? J Neurol Neurosurg Psychiat 2005; 76:617–619.
43. Dreier JP, Korner K, Ebert N. Nitric oxide scavenging by haemoglobin or nitric oxide synthase inhibition by N-nitro-L-arginine induces cortical spreading ischemia when K^+ is increased in the subarachnoid space. J Cerebral Blood Flow Metab 1998; 18:978–990.
44. Dorfman LJ, Marshall WH, Enzmann DR. Cerebral infarction and migraine: clinical and radiologic correlations. Neurology 1979; 23:317–322.
45. Castaldo JE, Anderson M, Reeves AG. Middle cerebral artery occlusion with migraine. Stroke 1982; 13:308–311.
46. Casas JP, Hingorani AD, Bautista LE, Sharma P. Meta-analysis of genetic studies in ischemic stroke. Arch Neurol 2004; 61:1652–1662.
47. Spence JD, Wong DG, Melendez LJ, et al. Increased prevalence of mitral valve prolapse in patients with migraine. Can J Neurol Sci 1984; 131:1457–1460.
48. Garnier P, Michel D, Antoine JC, et al. Myxoma of the left atrium with neurological manifestations: 8 cases. Revue Neurologique 1994; 150:776–784.
49. Lechat P, Mas JL, Lascault G, et al. Prevalence of patent foramen ovale in patients with stroke. N Engl J Med 1988; 318:1148–1152.
50. Overell JR, Bone I, Lees KR. Interatrial septal abnormalities and stroke. A meta-analysis of case-controlled studies. Neurology 2000; 55:1172–1179.
51. Bogousslavsky J, Garazi S, Jeanrenaud X, Aebischer N, Van Melle G. Stroke recurrence in patients with patent foramen ovale; the Lausanne Study. Neurology 1996; 46:1301–1305.
52. Del Sette M, Angeli S, Leandri M, et al. Migraine with aura and right-to-left shunt on transcranial Doppler: a case controlled study. Cerbrovasc Diseases 1998; 8:327–330.
53. Wilmshurst PT, Nightingale S, Walsh KP, Morrison WL. Effect on migraine of closure of cardiac right-to-left shunts to prevent recurrence of decompression illness or stroke or for haemodynamics reasons. Lancet 2000; 356: 1648–1651.
54. Sztajzel R, Genoud D, Roth S, Mermillod B, Le Floch-Rohr J. Patent foramen ovale, a possible cause of symptomatic migraine: study of 74 patients with acute ischemic stroke. Cerebrovasc Diseases 2002; 13:102–106.

55. Onorato E, Melzi G, Casilli F, et al. Patent foramen ovale with paradoxical embolism: mid-term results of transcatheter closure in 256 patients. J Interventional Cardiol 2003; 16:43–50.
56. Anzola GP. Clinical impact of patent foramen ovale diagnosis with transcranial Doppler. Eur J Ultrasound 2002; 16:11–20.
57. Morandi E, Anzola GP, Angeli S, Melzi G, Onorato E. Transcatheter closure of patent foramen ovale: a new migraine treatment? J Interventional Cardiol 2003; 16:39–42.
58. Yankovsky AE, Kuritzky A. Transformation into daily migraine with aura following transcutaneous atrial septal defect closure. Headache 2003; 43: 496–498.
59. Karttunen V, Hiltunen L, Rasi V, Vahtera E, Hilbom M, Factor V. Leiden and prothrombin gene mutations may predispose to paradoxical embolism in subjects with patent foramen ovale. Blood Coagulation Fibrinolysis 2003; 14:261–268.
60. Angeli S, Carrera P, Del Sette M, et al. Very high prevalence of right-to-left shunt on transcranial Doppler in an Italian family with cerebral autosomal dominant angiopathy with subcortical infarcts and leucoencephalopathy. Eur Neurol 2001; 46:198–201.
61. Wilmshurst PT, Pearson MJ, Nightingale S, Walsh KP, Morrison. Inheritance of persistent foramen ovale and atrial septal defect and the relationship to familial migraine with aura. Heart 2004; 90:1315–1320.
62. Bienfait HP, Moll LC. Fatal cerebral embolism in a young patient with an occult left atrial myxoma. Clin Neurol Neurosurg 2001; 103:37–38.
63. Kallela M, Farkkila M, Sajonmaa O. Endothelin in migraine patients. Cephalalgia 1998; 18:329–332.
64. Dreier JP, Kleeberg J, Petzold G, et al. Endothelin-1 potently induces Leao's cortical spreading depression in vivo in the rat: a model for an endothelial trigger of migrainous aura? Brain 2002; 125:102–112.
65. Fisher CM . Occlusion of the internal carotid artery. Arch Neurol Psychiatry 1951; 65:346–377.
66. Fisher CM. Transient migrainous accompaniments (TMAs) of late onset. Stroke 1979; 10:96–97 (Abstract II-4).
67. Fisher CM. Late-life migraine accompaniments—further experience. Stroke 1986; 17:1033–1042.
68. Peatfield RC. Can transient migraine attacks and classical migraine always be distinguished? Headache 1987; 27:240–243.
69. Al-Mefty O, Marano G, Raiaraman S, Nugent GR, Rodman N. Transient ischemic attacks due to increased platelet aggregation and adhesiveness. Ultrastructural and functional correlation. J Neurosurg 1979; 50:449–453.
70. Schwerzmann M, Seiler C, Lippe E, et al. Relation between directly detected patent foramen ovale and ischaemic brain lesions in sports divers. Ann Intern Med 2001; 134:21–24.
71. Grubb BP, Kosinski D. Current trends in etiology, diagnosis and management of neurocardiogenic syncope. Curr Opin Cardiol 1996; 11:32–41.
72. Mohan L, Lavania AK. Vasovagal syncope: an enigma. J Assoc Phys India 2004; 52:301–304.

73. Hainsworth R. Pathophysiology of syncope. Clin Autonomic Res 2004; 14: 18–24.
74. Lance JW, Anthony M. Some clinical aspects of migraine. Arch Neurol 1966; 15:356–361.
75. Basser LS. The relationship of migraine and epilepsy. Brain 1969; 92:285–300.
76. Hockaday JM, Whitty CWM. Factors determining the electroencephalogram in migraine; a study of 560 patients according to clinical type of migraine. Brain 1969; 92:769–788.
77. Bandinelli G, Cencetti S, Bacalli S, Lagi A. Disease-related syncope. Analysis of a community-based hospital registry. J Intern Med 2000; 247:513–516.
78. McHarg ML, Shinnar S, Rascoff H, Walsh CA. Syncope in childhood. Paediatr Cardiol 1997; 18:367–371.
79. Sicuteri F, Boccuni M, Fanciullacci M, D'Egidio P, Bonciani M. A new nonvascular interpretation of syncopal migraine. Adv Neurol 1982; 33:199–208.
80. Del Zompo M, Lai M, Loi V, Pisan MR. Dopamine hypersensitivity in migraine: role in apomorphine syncope. Headache 1995; 35:222–224.
81. Fanciullacci M, Alessandri M, Del Rosso A. Dopamine involvement in the migraine attack. Funct Neurol 2000; 15:171–181.
82. Lane RJM. Migraine and epilepsy. Megrim 1991; 4:8–12.
83. Sieveking EH. On Epilepsy and Epileptiform Seizures, their Causes, Pathology and Treatment. London, 1858. 2nd ed., 1861.
84. Montagna P, Gallassi R, Medori R, et al. MELAS syndrome: characteristic migrainous and epileptic features and maternal transmission. Neurology 1988; 38:751–754.
85. Durand-Dubief F, Tyvlin P, Mauguiere F. Polymorphism of epilepsy associated with the A3243G mutation of mitochondrial DNA (MELAS): reasons for delayed diagnosis. Revue Neurologique (Paris) 2004; 160:824–829.
86. Schon F, Blau JN. Post-epileptic headache and migraine. J Neurol Neurosurg Psychiat 1987; 50:1148–1152.
87. Forderreuther S, Henkel A, Noachtar S, Straube A. Coma associated with epileptic seizures: epidemiology and clinical characteristics. Headache 2002; 42:649–655.
88. Leniger T, von den Driesch S, Isbruch K, Diener HC, Hufnagel A. Clinical characteristics of patients with comorbidity of migraine and epilepsy. Headache 2003; 43:672–677.
89. Beauvais K, Cave-Riant F, De Barace C, Tardieu M, Tournier-Lasserve E, Furby A. New CACNA1A gene mutation in a case of familial hemiplegic migraine with status epilepticus. Eur Neurol 2004; 52(1):58–61.
90. Mateo I, Foncea N, Vicente I, et al. Migraine-associated seizures with recurrent and reversible magnetic resonance imaging abnormalities. Headache 2004; 44:265–270.
91. Andermann F. Clinical features of migraine-epilepsy syndromes. In: Andermann F, Lugaresi E, eds. Migraine and Epilepsy. London: Butterworths, 1987:3–31.
92. Olivier A, Gloor P, Andermann F, et al. Occipitotemporal epilepsy studies with stereotaxically implanted depth electrodes and successfully treated by temporal lobe resection. Ann Neurol 1982; 11:428–432.

93. Muller GE. Atypical early posttraumatic syndromes. Acta Neurologica Belgica 1974; 74:163–181.
94. Kempster PA, Iansek R, Bala JI. Impairment of consciousness in migraine. Clin Exp Neurol 1987; 23:171–173.
95. Fitzsimons RB, Wolfenden WH. Meningitic migraine with cerebral edema associated with a new form of autosomal dominant cerebellar ataxia. Brain 1985; 108:555–577.
96. Corbin DOC, Martyr T, Graham AC. Migraine coma. J Neurol Neurosurg Psychiat 1991; 54:744–749.
97. Ducros A, Denier C, Joutel A, et al. The clinical spectrum of familial hemiplegic migraine associated with mutations in a neuronal calcium channel. N Engl J Med 2001; 345:17–24.
98. Tottene A, Pivotto F, Fellin T, Cesetti T, van den Maagdenberg AM, Pietrobon D. Specific kinetic alterations of human CaV2.1 calcium channels produced by mutation S218L causing familial hemiplegic migraine and delayed cerebral edema and coma after minor head trauma. Journal of Biological Chemistry 2005; 280:17678–17686.
99. Schon F, Martin RJ, Prevett M, Clough C, Enevoldson TP, Markus HS. "CADASIL coma": an underdiagnosed acute encephalopathy. J Neurol Neurosurg Psychiat 2003; 74:249–252.
100. Bickerstaff ER. Impairment of consciousness in migraine. Lancet 1961; 2:1057–1059.
101. Frequin ST, Linassen WH, Pasman JW, Hommes OR, Merx HL. Recurrent prolonged coma due to basilar artery migraine. A case report. Headache 1991; 31:75–81.
102. Ganji S, Hellman S, Stagg S, Furlow J. Episodic coma due to acute basilar artery migraine: correlation of EEG and brainstem auditory evoked potential patterns. Clin Electroencephalogr 1993; 24:44–48.
103. Requena I, Indakeotxea B, Lema C, Santos B, Garcia-Castineira A, Arias M. Coma associated with migraine. Revue Neurologique 1999; 29:1048–1051.

Variants

CLASSIFYING PRIMARY HEADACHES

It has long been hoped that a definitive classification system for headaches might aid diagnosis, standardize and improve headache research, and lead to more rational treatments. However, our incomplete understanding of the fundamental nature of the primary headaches has hindered attempts to achieve this aim. Above all, the lack of biological markers for different forms of headache continues to cause controversy and frustrate progress.

Orthodoxy views primary headaches as comprising a large number of discrete entities with specific diagnostic criteria (1). The current International Headache Society (IHS) classification considers four main categories of primary headache:

- Migraine
- Tension-type headache
- Cluster headache and other trigeminal autonomic cephalalgias (TACs)
- Other primary headaches

The key issue however, is whether these individual primary headache syndromes are truly different disorders or, as we will argue, simply points on a continuum, representing commonly encountered aggregations of otherwise non-specific headache characteristics. As noted in Chapter 2, groups of patients can be identified with symptoms and treatment responses that are sufficiently stereotypic and coherent to constitute working diagnostic entities (2), but in practice it is often unclear where the boundaries of these conditions start and finish. *"Overlap"* cases with symptoms that seem to straddle different primary headache syndromes are common (see Chapter 6). In fact, there seems to be no single symptom that occurs in one form of primary headache that does not occur in any other, with the possible exception of premonitory symptoms in "migraine."

The extent to which primary headache syndromes can vary is impressive. At one extreme, there may be a single cataclysmic event suggestive of a subarachnoid hemorrhage, referred to as *primary thunderclap headache*. At the other extreme, primary headache may be constant from the outset— *new daily persistent headache*. The variation in frequency and duration of primary headache is also striking. *Primary stabbing headache* attacks last a few seconds or less and can occur hundreds of times a day, while attacks in *episodic* and *chronic paroxysmal hemicrania* are also brief and repetitive but less frequent and usually accompanied by trigeminal autonomic symptoms. In *short-lasting unilateral neuralgiform headache with conjunctival injection and tearing* (SUNCT) and *short-lasting unilateral neuralgiform headache attacks with cranial autonomic symptoms* (SUNA), the head pains are again frequent and repetitive, but are invariably associated with prominent trigeminal autonomic reflex activity. *Cluster headache* shares these trigeminal autonomic features but usually occurs only a few times a day, although there are repetitive and chronic forms, while *migraine* headache is more protracted, lasting 4 to 72 hours (according to IHC-2) and generally less intense, typically with little in the way of trigeminal autonomic features. Longer lasting headaches are generally milder than the paroxysmal forms. For example, chronic daily headache (CDH), which has heterogeneous origins, is mild-to-moderate in intensity but is present on most days to a greater or lesser extent. Recently, treatment responses have also been included in syndrome definitions, for example, in distinguishing chronic cluster headache from the indomethacin-responsive *"hemicrania continua."* However, as we shall discuss in Chapter 7, there is not necessarily a correlation between headache phenotypes and their response to a particular type of medication; one cannot reliably deduce pathogenesis from a treatment response.

Alongside the spectrum of primary headache syndromes, there can also be significant intrapatient variation. For example, patients may have headaches that conform to the definition of cluster headache on some occasions but are typical of migraine at other times, whereas classical migrainous visual auras, arguably the defining feature of a "migraine" attack, can also occur rarely in patients with cluster headache (3). Migraineurs can also sometimes experience other archetypical headache syndromes. For example, the various paroxysmal headache disorders, such as thunderclap headache and idiopathic stabbing headaches, are conspicuously more common in patients with previous or active migraine. Is it possible, therefore, that all primary headaches actually stem from a single, fundamental process? We will return to this theme in Chapter 6.

LOOKING BACK AT "VARIANTS"

As we saw in Chapter 1, Arateus was the first to recognize different forms of headache. In particular, he distinguished unilateral headache (heterocrania—our "migraine") from "cephalalgia" (briefer, more frequent but less severe than migraine headache) and "cephalea" (headaches lasting days or weeks without remission—presumably our "CDH"). Of course, in those times, it would have been almost impossible to distinguish primary headache from headache caused by disease ("secondary headache"), but this simple classification proved remarkably durable.

However, during the late nineteenth century and early twentieth century, a number of new headache syndromes were identified that seemed to be distinct from migraine. These were forms of severe, paroxysmal head and facial pain recognized by a bewildering number of names, often eponymous, which we would now recognize as forms of TAC. The term "cluster headache," the archetype of this group, was coined by Kunkle et al. in 1952 (4), but the first complete description of the condition as we now know it was provided in 1745 by Gerhard van Swieten, founder of the First Vienna School of Medicine (5). Interestingly, although this condition was initially believed to be distinct from migraine, and indeed is now believed by many authorities to be so, it was classified as a migraine subtype in the first, widely accepted headache classification system.

Chronic holocranial headache has been recognized for centuries, and until recently, was commonly but erroneously considered to be due to persistent pericranial muscular contraction ("tension headache") (6). In addition, terms such as "tension vascular headache," "combined headache," "combination headache," "mixed headache," and "vascular and muscle contraction headache" came to be used by various authorities over the years when referring to headache with features of both "migraine" and "tension" headache.

This then was the rather confusing picture of primary headache prior to 1962.

Early Attempts at Definitions and Classification

The first proposals for a new headache classification came in the 1960s, one from an ad hoc committee of the World Federation of Neurology and another, rather similar, from an ad hoc committee of the U.S. National Institutes of Health (7). The resulting classification was generally accepted in the U.S.A. and Western Europe (8). The scheme was based on the few headache disorders that were recognized at the time, from clinical observation and the prevailing understanding of pain mechanisms, together with "reasonable inference" (Table 1). It was recognized that the story was far from complete but it was

Table 1 1962 Summary of the Ad Hoc Committee Classification of Primary Headaches

Vascular headache of migraine type
 Classic migraine
 Common migraine
 Cluster headache
 Hemiplegic and ophthalmoplegic migraine
 "Lower half" headache
Muscle contraction headache
Combined headache

hoped that the classification could act as a framework for diagnostic criteria, and that "by emphasis on basic mechanisms, it would offer a logical approach to the planning of clinical trials."

In fact, it was a landmark in the study of headache. For the first time, it brought some order to headache syndromes and distinguished primary from secondary headaches. However, it had a number of weaknesses. In particular, it did not provide any diagnostic criteria for different primary headache types but rather differentiated them on the basis of presumed pathogenesis, using assumptions we now know to be almost completely erroneous. It also used terms such as "usually" or "sometimes," which were open to wide interpretation.

The classification did not include a definition of migraine, but considered migraine to be: *"Recurrent attacks of headache, widely varied in intensity, frequency, and duration. The attacks are commonly unilateral in onset; are usually associated with anorexia, and sometimes with nausea and vomiting; and some are preceded by, or associated with, conspicuous sensory, motor, and mood disturbances; and are often familial."*

Many have attempted a definition of migraine. Vahlquist (9) defined it as: *"Paroxysmal headache separated by free intervals, plus at least two of the following four points—unilateral headache, nausea, visual aura, and family history."*

Nat Blau, in a Lancet paper entitled "Towards a Definition of Migraine" (10), also supported the view that migraine characteristically occurred in attacks with pain-free intervals. He defined migraine as: *"Episodic headache lasting 2 to 72 hours with total freedom between attacks. The headaches must be associated with visual or gastrointestinal disturbances or both. The visual symptoms occur as an aura before, and/or photophobia during the headache phase. If there are no visual but only alimentary disturbances, then vomiting must feature in some attacks."*

Lance (11) had already foreseen the difficulty of separating migraine from "chronic migraine" (see below) when, in 1982, he wrote that migraine was: *"Episodic headache, cerebral disturbance or both, with intervening periods of relative freedom from headache and without evidence of primary structural abnormality."*

This definition however, did not prescribe specific manifestations essential to sustain the diagnosis.

Thus, by the early 1980s, three main forms of primary headache were recognized—migraine, cluster headache, and tension headache. These descriptors still cover the great majority of cases. However, it was appreciated that some uncommon but important headache syndromes were unaccounted for.

THE INTERNATIONAL HEADACHE SOCIETY (IHS) CLASSIFICATION OF HEADACHE DISORDERS

As research into migraine and other primary headaches progressed, the demand for generally accepted operational criteria for headache diagnosis increased. In 1985, the IHS proposed that such a system should be established, and in 1988 the recommendations of the Headache Classification Committee were published as the "Classification and diagnostic criteria for headache disorders, cranial neuralgias, and facial pain". The chairman of the committee for the first (and second) editions was Jes Olesen. He encouraged debate over the classification and invited proposals for change or additions. This classification was almost universally accepted and was translated into more than 20 languages. It was a major advance. Continuing research led to the current classification, published as the Second Edition (IHC-2) in a Supplement to the IHS journal *Cephalalgia*, in 2004 (1) (Appendix 1). Like the first edition, IHC-2 divides all headache disorders into primary headaches, and secondary headaches, due to definable pathology.

The main primary headache syndromes are shown in Table 2. Migraine, tension-type headache, and cluster headache are each considered to occur in both episodic and chronic forms and the system is hierarchical, allowing diagnoses with varying degrees of specificity, with up to four digits for coding.

IHC-2 did not change the principles of the classification or diagnosis of primary headaches established under IHC-1, and the body of evidence gained during the period that IHC-1 was used remains valid for most diagnoses made under IHC-2. However, a number of new primary headache entities were added, including the following:

- Chronic migraine
- Hemicrania continua
- New daily persistant headache (NDPH)
- Hypnic headache
- Trigeminal autonomic cephalalgias (TACs)—a term introduced to include cluster headache, PH, and the new headache syndromes SUNCT and SUNA

Table 2 Primary Headache Syndromes (IHC-2)

Migraine (for subtypes, see Chapter 2)
Tension-type headache
Cluster headache and other trigeminal autonomic cephalalgias
    Cluster headache
        Episodic cluster headache
        Chronic cluster headache
    Paroxysmal hemicrania
        Episodic paroxysmal hemicrania
        Chronic paroxysmal hemicrania
    Short-lasting unilateral neuralgiform headache attacks with conjunctival
       injection and tearing
    Probable trigeminal autonomic cephalalgia
Other primary headaches
    Primary stabbing headache
    Primary cough headache
    Primary exertional headache
    Primary headache associated with sexual activity
        Preorgasmic headache
        Orgasmic headache
    Hypnic headache
    Primary thunderclap headache
    Hemicrania continua
    New daily persistent headache

The IHS Headache Classification Subcommittee acknowledged that there were also a number of headache types that "have not been sufficiently validated by research studies" but were of the view that these were "believed to be real but for which further scientific evidence must be presented before they can be formally accepted." These included a number of poorly defined entities, such as "cluster-tic" and "cluster migraine."

In this chapter, we have adhered to the general structure and definitions of IHC-2 but have made minor changes to the hierarchical organization and categorization of syndromes, where we feel it is appropriate with regard to the thrust of our argument.

DIAGNOSING PRIMARY HEADACHE SYNDROMES

In practice, primary headache syndromes are defined and recognized by the following:

- Duration of attacks, especially pain duration
- Frequency of attacks
- Severity of attacks

- Site of pain in attacks, especially unilaterality
- Repetition and stereotypy
- Presence or absence of
  - Premonitory symptoms
  - Aura
  - Nausea and/or vomiting
  - Hypersensitivity to sensory inputs such as light, sound, and odors
  - Presence of cranial autonomic symptoms (ipsilateral ptosis, conjunctival injection, epiphora, nasal blockage and/or discharge, etc.)

From a historical perspective, we might consider resurrecting the distinction between the classical "unilateral" headache of "megrim" and "holocranial" headache, but we are now aware that otherwise typical migraine can be accompanied by "atypical" headache, a point fully acknowledged in IHC-2. Other etymological considerations might include the characteristics of triggers, premonitory symptoms, aura symptoms, the features of the recovery phase, or even treatment responses to triptans or indomethacin. However, none of these is sufficiently consistent or discriminating to be used as the basis of classification and there is a danger of producing so many artificial categories that one can miss "the big picture."

International Headache Society Migraine Subtypes

We have previously defined and discussed the typical characteristics of migraine with and without aura (MA and MO). Table 1, Chapter 2, summarizes the IHC-2 classification of migraine subtypes. The current classification is somewhat inconsistent in the way it groups migraine variants. For example, "retinal migraine" is classified in the migraine group, whereas "ophthalmoplegic migraine" is now grouped with the "cranial neuralgias and central causes of facial pain," because it has been suggested that this very rare condition might be caused by episodes of recurrent cranial nerve demyelination (12). However, we have observed cases that seem entirely consistent with migraine (see p. 215).

Facial Migraine

Facial migraine has not been included in the current IHS classification. We feel facial migraine deserves to be restored because it acknowledges that migraine can present as a recurrent facial pain, often misdiagnosed and indeed treated as "sinus." Facial migraine can be unilateral or bilateral and is usually of the "without aura" type, as the following cases illustrate.

CASE 161: FACIAL MIGRAINE

A 35-year-old accountant was referred from the ear, nose, and throat department with a four-year history of stereotyped attacks of facial pain occurring initially every couple of months but lately up to once a week. She had previously also seen a dentist but no diagnosis had been made. The attacks of facial pain could be triggered by sudden change in temperature, such as emerging from the ice rink into a warm car. She would experience increasing pain radiating up the nostrils and gums bilaterally, spreading into the nose and both eyes. When this happened, the nose tended to block up and then run, on either side or both sides. The pain could be so intense it would make her cry. On occasions she would experience nausea. The sclera would not redden nor the eyelids droop.

She had previously suffered from typical MO. A diagnosis of facial migraine was made, and she found that the attacks responded very well to zolmitriptan.

CASE 162: FACIAL MIGRAINE

A 35-year-old man described MO attacks starting at about five years of age and continuing until around the age of thirteen. He recalled that the headache was severe and associated with photosensitivity. At the age of 20, he developed different symptoms. He described episodes of severe pain localized to the face, sparing the head, and typically lasting a day, associated with nausea and photophobia.

Status Migrainosus, Chronic Migraine, and Chronic Daily Headache

Status migrainosus and chronic migraine are designated as "complications" of migraine under IHC-2 (see Chapter 4), but we consider them to be variants in which, for some reason, the migraine mechanism has failed to "switch off" or has become recurrent. Although IHC-2 does not use the term chronic daily headache, it is in common clinical use and has a number of causes (see below) one of which is "chronic migraine." In that condition, the symptoms are suggestive of migraine but they occur on 15 or more days each month.

Status migrainosus: Status migrainosus is defined under IHC-2 as a debilitating migraine attack of severe intensity, unremitting for more than 72 hours. We do not think this is a particularly useful definition because migraine headache and migraine-related symptoms quite commonly persist for longer than 72 hours. The diagnosis should in our view be reserved for single attacks of more than three days duration causing total incapacity, or rapidly recurrent attacks without recovery between exacerbations, by analogy to status epilepticus. Medication overuse often clouds the picture. In contrast, we have encountered a patient with what we can only describe as "cluster status" although no such term exists in IHC-2!

CASE 163: CLUSTER STATUS

A 52-year-old woman developed "persistent and severe" right temporal and periorbital headaches, lasting up to an hour at a time. She was diagnosed as having "sinusitis" but failed to respond to antibiotics or nasal decongestants. She eventually had bilateral antral washouts, despite the fact that a computed tomography (CT) scan of the sinuses showed no significant abnormalities. The headache settled. Six years later it recurred. She was again treated with courses of antibiotics, inhalations, and analgesics but without lasting benefit. After six months, the pain at times was unbearable and she was described as "pacing the garden between 3 and 4 A.M." However, by the time she was seen in the neurology clinic three months later, the headache had resolved. On specific inquiry, she gave a history of occasional migraine with visual aura attacks as a young woman but also mentioned that the more recent right-sided headache had been associated with some reddening of the eye on occasions.

She was then asymptomatic until three years later when the attacks recurred. During an admission for unrelated issues, some three months after onset, she had a severe attack witnessed on the ward and, on this occasion, was observed to have clear-cut reddening of the right eye and ipsilateral epiphora. She described the pain as knife-like, and sometimes associated with nasal obstruction, and said it would wake her in the early hours of the morning, every day. However, as the attacks became more severe, she also had attacks during the day. A diagnosis of cluster headache was made, but this cluster resolved without specific treatment shortly afterwards.

Some 18 months later, she had her fourth cluster. On the basis of previous advice, her GP treated her successively with lithium and verapamil without benefit but individual attacks responded to 100% oxygen (actually prescribed to her husband who was crippled with obstructive airways disease!). A trial of oral steroids was also unsuccessful. As before, the cluster resolved after some three months.

She continued to have cluster periods, but the intervals between them became progressively shorter. The attacks seemed refractory to intervention. She was eventually re-referred, and a trial of ergotamine suppositories (and oral domperidone to prevent nausea) taken on retiring was instituted and this was immediately successful. When she stopped using them, the attacks returned but could be aborted with 100% oxygen. At the onset of the next cluster a few months later, nausea induced by the ergot became an increasing problem and precluded its use but zolmitriptan nasal preparation proved very effective. However, the attacks had lost their previous periodicity, and she now had secondary chronic cluster headache.

The attacks became increasingly frequent during the night and daytime as well. Eventually, the attacks crescendoed until she was having them every few hours throughout the day, with a residual dull headache in the same area between acute events. She felt nauseated and completely disabled, and was admitted for further evaluation. Magnetic resonance imaging (MRI) brain scan was normal. She was treated with subcutaneous sumatriptan and regular topiramate and the attacks slowly resolved, and to date have not returned.

Chronic migraine: Persistent and frequent headache is a common problem in neurological clinics. As noted, if headache occurs on more than 15 days per month, it is (somewhat arbitrarily) referred to as CDH. CDH often evolves from a background of episodic "migraine" or "tension-type" headache, and may then be referred to as "chronic migraine" or "chronic tension-type headache," respectively. A discharge summary from the 1960s concerning one of our patients, evaluated at a nearby center of excellence, referred to this situation rather quaintly as "migraine spread out thin"— which in our view is exactly what it is! Sometimes, however, headache can be chronic from the outset. The term "new daily persistent headache" was introduced under IHC-2 to denote new onset headache occurring on more than 15 days per month without a background of previous headache.

IHC-2 defines chronic migraine as: "Migraine headache occurring on 15 or more days per month for more than three months in the absence of medication overuse." The only other requirements are that the headache is like migraine without aura and cannot be attributed to another disorder. Most cases of chronic migraine start as MO, although it may, of course, develop in patients with previous MA. It is, in our view, rather surprising that this entity, hidden for so many years, is now such a widely recognized and accepted disorder. Chronic migraine is one of the most common presentations in neurological and headache clinics, and only a few illustrative cases are presented here.

CASE 164: CHRONIC MIGRAINE EVOLVING FROM MIGRAINE WITHOUT AURA

A 34-year-old woman was referred with recurrent headaches that had started about 18 months earlier, after a pregnancy. They were rather nonspecific in quality but were associated with nausea and photophobia. Eating chocolate could precipitate them. In addition, she had intermittent head pain in the right frontal region during which she felt her nose was blocked on that side. CT brain scan was normal. Her father suffered from migraine.

These headaches barely troubled her initially, but about eight years later she suddenly experienced a marked increase in severity and frequency of the attacks. The headaches, which now occurred on most days, were preceded by a premonitory feeling of well being for a few hours and comprised a right-sided, throbbing headache followed by nausea, photophobia, and looseness of the bowels, the whole attack lasting about four hours.

CASE 165: CHRONIC MIGRAINE EVOLVING FROM MIGRAINE WITH AURA

A 49-year-old woman developed typical attacks of MA beginning at the age of 32. The attacks, which occurred once every three months, comprised a premonitory stiffness in the neck, with nausea followed by typical scintillating scotoma and then hemianopia to the right. The aura phase could last six to seven hours before bitemporal headache began. The headache would last for two or three days. She would sometimes vomit at the onset of an attack and then again at the zenith of the headache on the second day. The attacks became progressively more frequent following a pregnancy six years later, and at the age of 48, the attacks occured on almost a daily basis. She described persistent throbbing headache with frequent nausea and vomiting, not helped by medication. Her sister suffered from migraine. Investigation showed no abnormalities.

CASE 166: CHRONIC MIGRAINE EVOLVING FROM MIGRAINE WITH AND WITHOUT AURA

A 17-year-old girl was referred because of "chronic persistent headache." She had a history of typical migraine with aura dating from puberty. Attacks comprised left-sided visual disturbance over some 30 minutes followed by right-sided throbbing headache without nausea. MA attacks would occur weekly, but she would also get MO, with nausea and vomiting, and occasionally migrainous syncope. The MO attacks would occur about twice a week and last for 12 to 24 hours. She also had a mild but constant right-sided throbbing headache, such that she was hardly ever free of headache of some description. Simple analgesics were ineffective, and she was not overusing rescue medication. The constant background pain was helped by amitryptiline, and rizatriptan proved effective for the acute exacerbations.

Chronic daily headache: Although it is a rather arbitrary benchmark, CDH has proved to be a popular and useful label. However, it should be only the first step in elucidating the underlying mechanism. For example, we suggest that CDH of "tension-type" is heterogeneous and includes cases of migraine, cervicogenic headache, and psychogenic headache. Table 3 lists headache diagnoses that can come under the CDH umbrella.

Medication-Overuse Headache. Many patients with CDH in fact have "medication-overuse headache" (MOH) due to repeated use of rescue medications, particularly opiate-based analgesics. This condition is sometimes referred to as "analgesic abuse headache," although drugs other than analgesics, including triptans, may be culpable. MOH is excluded under IHC-2 if there is no improvement two months after rescue medication has been withdrawn. We will consider this problem further in Chapter 7.

Basilar Type Migraine

"Basilar type migraine" is a good example of how names change as we get a better understanding of a condition. Originally termed basilar *artery* migraine by Bickerstaff (see p. 190), the name changed first to *basilar migraine* under IHC-1, to avoid the implication that the syndrome was of vascular origin and involved only the basilar artery and its vascular

Table 3 Causes of "Chronic Daily Headache"

Primary headache syndromes
   Chronic migraine
   Chronic tension-type headache
   Chronic cluster headache
   Chronic paroxysmal hemicrania
   Short-lasting unilateral neuralgiform headache attacks with conjunctival injection
     and tearing (SUNCT)
   Hemicrania continua
   Hypnic headache
Secondary headache syndromes
   Medication-overuse headache
   Headache of cervical origin
   Headache associated with head trauma
   Temporomandibular disorders and headache
   Raised cerebrospinal fluid pressure headache
   Low cerebrospinal fluid pressure headache

---

territory, and then to "basilar type" migraine under IHC-2, because the syndrome may include symptoms that are of hemispheric as well as of brainstem origin. The essence of the condition is encapsulated by the IHC-2 description: "Migraine with aura symptoms clearly originating from the brainstem and/or from both hemispheres simultaneously, but no motor weakness."

There must be at least two of the following qualifying aura symptoms:

- Dysarthria
- Vertigo
- Tinnitus
- Decreased hearing
- Diplopia
- Ataxia
- Decreased level of consciousness
- Visual symptoms simultaneously in both temporal and nasal fields of both eyes
- Simultaneous bilateral paresthesiae.

We have described a number of examples of patients with bilateral blindness in basilar type migraine in Chapter 3 (see p. 100), and we have also discussed impaired consciousness and coma in basilar type migraine in Chapter 4 (see p. 190). Vertigo can be a conspicuous feature of basilar type migraine but more often occurs in isolation, in "migrainous vertigo" (see p. 113).

In our experience, basilar type migraine is not common, at least in adults. Difficulties can be encountered in trying to distinguish from the patient's account, dysarthria from dysphasia, near syncope from vertigo, ataxia from clumsiness associated with sensory dysfunction, and decreased level of consciousness from sleepiness. Basilar type migraine attacks are often interspersed with migraine with more common characteristics.

Basilar Type Migraine with Vertigo as the Predominant Symptom

CASE 167: VERTIGO IN BASILAR TYPE MIGRAINE
A 67-year-old woman was referred because of recurrent headaches that had troubled her most of her life. These were non-specific in character, with a tight sensation over the occipital and nuchal areas lasting up to 24 hours a day, and were not associated with nausea, photophobia, or phonophobia. There was a strong family history of migraine in the patient's mother and her two daughters. At the age of 14, she began to experience stereotyped auras prior to some of these headaches, comprising diplopia followed by rotatory vertigo, nausea, and vomiting. These aura symptoms had stopped many years previously, until a few months before referral when they recurred and were accompanied by oscillopsia and ataxia. Neuroimaging showed no abnormality.

CASE 168: VERTIGO IN BASILAR TYPE MIGRAINE
A 67-year-old man was referred because of a five-week history of almost daily recurrent episodes comprising a dull frontal headache with nausea, rotatory vertigo, diplopia, occasionally a right hemianopia, severe diaphoresis, numbness and

tingling of the tongue, altered taste sensation, and sometimes weakness of all four limbs. These attacks would last from 10 to 30 minutes after which he would recover completely. He had suffered similar attacks 12 years previously, attributed to transient ischemic attacks (indeed, he had been enrolled in a clinical trial of aspirin in TIA, and had taken 75 mg daily ever since!), and in that year, he suffered an episode of migraine with visual aura also. CT brain scan and extracranial ultrasound studies were normal, and the attacks settled with atenolol.

Basilar Type Migraine with Mixed Hemisphere and Brainstem Symptoms

CASE 169: MIXED HEMISPHERE AND BRAINSTEM SYMPTOMS

A 44-year-old woman with a history of typical migraine with visual auras was referred because of new stereotyped acephalalgic attacks. These had begun when she was about nine years of age and had recurred at intervals of between two to seven years. Each began with paresthesiae in the toes of both feet, which spread slowly up the body to the face over some 15 minutes. The tongue would become numb on one side. After this, she would get a combination of symptoms including unilateral facial weakness, sensorimotor impairment of the left arm, and mild dysphasia with confusion in which she did not seem to know who or where she was, and was unable to answer questions rationally. These additional symptoms lasted about half an hour, and the sensory symptoms would then gradually wear off "like a dental anesthetic." In a recent attack, her left arm had become totally paralyzed for some nine hours, but she had recovered completely. Her mother had occasional migraine attacks. Neuroimaging was normal. On follow-up three years later, she had had no further significant symptoms.

CASE 170: MIXED HEMISPHERE AND BRAINSTEM SYMPTOMS

A 61-year-old woman was referred with a history of about a dozen attacks over a three-year period, during which, without warning, she would first experience discomfort in the head associated with some disturbance of eye movements. She would be afraid to open the eyes and may have been experiencing oscillopsia. She would feel unsteady. These symptoms were initially short-lived, lasting only a few minutes, but she was referred after an attack that lasted at least 90 minutes during which she also experienced paresthesiae in the tongue, around the mouth, and in both arms. She had a past history of MO and her daughter had migraine. Investigation revealed no significant abnormalities. On review seven years later, these attacks had resolved completely.

CASE 171: BASILAR TYPE MIGRAINE ON A BACKGROUND
OF MIGRAINE WITH AURA

A 32-year-old man described an attack in which, while watching television, he suddenly developed paresthesiae of both knees, and then weakness of the legs such that he was unable to stand. Within minutes, the sensory symptoms affected his right arm, which then became so limp and weak that he could not use it. The sensory disturbance continued its gradual march to the right side of the face. He then developed a right hemicranial headache with vague visual blurring, and subsequently had difficulty in speaking. The neurological symptoms resolved completely after about two hours, but the headache persisted and he subsequently had a bout of nausea and vomiting. He had recovered completely the next day. He had a past history of migraine with visual aura, sometimes with diplopia.

CASE 172: BASILAR TYPE MIGRAINE AND MIGRAINE WITH AURA

A 46-year-old lady presented with a year's history of brief monthly attacks comprising mild faintness followed by loss of function of both arms, which became cyanosed and then white and tingly. She would have difficulty communicating, but retained full consciousness. Subsequently, she had recurrent episodes that were similar but affected only the left side. She was examined after a particularly severe left-sided attack that prompted urgent referral to hospital. CT brain scan and extracranial ultrasound were normal.

She a 20-year history of migraine with visual aura. She had also experienced independent episodes of vertigo, nausea, and abdominal pain lasting one to three days in her teens.

The presenting episodes were interpreted as aura without headache, the first form being due to basilar type migraine. She was re-referred six years later because of recurrent syncopal and presyncopal attacks related to her migraine, and further left-sided sensory and hemiparetic attacks with speech arrest. MRI brain scan and magnetic resonance angiogram (MRA) were normal.

Childhood Migraine Syndromes

Migraine manifestations in childhood may differ significantly from the typical symptoms of migraine in adults. In particular, headache is frequently not a feature. A detailed consideration of these conditions is beyond the scope of this book, but it is always worth asking headache patients about relevant symptoms during childhood, such as unexplained recurrent vomiting, "grumbling appendix," fainting, and recurrent vertigo.

Abdominal migraine: IHC-2 includes "cyclical vomiting, benign paroxysmal vertigo of childhood and abdominal migraine" under this rubric. The latter is defined as: "An idiopathic recurrent disorder seen mainly in children, of episodic midline abdominal pain manifesting in attacks lasting 1–72 hours with normality between episodes. The pain is of moderate to severe intensity and associated with vasomotor symptoms, nausea, and vomiting."

Note that concurrent headache is not required for this diagnosis, although it may, in fact, occur. Abdominal migraine can sometimes be encountered in young adults.

CASE 173

A 15-year-old boy was referred with weekly, disabling migraine headaches preceded by vague auras of blurred vision. At the age of seven, he had developed severe recurrent colicky abdominal pains, with fever, nausea, and vomiting, lasting up to two days during which he was extremely pale. He eventually had an elective appendicectomy at the age of 14, but the attacks continued. Subsequently, it became clear that these abdominal pains were increasingly associated with or preceded by headache. The abdominal symptoms were eventually replaced by the more typical recurrent migraine headaches. His father was a migraineur.

CASE 174

A 16-year-old girl was referred with recurrent headache attacks. She evidently began to suffer migraine without aura as a child, with episodes of severe, unilateral thumping headache with nausea. Independently, she had been seen in hospital on a number of occasions with abdominal pain. These pains were sometimes excruciating, constant, midline, and associated with a degree of constipation. They were not associated with headache, but she would be nauseous, and would often vomit with the attacks, which lasted 10 minutes to an hour. More recently, she had developed symptoms suggestive of basilar type migraine, with an aura of total blindness for some 15 seconds followed by a two-hour interval during which she said she felt as though "my spirit had left my body." She might then develop other neurological symptoms, including ataxia, amnesia and mild confusion, speech arrest, and diplopia, together with the familiar thumping headache. Her mother had a life-long history of migraine, including an episode of bilateral blindness at age 21.

CASE 175
A 16-year-old girl was referred with a complex migraine history including MO from childhood, abdominal migraine, and seizures followed by migraine headache. The abdominal attacks comprised central or right iliac fossa pain lasting up to a day, often associated with nausea and vomiting, but without headache. They occurred about once monthly and a diagnosis of mittelschmerz was considered initially, but her mother was a migraineur and had also had mittelschmerz as a child. The girl also had two grand mal seizures, both followed by severe migraine headache, the first six years earlier and the second, the year before referral. Investigation revealed no abnormalities.

Retinal Migraine

With migraine firmly established as a disturbance of the brain, it would not be surprising if the retina, embryologically a cerebral outgrowth, was also sometimes subject to the affects of the migraine mechanism. Indeed, chick retina is sometimes used to study spreading depression (SD) and in particular, the underlying neurochemical processes, because the tissue is avascular. For example, sumatriptan was shown to block SD in this system independent of its vascular effects (13).

Some headache specialists did not accept the existence of retinal migraine at first, and it can be difficult even for a good witness to be quite sure that a transient visual hallucination or obscuration is truly monocular. IHC-2 defines retinal migraine as: "Repeated attacks of monocular visual disturbance, including scintillation, scotoma or blindness, associated with migraine headache."

The diagnosis requires that either the patient is examined during an attack, or after proper instruction, the patient's drawing of the field defect during the attack confirms it to be monocular. The headache phase must fulfill the criteria for migraine and begin during the visual aura phase or follow it within 60 minutes. No duration for the visual disturbance is specified. Of course, the symptoms must not be attributable to another disorder.

This definition may be too restrictive. We have encountered examples of what we believe to be isolated attacks of retinal migraine in patients with a history of otherwise typical migraine, persistent monocular aura, and permanent monocular visual impairment. Blindness due to retinal migraine has been described previously (14). We have also encountered instances of what we can only assume are attacks of "acephalalgic" retinal migraine.

It is suggested that the more protracted symptoms result from retinal artery vasospasm, which has been observed in some instances (15). It is conceivable that this could indeed result in ischemic optic neuropathy if there was significant underlying arteriosclerosis. Interestingly, in keeping with this, it was observed in one study that vascular disorders such as myocardial infarction and central retinal vein thrombosis were almost four times as common in migraine patients with monocular visual symptoms than with the more typical hemianopic form (16).

CASE 176: ISOLATED EPISODE OF RETINAL MIGRAINE
A 52-year-old man was referred following an episode of "amaurosis fugax" in the right eye. He had suffered typical migraine with visual aura since childhood. His habitual attacks comprised scintillating scotoma usually in the right hemifield but sometimes in the left, and these had recently increased from once every three months or so to monthly. One recent attack had been different, however. Early one morning, he suddenly went almost completely blind in his right eye. He described a dense but misty white scotoma, which he carefully confirmed was not present in the left eye. This lasted about 15 minutes and faded from the top downwards to be followed by a moderate headache. He recovered completely. No abnormalities were disclosed on full ophthalmological and neurovascular investigation.

CASE 177: PRESUMED ACEPHALALGIC RETINAL MIGRAINE
A 54-year-old man began to experience increasingly frequent episodes of visual blurring in the left eye, until they were occurring weekly. The vision in the right eye was normal at all times. Attacks would start on waking. At best, he found difficulty reading words with the left eye and at worst, even substantial objects such as cars and office blocks were difficult to see. On one occasion, he had consulted his optician on three occasions during a single day when the vision in his affected eye was so blurred he couldn't locate the Snellen chart! Usually an attack would last a day and would resolve completely after a night's sleep. There were no other significant symptoms, although direct questioning revealed that he had experienced photophobia in the left eye during attacks, together with some vague headache that he had attributed to "eye strain." He was asymptomatic between attacks and had no previous or family history of headache. MRI brain scan, MRA, perimetry, and visual-evoked responses were normal.

CASE 178: PRESUMED RETINAL MIGRAINE
A 42-year-old man was referred because of recurrent attacks of "optic neuropathy" in the right eye. On each occasion, he had first developed a severe headache over the right eye, worsened by eye movement, with impairment of acuity down to around 6/24. The attacks were infrequent, the first two attacks being some eight years apart. Four years after the second attack, he had a third episode of monocular visual impairment, this time with a severe migrainous headache over the preceding two days. This was so severe that at one point, he had a migrainous syncope. On examination, he had a right afferent pupillary defect and the corrected acuity 6/12, the left being normal. The optic disc was pale. MRI brain scan showed no significant abnormalities and no other cause could be found.

[We cannot exclude the possibility that this patient had in fact, suffered recurrent attacks of demyelinating optic neuropathy, which may on occasions be very painful, although his headaches were compatible with IHS migraine and he did not develop any other features of demyelinating disease over the period of observation].

Ophthalmoplegic Migraine

As already mentioned, ophthalmoplegic migraine was included in the "migraine" section in the 1988 IHC classification but changed its designation under IHC-2. It is now defined as: "Recurrent attacks of headache with migrainous characteristics associated with paresis of one or more ocular cranial nerves (commonly the third nerve), in the absence of any demonstrable intracranial lesion other than MRI changes within the affected nerve." Although very rare, we have encountered a few instances that broadly conform to this definition. However, it is difficult to distinguish such cases from restricted manifestations of basilar type migraine.

CASE 179: OPHTHALMOPLEGIC MIGRAINE

A 42-year-old man was referred because of "transient ischemic attacks." Six months previously, he had suddenly felt strange, with unsteadiness and slurring of speech. He then developed kaleidoscopic tunnel vision. By then, he was frankly dysarthric and ataxic, and noticed that his left eyelid was drooping. These symptoms lasted about 30 minutes and were then followed by a vertical band-like headache with nausea and photophobia, which lasted about two hours. He then recovered completely. He had no previous or family history of migraine.

Over subsequent days, he began to have brief, recurrent vertical headaches and then had a recurrence of the original symptoms, except that on this occasion he developed frank diplopia. When he looked in the mirror, he had a clear strabismus, the left eye being fully abducted. The ophthalmoplegia lasted some 40 minutes and was followed by a typical migrainous headache. MRI brain scan and MRA were normal, as was a transthoracic echocardiograph.

CASE 180: OPHTHALMOPLEGIC MIGRAINE

An 11-year-old boy was first seen at the age of three as a ward consult when he was admitted with fever and a possible febrile convulsion. On the second day of this episode, it was noted that his left eye was closed and that he had developed a squint. He had had a febrile convulsion a year previously. On examination, he had marked meningism with mild fever. His head was inclined to the right. There was a partial left-sided ptosis with limited up gaze in the left eye. A CT head scan and lumbar puncture were both normal. His symptoms resolved completely over a number of days except that since that time, he had been somewhat troubled by his left eye, which he tended to close because of persistent light hypersensitivity.

At the age of seven, he was continuing to get episodes of diplopia and discomfort around the left eye. Examination when symptomatic suggested a partial left third nerve palsy. CT scans were again normal. A professor of neurology who had a particular interest in eye movement disorders reviewed him, and suggested a diagnosis of ophthalmoplegic migraine. Since then, he had continued to experience episodic headache with nausea compatible with migraine but not associated with ophthalmoplegia.

OTHER PRIMARY HEADACHES

There remain a number of other primary headache syndromes that differ from typical migraine in terms of symptoms and chronology. However, a notable feature of some of these syndromes is their tendency to occur most commonly in individuals who have a current or previous history or migraine, or who subsequently develop migraine. We, therefore, believe that these syndromes represent *"migraine fragments."* We would emphasis, however, that headaches of this type can be manifestations of cranial pathology. Full investigation is always required, although the yield is low.

We have divided these syndromes into two broad groups: "paroxysmal headaches and head pains," occurring either as single episodes or repeatedly during a day; and the TACs, which include cluster headache. The TACs are distinguished by marked reflex trigeminal parasympathetic activity, and sometimes features of cranial sympathetic paralysis, ipsilateral to the head pain. All these syndromes are relatively rare, with the exception of cluster headache.

Paroxysmal Headaches and Head Pains

A number of headache syndromes occur as paroxysmal attacks of extremely severe intensity. These include *thunderclap headache*, a spontaneous cataclysmic attack that is usually but not invariably a single event; and recurrent headaches induced by a variety of inputs and activities—the *exertional cephalalgias*, *Valsalva-induced headaches* (including *cough headache* and *coital cephalalgia*), and the *reflex cephalalgias*.

Thunderclap Headache

Thunderclap headache is an excruciating headache of instantaneous onset, reaching maximum intensity within a minute. Such headache is typical of subarachnoid haemorrhage (SAH). In the absence of other manifestations of SAH, it may still represent a warning leak from an aneurysm ("sentinel headache"), and this presentation always requires full investigation, by CT brain scan followed by lumbar puncture at least 12 hours after the ictus, to look for cerebrospinal fluid (CSF) xanthochromia by spectroscopy (17). We will mention this again in Chapter 7. Thunderclap headache can also be a manifestation of other serious intracranial disorders, including intracerebral hemorrhage, cerebral venous thrombosis, arterial dissection (both intra- and extracranial), cerebral angiitis, pituitary apoplexy, acute hydrocephalus (due, for example, to ventricular obstruction by a colloid cyst of the third ventricle), and spontaneous intracranial hypotension. "Primary" thunderclap headache, first delineated by Day and Raskin in 1986 (see below), can only be diagnosed when all other causes have been excluded, but is by far the most common explanation for this clinical presentation.

It is benign, but patients who have experienced an episode have often had headaches previously, or go on to experience recurrent primary headaches, usually of migrainous type (18).

CASE 181: THUNDERCLAP HEADACHE WITHOUT PREVIOUS MIGRAINE

A 33-year-old man suddenly suffered an excruciating vertical headache radiating down the back of the neck followed by severe nausea and vomiting. This resolved after a few minutes but then recurred. He did not experience a change in consciousness but felt his neck was a little stiff. He was noted to be pale. He had no previous history of significant headache, but his mother was a migraineur. He was taken to a local emergency room, where the headache continued, and he vomited for the next 10 hours. MRI brain scan and MRA were normal and no serious disease could be defined. The headache gradually resolved over a few days.

CASE 182: THUNDERCLAP HEADACHE IN A MIGRAINEUR

A 31-year-old man had a long history of infrequent MO. He would experience headache attacks, usually in the region of the right eye, perhaps once every couple of years and his mother and sister were also migraineurs. While living abroad, he had been working out in a gym on a "lats" machine, when he suddenly had an explosive headache, "like a bang in the head," followed by visual blurring, nausea, and slight neck stiffness but no alteration in consciousness. There were a number of medically trained people in the gym, but he was not encouraged to go to hospital! The headache persisted in a severe form for about four days and then settled to a persistent background, band-like headache, which would worsen with exertion. He was eventually evaluated on his return home some three months after the event. Neurological examination was normal and MRI brain scan and MRA showed no abnormality.

Occasionally, primary thunderclap headache can occur serially.

CASE 183: RECURRENT THUNDERCLAP HEADACHE

A 30-year-old receptionist was perfectly well until three weeks prior to consultation, when she developed intermittent tingling in the right arm and occasionally in the left leg. About three days later, she suddenly suffered the most severe headache she had ever experienced. She described it as "like an explosion" located in the occipital area, and it was associated with severe nausea, but no vomiting. She mentioned that her neck went stiff and tight. She went to an emergency room where a "viral infection" was diagnosed. She was left with some mild paresthesiae, and every time she bent down she felt sick and vertiginous and would vomit. Just before being seen in the Neurology clinic, she had a further attack of sudden-onset, severe headache, although it was not quite as severe as the first. This was bitemporal and frontal with no neck pain. Again she felt very nauseous. There was no photophobia or phonophobia. There was no past or family history of note. Neurological examination and subsequent CT brain scan were both normal.

Exertional Cephalalgias

Some primary headaches are precipitated reproducibly and almost predictably by exertion of one sort or another. The pathogenesis is not well understood but at least half of all cases have a migraine history. All patients with exertional headache must be investigated to exclude underlying pathology such as Chiari malformation and other causes of ventricular obstruction, but it is actually rare to find causative pathology (19).

Primary exertional headache: The most common of these disorders is "primary exertional headache" (previously known as "benign exertional headache"). According to IHC-2, primary exertional headache is: "A throbbing headache lasting from 5 minutes to 48 hours brought on by and occurring only during or after physical exertion but not at other times, and not attributable to another disorder."

Any form of exertion can precipitate attacks, and in our experience the headache duration in true primary exertional cephalalgia tends to be short, usually minutes and always less than an hour. However, exertional cephalalgia is easily confused with *exercise-triggered migraine*, which causes more protracted headache that develops in the postexercise period. This was discussed in Chapter 2, in the general context of migraine triggers, and we provide some further examples here. The fact that primary exertional cephalalgia and exercise-triggered migraine can coexist supports the view that they are manifestations of the same fundamental mechanism.

Primary exertional headache tends to be more prominent in high temperatures or at high altitude. Caffeine, hypoglycemia, and alcohol use have been described as contributing factors (20). It can sometimes be prevented by ergotamine and also by β-blockers or indomethacin (see Chapter 7).

CASE 184: PRIMARY EXERTIONAL HEADACHE

A 31-year-old man had started to experience exertion-related headaches over the previous year. He was in the habit of going to the gym two or three times a week. He remembered that on one occasion after doing about 15 push-ups, he suddenly experienced severe, throbbing, occipitonuchal headache. At the same time he felt a little light-headed. All the symptoms settled after a few minutes, but subsequently he found that whenever he was lifting heavy weights or doing a particularly strenuous exercise, the same headache would recur. These were, however, the only occasions that he would experience the headache.

He had experienced 20 or 30 of such headaches by the time of presentation. Although he gave no personal history of migraine, his father suffered severely. No abnormalities were found on examination, and a CT brain scan was normal. He was started on propranolol 40 mg/day. Follow-up some years later revealed that he was now a migraine sufferer, and he was still getting headaches whenever he lifted heavy weights. MRI brain scan was normal.

CASE 185: PRIMARY EXERTIONAL HEADACHE

A 27-year-old man gave a two- to three-year history of symptoms compatible with benign exertional cephalalgia. He would experience headache when he carried out any form of strenuous activity, such as tightening bolts up on cars, doing household chores, and during weight lifting, which he did to competition level despite the symptom! Pain would usually begin in the nuchal area and spread occipitally, becoming pounding in quality. There was no associated nausea or photophobia, nor did he lose consciousness. Pain severity was maximal at the peak of exertion and declined as he relaxed. Examination and CT brain scan (looking particularly at the hind brain) were both normal. He found ibuprofen 800 mg, taken twice daily, to be completely effective in abolishing his attacks of headache, although he would get occasional dyspepsia that prevented him from using ibuprofen as often as he would have liked.

CASE 186: EXERCISE-TRIGGERED MIGRAINE EVOLVING TO CHRONIC DAILY HEADACHE

A 32-year-old man suddenly developed a severe headache following (not during) sexual intercourse. It began in the occipital area and spread rapidly over the head, but there was no neck stiffness, nausea, or alteration in consciousness. The headache had a throbbing quality. It lasted about an hour, after which he slept and awoke the next day entirely well. He had no previous or family history of headache. However, he subsequently had similar headaches following intercourse and also with exertions such as jogging and lifting heavy objects, but never spontaneously. However, these headaches later became spontaneous, and he would often wake up with one. By the time he was seen, they were occurring on a daily basis. Neurological examination and CT brain scan were normal.

CASE 187: EXERCISE-TRIGGERED MIGRAINE EVOLVING TO CHRONIC DAILY HEADACHE

A 34-year-old man had a history of headaches dating back to his teens. At the outset, these were exclusively post-exertional. Following most sporting events, he would develop a modest generalized headache lasting an hour or so. As he got older, the post-exertional headaches continued, but he also began to experience similar headaches with work stress. These were more protracted, with a pressure-like quality, around the head, consistent with "tension-type" headache and sometimes accompanied by nausea. A year prior to presentation, these headaches became increasingly frequent and severe, constituting CDH. Following a recent rowing competition, he had developed his customary post-exertion headache but it persisted. The following day, he awoke with severe headache accompanied by vertigo, nausea, and vomiting, which took a day to resolve. He also remembered a curious episode following a day's skiing. Lying on his bunk, he suddenly developed uncontrollable jactitation and bit his tongue. He was unable to speak, but there was no change in consciousness and he had no further events of this type. MRI brain scan was normal.

Valsalva-Induced Headache

Headache can also be induced by activities such as coughing, sneezing, laughing, or straining, which all produce a Valsalva response.

Cough headache: Cough headache may be primary but about half of all cases are caused by structural pathology, so neuroimaging is mandatory.

"Primary cough headache" occurs in both sexes, often in middle age. It is usually bilateral and brief, lasting up to 30 seconds, but can sometimes be unilateral and more protracted. Generally there are no additional symptoms. It can be very debilitating. The pain may be severe, and avoiding triggers completely is difficult and inconvenient. Some patients, when they realize a cough or sneeze is inevitable, hold their head in anticipation of the pain.

The mechanism is obscure, although it probably relates to acute venous distension. Use of indomethacin, propranolol and lumbar puncture seem to be effective treatments, but the condition often subsides spontaneously after some months. Cough, or other Valsalva-induced headache, has been linked recently to cystic dilatation of the cavum septum pellucidum (21) and may progress to CDH.

Hindbrain hernia headache: Chiari malformation is a particularly important cause because surgical treatment can be curative. However, "hindbrain hernia headache," typical of this condition, is said to differ from classical primary cough headache in that headache occurs at the zenith of exertion in cough headache whereas in hindbrain herniation, the headache is typically delayed by a few seconds (22). However, this is not axiomatic in our experience. We would note that this condition might be more appropriately considered to be a "secondary headache" but is included here because of its close similarity to primary exertional headache.

Downbeat nystagmus may also be present in patients with Chiari malformation, which can also be associated with radiological and sometimes clinical features of syringomyelia, as illustrated by Case 189. We have also seen a case of stabbing headaches associated with this structural abnormality (Case 190, below).

CASE 188: COUGH HEADACHE
A 52-year year-old man complained of episodic headache occurring only in relation to activities such as coughing, sneezing, lifting, and bending. He did not suffer from other headaches. The pain was bilateral and mainly occipital, would occur within a second or so of the activity, and last for 30 seconds to a few minutes. Most disabling was the pain occurring with stooping, because his job as a carpenter involved a lot of bending down. Neurological examination and MRI brain scan were normal. Prophylaxis was tried with indomethacin, propranolol, and methysergide without significant benefit. Lumbar puncture, a procedure that has been reported to help alleviate cough headache, did not help, and he was lost to follow up.

CASE 189: HINDBRAIN HERNIA HEADACHE
An 18-year-old girl presented with a one-year history of occipital headache. The headache was exclusively related to coughing and straining. However, the headache started *after* the exertion and built to maximum intensity over about 30 seconds. There were no neurological abnormalities on examination, but the cervical MRI showed a Type 1 Chiari malformation, with extension of the cerebellar tonsils below the foramen magnum and a small cervical syrinx cavity. Her headache problem was completely relieved following decompression of the foramen magnum (Fig. 1).

CASE 190: HINDBRAIN HERNIA HEADACHE
At first presentation, this 36-year-old woman gave a rather nonspecific headache history. Over the previous winter, she had suffered a number of presumed viral upper respiratory tract illnesses. With these, her head had become "stuffy" and

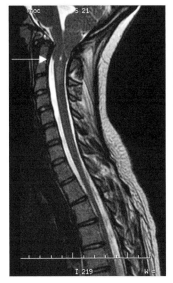 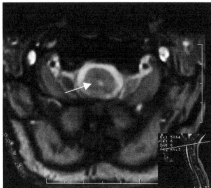

Figure 1 Case 189: Hindbrain hernia headache. *Left panel*—Marked Chiari Type I malformation, with herniation of the cerebellar tonsils below the level of the foramen magnum (*arrow*). *Right panel*—The small syrinx cavity visible on the saggital view (*arrow*) is seen more clearly on the axial view.

she developed persistent occipital headache, occasionally shooting up to the top of her head. She experienced right-sided tinnitus and episodes where she would feel faint and nauseous, and would experience what sounded like true vertigo. She had had unsuccessful antibiotic and nasal decongestant treatment from her general practitioner. Neurological examination was unremarkable. No diagnosis was made at the time, but on subsequent investigation, MRI brain scan demonstrated a Chiari Type 2 malformation without hydrocephalus or syrinx formation.

On reviewing the history, it became clear that she had been experiencing a significant cough headache with the characteristics of hindbrain hernia headache. When she coughed or strained, she would experience a severe occipital headache that reached a crescendo just after the maximum rise in intrathoracic pressure. This history had not been forthcoming when she had first been seen but she had recently had a cold and had been coughing a lot, and as a result has been experiencing a good deal more paroxysmal headache.

A foramen magnum decompression was performed. She was essentially asymptomatic at the follow-up appointment four months postoperatively.

Coital Cephalalgia

Referred to in IHC-2 as "primary headache associated with sexual activity," coital cephalalgia is a fairly common condition and many cases probably go unreported. However, it should always be borne in mind that onset of severe headache during intercourse can be due to SAH or arterial dissection, and patients presenting after a first or second episode should be investigated accordingly. It should also be noted that postural headache following intercourse has also been described, caused by spontaneous intracranial hypotension (see p. 292). This is very rare and should be regarded as a secondary headache (23).

The IHC-2 describes "pre-orgasmic" headache as starting as a dull bilateral ache, with awareness of neck and/or jaw muscle contraction, increasing as sexual excitement increases, and suddenly becoming intense at orgasm. This can last minutes to hours. "Orgasmic" headache (the most common form) is described as a sudden, severe or explosive headache at climax, subsiding within minutes. The relationship between coital amnesia and sexual headache was discussed in Chapter 3.

Whether this condition should be grouped with "exertional cephalalgias" or "Valsalva headache" is a matter of opinion (or technique?), but coital cephalalgia can also be a feature of a more generalized exercise-induced headache problem.

Isolated coital cephalalgia

CASE 191: RECURRENT COITAL CEPHALALGIA

A 33-year-old woman gave a history of three episodes of coital cephalalgia. The first had occurred three years previously and the second and third attacks were more recent. On each occasion, headache had come on without warning at the point of orgasm. She described the pain as terrifying and paralyzing. The pain was in the occipital and vertical areas and defervesced over a few minutes. She was left with a dull headache that persisted for hours on each occasion. She denied having associated nausea, vomiting, or other neurological symptoms.

She had not suffered migraine, exertional headache, or other significant headaches previously. Examination, MRI brain scan, and MR cerebral angiogram were all normal. At follow-up, she had had no further coital headaches but felt she was more "headache prone" than she used to be.

CASE 192: RECURRENT COITAL CEPHALALGIA

A 42-year-old -man said that after drinking heavily one evening, he had experienced "the worst headache" he had ever encountered, during sexual intercourse. The head pain had developed suddenly in the occipital region, but there was no alteration of consciousness, nausea, or symptoms of meningism. The occipital headache lasted for about 24 hours, and he was left with a dull, vague ache in the same region for the next few weeks. All his symptoms resolved, and he had intercourse subsequently without problems, before consultation.

He had, in fact, experienced coital cephalalgia previously, although the symptoms had been much milder. He had not experienced other forms of exertional headache and there was no history of migraine. He drank at least five pints of beer a day. On examination, he had an alcoholic fetor and was obese, but neurological examination and subsequent CT brain scan were normal. At follow-up, he denied further coital headache.

CASE 193: RECURRENT COITAL CEPHALALGIA

A 63-year-old man was seen urgently at his general practitioner's request. He had experienced two episodes of headache during sexual intercourse. The first had been about nine months previously and was relatively mild. Further episodes of sexual intercourse were uncomplicated until the more recent attack four days before consultation. At the point of orgasm, he had developed extremely severe holocranial headache, but no other symptoms such as alteration in consciousness, nausea, or vomiting. Neurological examination and subsequent CT brain scan were normal. At follow-up 14 years later, he reported no further episodes.

CASE 194: RECURRENT COITAL CEPHALALGIA

A 35-year-old man presented with a three-year history of headache exclusively related to sexual intercourse. He had put up with this until he heard that a friend with a similar problem of some nine months duration had suffered an SAH and had undergone clipping of an aneurysm!

The patient's headache occurred during most sexual encounters. Toward climax and at orgasm, he would experience a "staggeringly severe" holocranial headache "like an explosion in the skull", associated with a scintillating scotoma and followed by nausea and photophobia. The symptoms would gradually resolve over 5 to 20 minutes. He had no previous history of headache, but his brother and sister suffered from migraine. MRI brain scan and MRA showed no clinically significant abnormalities.

Mixed Coital Cephalalgia and Exertional Cephalalgia

CASE 195: COITAL CEPHALALGIA WITH EXERTIONAL CEPHALALGIA

A 30-year-old woman developed, for the first time, severe occipitonuchal headache during sexual intercourse. For the first 10 minutes it was so severe she thought she was going to die. It took 30 minutes to resolve, but she then had a persistent dull headache for the next two days. Shortly afterwards, she had a very similar headache at work, but this time it came on when she had to run quickly to a different location. She was admitted to hospital and had a CT brain scan and lumbar puncture, which were both normal. She was discharged home. A week later she had another episode of coital cephalalgia, with pain very similar to the previous two severe episodes.

CASE 196: RECURRENT COITAL CEPHALALGIA WITH EXERTIONAL CEPHALALGIA

A 36-year-old man had experienced a severe right occipital headache six days previously, just before orgasm during sexual intercourse. There were no associated symptoms, and the pain gradually eased over half an hour. Subsequently, he had a continuous, very slight, background headache, increased by postural maneuvers and by exertion, for example, on using his ski exercise machine. He had a further, very similar headache during sexual intercourse two days after the first event. He suffered other headaches rarely, but also in the right occipital region. There were no additional migrainous symptoms with these headaches, which were readily responsive to simple analgesics, and there was no family history of headache. Neurological examination and subsequent MRI brain scan were normal.

CASE 197: COITAL AND EXERTIONAL CEPHALALGIA

A 41-year-old man reported headaches during sexual intercourse. They occurred in a very stereotyped way. As climax approached, he began to experience severe pain in and around the left eye and in the left frontal region, which reached its maximum at climax and then gradually eased over the next half hour. There were no associated symptoms. He also described one episode of similar headache, caused by carrying heavy bags of shopping. There was no other past history of note. His mother suffered from migraine.

Sex-triggered migraine: As noted, sexual intercourse can occasionally trigger migraine, just as other forms of exertion can (see p. 75). This should not be confused with coital cephalalgia, although in the following case the patient also later developed benign exertional cephalalgia.

CASE 198: MIGRAINE TRIGGERED BY SEXUAL INTERCOURSE
A 36-year-old man requested review because of recurrence of headaches. He had been seen two years previously because of CDH. CT brain scan at that time was normal, and the headaches settled after six months. Two months before review, he developed headaches following sexual intercourse. He would develop a severe occipitonuchal headache between two and six hours after sexual intercourse on virtually every occasion, but at no other time. As a result, he had begun to avoid sex. The headache could be associated with nausea and slight dizziness, and also with mild photo and phonophobia. The headache would last about two or three hours. On follow-up, he had begun to develop some sharp head pains on lifting heavy objects into lorries. Neurological examination and subsequent MRI head scan were both normal.

The mechanism of thunderclap headache and of coital and other forms of exertional cephalalgia is not known, but a common feature reported in investigated cases is the presence of "focal cerebral vasospasm." In Chapter 2, we noted that secondary vascular responses in the migraine mechanism can occasionally be sufficiently marked to produce vasospasm visible on angiography, and we would suggest that this supports our contention that these paroxysmal cephalalgias are "fragments" of this process. Indeed, Miller Fisher called thunderclap headache "crash migraine" (24) and a patient of Day and Raskin had recurrent primary thunderclap headache associated with diffuse vasospasm on each occasion (25). They attributed the syndrome to the presence of an unruptured posterior circulation aneurysm (25), but vasospasm has also been reported in a number of cases of benign headache induced by sexual intercourse and masturbation (26). The vasospasm often persists long after the headache has resolved, so it is presumably not the direct cause of the headache. However, it may be associated with appropriate focal neurology due to ischemia, and even cerebral infarction (27).

Reflex Cephalalgias

Occasionally, severe paroxysmal headache can be precipitated by exposure of the head to some external stimulus, commonly intense cold or heat. This has been described most often in association with eating cold foods such as ice cream (*ice-cream headache*, or *cold stimulus headache*). Headache usually develops in the mid-frontal region when ice cream or similar very cold food is eaten quickly. The condition seems to be more prevalent in migraineurs, in which case the headache tends to occur at the usual site of the migraine headache (28).

CASE 199: ICE CREAM HEADACHE AND MIGRAINOUS VISUAL AURAS

A 15-year-old boy described three attacks of typical scintillating scotoma. Each had been precipitated by strenuous activity, such as playing hockey. He described the sudden development of a "white hole" in the middle of his vision in both eyes, which gradually cleared over about 15 minutes, during which he felt vaguely "spaced out." These events were not associated with headache, however, and he would manage to continue his activity despite the symptoms. Although there was no personal or family history of typical migraine, he had for years been susceptible to "ice cream headache." Ingesting a dollop of ice cream or similar very cold food would inevitably elicit a severe, piercing pain in the right eye, lasting up to 10 seconds. On review 10 years later, he had not developed typical migraine or further auras but the "ice cream headache" problem had continued, although it was much less frequent or reproducible.

CASE 200: COLD WIND–INDUCED HEADACHE

A 37-year-old man complained of recurrent headaches approximately monthly for the previous seven years. There was no premonition to these attacks, which developed as a vise-like, constant bi-temporal pain accompanied by mild photophobia but no phonophobia or nausea. These headaches were typically triggered by cold air blowing on his head, for example, when riding in a car with the window down, but not by low ambient temperature per se. He denied symptoms of ice-cream headache. The headache once started would continue for about four hours. There was no other personal or family history of relevance.

Bath-related headache: An unusual variant of this phenomenon, referred to as "bath-related headache," has been described, so far exclusively in oriental women (29). This is a severe headache, lasting 3 to 30 hours, which is precipitated reproducibly by exposure to hot water, as when bathing or showering, although on occasions susceptible patients also experience the symptom when swimming or on exposure to cold wind. Multisegment vasoconstriction has been seen on angiography following attacks, in occasional cases (30). This benign syndrome appears to remit spontaneously in about three months.

Hypnic headache: Although cluster headache is well known for waking sufferers from their slumber at a particular time of the night, attacks can also occur during waking hours. Migraine also often starts during sleep, so that patients awake in the middle of an attack. Most migraine attacks occur between 6 A.M. and 10 A.M. However, only one headache syndrome, hypnic headache or "alarm-clock headache," occurs *exclusively* during sleep.

Raskin first described this syndrome in 1988 (31), and its prevalence is estimated to be 0.07%. It affects the middle-aged to elderly and is more common in women than in men, in a ratio of about 3 to 1. The pain is bilateral in about two-thirds of sufferers. The headache usually wakes the patient between 1 A.M. and 3 A.M., often with clock-like regularity, lasts at least 15 minutes and typically about an hour, and is dull in character, certainly less severe than cluster headache. It occurs with a highly variable frequency, between once and six times a night, and generally four or more times a week (32).

Hypnic headache is associated with rapid eye movement (REM) sleep, and it has been suggested that it might be a REM sleep disorder in which the sleep-controlling areas of the brain stem intrude into the antinociceptive system, thereby causing pain (33). Migrainous symptoms such as nausea, photophobia, and phonophobia may occur rarely, but there are usually no autonomic features. Like cluster headache, it may respond to lithium.

CASE 201: HYPNIC HEADACHE

A 65-year-old woman was referred by her general practitioner when she began to have a new pattern of headache. She had suffered MO very occasionally over many years, but for the previous two years she had experienced headaches exclusively from sleep. She would be woken consistently between 2.30 A.M. and 3 A.M. by a left-sided, moderately intrusive headache that would last about an hour. She had attributed the attacks to arthritis in her neck and would prop herself up on a third pillow, which she thought was helpful. Occasionally, if she had a nap during the day she would awaken with a similar type of headache. She had tried a slow-release anti-inflammatory preparation and amitriptyline without success. There were no neurological abnormalities on examination.

Exploding head syndrome: Coincidentally, the same year that Raskin described hypnic headache, the term "exploding head syndrome" was coined by the British neurologist John Pearce to describe another paroxysmal disorder that, although not a headache as such, probably represents a similar disturbance in sensory control in relation to sleep (34). Patients typically report a terrifyingly loud but fleeting noise, usually on falling asleep but occasionally on waking. Some also report a simultaneous flash of light, and less commonly a strange sensation as though they had stopped breathing. This often leads to acute anxiety, which may be the most prominent symptom. As with hypnic headache, patients tend to be middle aged or elderly, but it can occur at any age. Attack frequency is variable. Some report an attack or two followed by prolonged or total remission, whereas some can have up to seven attacks in one night for several nights each week. Investigation reveals no causative pathology. It is not yet clear whether this entity is related to the migraine mechanism.

CASE 202: EXPLODING HEAD SYNDROME

An 82-year-old man presented with a year-long history of being woken by "electric shock"–like feelings in the head. He would experience one to three attacks in a night, but sometimes he could go a night or two without it happening. They would occur at any time of the night and would last a second or two. He was quite frightened by them. There was no other history of note, and he was otherwise healthy. Examination was normal. He was treated with clonazepam 0.5 mg. At review two months later, he was much improved.

Primary stabbing headaches (Cephalalgia fugax): Another form of paroxysmal headache occurs as a single stab or a series of stabs, each lasting a second or so. These are typically felt in the periorbital, temporal, or parietal area in the distribution of the first division of the trigeminal nerve, but can occur elsewhere in the head. The stabs are unilateral but the site of the pain often moves within the hemicranium, and can switch sides. They often recur unpredictably with irregular frequency, sometimes very many times a day over a number of days. Raskin and Schwartz (35) first described these sharp, jabbing pains about the head as "ice pick–like," and they have often been referred to as "ice pick pains" or "jabs and jolts" in the literature. We are taken with the epithet "cephalgia fugax"—fleeting head pains.

They are clearly linked to the migraine mechanism and are uncommon in patients without active migraine. For example, Selby and Lance (36) obtained a history of ice pick pains in 200 out of 530 patients with migraine. The site of the stabbing pain usually coincided with the site of the patients' usual headache. Such pains have also been described in conjunction with cluster headaches, most common as the attack subsides, and again generally in the same area as the cluster pain. However, stabbing headaches are not usually associated with other migrainous or cranial autonomic symptoms.

As noted, this syndrome can rarely occur as a feature of headache related to structural pathology [see below, (37)].

CASE 203

A 17-year-old girl was followed over a three-year period after she presented with stabbing head pains. The stabs would occur up to 40 times a day, exclusively in the left occipital area. Each stab would last between 2 and 6 seconds and there were no associated symptoms. They could occur at any time, but she felt they were more likely to occur at times of stress. Between episodes she was fine. Remissions would occur lasting up to 6 months. Follow-up by letter, some three years after she was last seen, disclosed that no remission had occurred. Pain was occurring to some degree every week. Although she did not suffer migraine, her paternal grandmother did. There were no abnormalities on examination. An MRI head scan was normal.

CASE 204

A 29-year-old woman had experienced head pains over the previous seven years. They had always been in the right temple and were excruciating to the extent that they would make her wince. Each stab would last less than a second. At first they were infrequent, occurring perhaps every six months or so for no obvious reason. Over the month before she was seen, the pains had become more frequent, although they seemed to be less intense. At one point she was having 30 stabbing pains each day. There were no associated symptoms such as ptosis, conjunctival injection, or epiphora. No abnormality was found on investigation.

TRIGEMINAL AUTONOMIC CEPHALALGIAS

Cluster headache is the archetype of a group of primary headache syndromes that are usually strictly unilateral and have very prominent cranial autonomic features. These headaches have now been grouped together under IHC-2 as the *trigeminal autonomic cephalalgias*, or TACs.

Cluster Headache

The features of cluster headache, sometimes referred to as "periodic migrainous neuralgia," are typically precise and dramatic. The pain is nearly always unilateral (although patients with bilateral attacks have been described) and centered around one eye. The headache is often extremely severe (it has been referred to as "suicide headache") and typically lasts 20 to 30 minutes at this level, although the total duration can be between 15 and 180 minutes. Unlike the migraineur, who will usually seek solace by keeping still in a dark, quiet environment, the cluster sufferer is typically restless, pacing the room or kneeling on the floor holding the head, rocking to and fro. Some patients even strike the affected area of the head.

Usually only one attack occurs, most often during the night, typically waking the patient at around 2 or 3 A.M., but there can be up to eight attacks in a day and sometimes the pain does not settle completely between attacks. Most patients experience attacks only from sleep, others only when awake. Provocation by alcohol is a common feature. The condition is reviewed in reference (38).

One or more cranial autonomic symptoms usually occur during the headache attack. The most common result from activation of the trigeminal parasympathetic reflex (see Chapter 2). The eye ipsilateral to the head pain "goes red" (conjunctival injection) and "runs" (lacrimation or epiphora), and there may be eyelid edema. The ipsilateral nostril may feel blocked or may discharge (nasal congestion and rhinorrhea), and there may be excess sweating over the forehead and face on the affected side. In addition, there may be secondary sympathetic paresis, thought to be the result of neuropraxial injury to the sympathetic fibers in the outer layers of the walls of the ipsilateral carotid artery. Repeated attacks can cause permanent Horner's syndrome.

The mean age of onset, taken from a number of series, is about 30 years. It may appear at any age, although it is uncommon in children. Women represent only 10% to 30% of those affected.

Cluster headache is frequently misdiagnosed as "sinus," or an ophthalmological disorder, or a dental disease. Some patients experience severe pain in the face or in the jaw rather than the typical periorbital area, and may demand that their dentist removes some teeth —a suggestion that the dentist may acquiesce to! Some also find that the pain radiates into the neck or shoulder, indicative of extensive allodynia as in migraine (Chapter 2). There may also be considerable variation on these typical clinical features. In addition to reports of rare bilateral attacks, some cluster patients neither get autonomic features nor find alcohol to be a trigger in the cluster period. Finally, it may be difficult (or perhaps unnecessary—see Chapter 6) to distinguish individual attacks from episodic migraine with prominent trigeminal parasympathetic reflex symptoms.

The following cases illustrate the extent of variation that can occur in this syndrome.

CASE 205: IDIOPATHIC CLUSTER HEADACHE IN A YOUNG WOMAN

A woman in her early 20s gave a history of recurrent and stereotyped headache attacks starting from age 17. These would occur in distinct periods lasting seven to nine weeks during which she would get a single attack each day, at around 2 A.M. She would be woken from sleep with an excruciating left-sided head and face pain associated with ipsilateral nasal blockage and conjunctival injection, and symptoms of a possible Horner's syndrome. Occasionally, she would have nausea and vomiting. The symptoms would subside over three to four hours. She had been treated for "sinus" for years. Her father had suffered from precisely the same sort of attacks, but his attacks stopped when he reached his 40s. She was examined shortly after a cluster attack had occurred, and there were no abnormalities on examination. Investigations, including MRI brain scan, were negative.

CASE 206: RECURRENT DAYTIME CLUSTER ATTACKS

A 34-year-old electrician presented with a 10-year history of stereotyped headaches that only occurred when awake. Each attack occurred without warning, was always localized to the left orbital region, and comprised extremely severe pain associated with facial heat, ipsilateral nasal blockage, epiphora, and injection of the ipsilateral conjunctiva. There were no features of Horner's syndrome. Each attack would last 10 to 15 minutes, but he would experience several attacks daily during cluster periods that would typically last two to three weeks. Clusters would occur about once a year.

CASE 207: CLUSTER HEADACHE WITH HORNER'S SYNDROME

A 46-year-old man suddenly developed "catarrh" associated with a rapidly progressive head pain in the left periorbital and malar area. The pain was so severe that he felt compelled to press hard on the eye to gain some relief. The symptom subsided after about 10 to 15 minutes, but then recurred in an identical fashion every other day or so for the next couple of weeks, after which the attacks ceased. He had no further headache or neurological problems until some four years later when the symptoms recurred. This time, however, the pain was much worse and he likened it to being "slowly stabbed through the eye." He was left with a constant background ache between attacks and then had further acute exacerbations on a daily basis, each lasting about an hour. Others noted that his left pupil had become smaller compared to the right and the left eye seemed "more narrow." There was no previous or family history of headache. Examination was normal except for a left-sided Horner's syndrome. CT scan of the brain and sinuses was normal. The cluster resolved after about a month.

Chronic Cluster Headache

The defining feature of typical cluster headache is not, in fact, the clinical phenomena that occur in individual attacks, because none is exclusive to cluster headache, but rather the *periodicity* of the attacks. Patients typically experience attacks at about the same time each day on a daily basis for weeks or months, and are then free of symptoms for protracted periods, often a year or so. The attacks therefore "cluster" chronologically at intervals referred to as "cluster periods." We will discuss this phenomenon in detail below.

Cluster headache occurring for more than one year without remission, or with remissions lasting less than a month, is defined as "chronic cluster headache." If no previous clusters have occurred, it is called "primary" chronic cluster headache; if there have been previous episodes of cluster, it is termed "secondary" chronic cluster headache. Secondary chronic cluster headache can revert to the episodic form.

CASE 208: CHRONIC CLUSTER *AB INITIO*, DIAGNOSED FOLLOWING MULTIPLE SINUS OPERATIONS

A 50-year-old man gave a history of symptoms typical of cluster headache on an almost daily basis from age 18! The maximum period free of attacks had been about a week. The attacks were exclusively left-sided and would wake him from sleep at around 2 A.M. to 3 A.M., although he also had two attacks in the daytime. During the attacks, which would typically last 30 to 90 minutes, he would feel that the left side of his nose was blocked up, and his eye would water occasionally, but he had not noted conjunctival injection. He would sometimes feel nauseous during the attacks and had vomited on rare occasions.

In the past, he had been treated for "sinusitis" on numerous occasions and was eventually referred following septoplasty and endoscopic sinus surgery undertaken a year earlier, which had failed to improve matters. Interestingly, his mother had also undergone multiple sinus procedures for similar symptoms, and his brother suffered from severe migraine. On examination, he had a partial left-sided Horner's syndrome. CT scan of the brain and sinuses was normal. The attacks responded to sumatriptan and reduced dramatically in frequency on high-dose verapamil.

Occasionally, cluster headache can be surprisingly mild, as the following case illustrates.

CASE 209: MILD CLUSTER HEADACHE

A 30-year-old man had suffered with what was diagnosed as episodic cluster headache over a six-year period. He would experience dull persistent pain, always in the right temple, periorbital area, and retro-orbital area, lasting two to three hours. There were no associated symptoms and, in particular, no autonomic symptoms, and drinking alcohol would not provoke attacks. The headaches were not particularly disabling. They would occur in clusters every eight months. In a cluster, he would get between one and three attacks every day, usually around midday. Clusters would last between four and five weeks, occasionally up to three months. MRI brain and MR cerebral angiogram were both normal.

Cluster Migraine

Case 208 might reasonably have been diagnosed as "chronic migraine with prominent trigeminal autonomic symptoms" rather than primary chronic cluster, whereas Case 209 might be considered an example of clustering chronology in migraine but for the "short" duration of the attacks ("migraine" lasts between 4 and 72 hours under IHC-2). We consider such cases to be examples of primary headache "overlap." The triumvirate of migraine, "tension-type" headache, and cluster headache comprises the vast majority of primary headaches observed in clinical practice, but in Chapter 6, we will discuss the extent to which these and other primary headache syndromes resemble and differ from each other, and advance the hypothesis that they may all be driven by the same basic neural process—the migraine mechanism.

Is cluster headache really different from migraine? At first glance, they are very different.

- A typical cluster attack is shorter in duration and more stereotyped and coherent than most migraine headaches.
- Migraine features such as premonitory symptoms, aura, nausea, and vomiting are uncommon.
- Cluster headache is also the only primary headache disorder that is more common in men (the male:female ratio is about 5:1).
- Cluster headache generally starts in the 20s or 30s, a decade after the peak incidence of migraine onset.
- Unlike migraine, it is extremely uncommon in children.

On the other hand, as noted above, there have been a number of reports of typical migraine aura in cluster headache, and some patients with otherwise typical cluster headache never experience cranial autonomic symptoms with attacks. Conversely, cranial autonomic symptoms do sometimes occur in otherwise typical migraine attacks, as indeed would be anticipated from our understanding of the migraine mechanism (see p. 62).

The IHC-2 recognizes that some patients may experience different forms of primary headache at different times of life and even from one event to another. Clinical experience confirms that whereas clear examples of stereotypic cluster headache and migraine are common, individual patients with headaches having features of both migraine and cluster headache are encountered quite often, and we refer to such cases in general as "cluster migraine," although this term has pointedly not been included in the IHS classification. We view the existence of such cases as evidence against individual primary headache syndromes as immutable, discrete entities.

A number of cluster or migraine patterns emerge. The most common situation is where patients with a previous personal or family history of migraine later develop marked autonomic symptoms as a component of their migraine attacks. This might reasonably be referred to as "migraine with cranial autonomic symptoms." Less often, typical migraine attacks occur in temporal patterns reminiscent of the chronology of cluster headache, or patients with typical cluster headache develop concurrent typical migraine attacks.

Migraine with Cranial Autonomic Symptoms

CASE 210: MIGRAINE WITH CRANIAL AUTONOMIC SYMPTOMS AND WITH PREVIOUS HISTORY OF MENSTRUAL MIGRAINE WITHOUT AURA

A 65-year-old woman had developed menstrual MO some 20 years prior to consultation. This stopped after hysterectomy but in the last eight or nine years, headaches of a different type had developed. These stereotyped attacks would develop without warning, sometimes waking her from sleep. She experienced severe pain in and around either eye but never both. The affected eye would water and become reddened and she would get either nasal blockage or discharge on the same side. Severe nausea and vomiting would occur frequently. She had attacks once or even twice a week, lasting up to three days. Red wine and colored liqueurs could precipitate attacks. Her mother had had "bad headaches" during menopause.

She was treated successfully with pizotifen as prophylactic and inhaled ergotamine and metaclopramide suppositories for attacks. On inquiry 13 years later, she reported a gradual reduction in the attack rate to three or four events per year, and resolution of the autonomic features.

CASE 211: MIGRAINE WITH CRANIAL AUTONOMIC SYMPTOMS AND PREVIOUS HISTORY OF MIGRAINE WITH AURA

A 52-year-old woman had suffered migraine with typical auras (scintillating scotoma and hemisensory disturbance) once or twice a year from the age of 11. The attacks could be precipitated by cheese, chocolate, citrus fruit, and eggs. There was an equivocal family history of migraine in a cousin. She was referred when the attacks became more frequent after her menopause. Recent attacks had been increasingly complicated by severe ipsilateral epiphora and nasal blockage and discharge at the height of such attacks. She responded to atenolol and inhaled ergotamine, together with prochlorperazine suppositories.

CASE 212: MIGRAINE WITH CRANIAL AUTONOMIC SYMPTOMS

A 19-year-old woman began to have recurrent but rather nondescript holocranial headaches. After some two months, the episodes became stereotyped with single daily attacks of excruciating right periorbital pain radiating into the cheek and jaw and subsequently the right neck, shoulder, and arm. This would persist for some 30 to 40 minutes, during which she felt unable to move. She would feel nauseous and also noted swelling and slight drooping of the right eyelid, and epiphora, but there were no nasal symptoms and the eye did not redden. All the symptoms would resolve within an hour, but she felt unwell for the rest of the day and was left with a persistent and unpleasant allodynia over the right forequarter between attacks, which occurred every two or three days.

Two years earlier, she had suffered a sequence of very severe "sinus headaches." She described agonizing attacks of facial pain during which her nose seemed to be blocked on one side. She was treated with inhalations, and the symptoms resolved over a period of weeks. Her mother and sisters all suffered severe recurrent fsheadaches. MRI brain scan and MRA were normal and the symptoms settled with topiramate.

CASE 213: MIGRAINE WITH CRANIAL AUTONOMIC SYMPTOMS EVOLVING FROM MIGRAINE WITHOUT AURA AND FAMILY HISTORY OF CLUSTER HEADACHE

A 49-year-old woman was referred because of a change in the character of her headaches. When seen 13 years earlier, she gave a history of typical recurrent attacks of

MO (diagnosed during childhood as "sinus headache"), and there was a strong family history of this disorder. More recent attacks had not been associated with nausea and had become localized to the face and periorbital area on the right. Attacks would also be associated with nasal blockage and ipsilateral tearing and would last up to four days. Her brother, ten years her junior, had recently developed classical "cluster headaches."

CASE 214: PREMONITORY TRIGEMINAL AUTONOMIC SYMPTOMS IN MIGRAINE

A 19-year-old shop assistant gave a three-year history of recurrent stereotyped attacks occurring every two to three weeks. Each would start with a tingling numbness above and around the left eye, and she would notice "bruising" in this area. (In fact, this was erythema localized to the first and second divisions of the trigeminal nerve.) About 45 minutes later, she would experience a sharp stabbing pain in that area on top of a background pain. As the pain became severe, she would feel nauseated and on occasions she would vomit. She would also feel "dizzy" and photophobic. The pain was worse with movement, and she would have to go and lie down. If at work, her mother would come and bring her home to bed. An attack would last one to two days.

CASE 215: BILATERAL AUTONOMIC FEATURES IN MIGRAINE

A 31-year-old woman gave an eight-year history of stereotypic attacks, two or three times monthly, comprising frontal head pain with photophobia and bilateral bloodshot conjunctivae, epiphora, and nasal discharge. There was no nausea, vomiting, ptosis, or pupillary changes. Attacks could last up to a day but would often remit after a short sleep.

The attacks could be precipitated by alcohol, particularly white wine and vodka, and there was a history of headaches and recurrent facial pain in a younger sister, a maternal aunt, and maternal grandfather (who had undergone sinus operations for the symptoms, without success).

Cluster headache evolving from migraine: Sometimes the character of the commonest current headache type is more typical of cluster headache, but there is a previous or family history of migraine, or the headaches have additional typically migrainous qualities.

CASE 216: CLUSTER HEADACHE EVOLVING FROM MIGRAINE WITH AURA

A 43-year-old woman presented with a change in the character of her long-standing headache attacks. During childhood, she had suffered episodes of typical visual and hemisensory migrainous auras without headache. Later, she developed attacks of similar symptoms followed by severe unilateral headache, but nausea and vomiting were not prominent. Attacks could be precipitated by a variety of factors, including cheese, chocolate, bright lights, stress, starvation, and sleep deprivation. She could not tolerate the oral contraceptive pill, because this would also trigger attacks. Her father suffered from migraine.

Six years previously, the attacks had largely stopped when she was put on high-dose dothiepin for depression. As the dose was slowly reduced, the attacks returned. Eighteen months before referral, she began to experience a completely new type of headache. She would be woken at 4 A.M. each day, with intense pain around the right temple and periorbital region, together with ipsilateral nasal obstruction and discharge, epiphora, and, occasionally, right ptosis. An attack would last four to five hours and would recur daily for a week, followed by two or three weeks free of symptoms before the attacks started again. In addition, she described another headache form. On most days, she would wake up with pain over the head and eyes, radiating into the temples and into the neck and shoulders, and she experienced marked photophobia.

CASE 217: CLUSTER HEADACHE WITH MIGRAINE FEATURES
A 71-year-old woman presented with a history of increasingly frequent and troublesome headaches, beginning some 30 years earlier. A typical attack would wake her up at 3 A.M. or 4 A.M., with severe pain in the right eye that would continue for up to a day. Nausea, anorexia, and occasional vomiting would occur, and on some occasions, she had also experienced a visual aura of a fortification spectrum. Both eyes would water, and on occasions, the ipsilateral eye had become bloodshot, but there was no ptosis. She would lie still in bed and spend the day avoiding noise and other stimuli.

CASE 218: CLUSTER HEADACHE WITH FAMILY HISTORY OF MIGRAINE
A 22-year-old man began to suffer daily attacks of headache. The pain would start at about 8 P.M. each day and last anything from one hour to throughout the night. The pain was localized to the right eye, and at its height was associated with reddening of the eye, epiphora, and ptosis. He would feel nauseous but never vomited. He had found paracetamol helpful. There was a strong family history of typical MO.

Temporal clustering of migraine attacks: Less often, recurrent headaches with clinical characteristics of migraine will show chronological clustering of attacks.

CASE 219: MIGRAINE BEHAVING AS CLUSTER HEADACHE, WITHOUT CRANIAL AUTONOMIC SYMPTOMS
A 35-year-old man presented with a four-year history of stereotyped attacks. Each began with a feeling of stiffness and tightness in the right side of the neck and shoulder, followed by excruciating pain spreading over the right side of the head into the temple, then the jaw, right orbit, and cheek. The head pain would last between 10 minutes and one hour. He did not experience photophobia or nausea but would be markedly phonophobic during attacks. Although there were never any cranial autonomic symptoms, the attacks would occur every day for three to four weeks and then resolve completely, only to recur about a year later. He had noted that alcohol could precipitate attacks, but he also suffered from typical ice cream headaches, and his mother was a migraineur.

On inquiry three years later, the patient reported that these bouts of headache had continued but he had found that they now responded to simple analgesics, although they had not done so in the past.

CASE 220: MIGRAINE WITH CLUSTER PERIODS
A 20-year-old woman gave a history of MA attacks dating from age 15. These would begin with nausea, and after 30 minutes, she would develop left-sided ptosis, facial numbness, and ipsilateral nasal blockage, rapidly followed by a pounding left occipital headache and scalp tenderness. Vomiting might occur at the outset, and she would often vomit repeatedly throughout the attack. Photo and phonophobia were

invariable, and she would have to lie still in a quiet, dark room. The attack would largely resolve with sleep but a dull headache would persist for some two days, and she would remain unusually sensitive to sensory inputs over this time. These headaches would occur in clusters of three to four separate attacks over two or three days, separated by many weeks free of symptoms. Her sister had MO.

CASE 221: MIGRAINE WITH CLUSTER HEADACHE CHRONOLOGY

A 38-year-old man had experienced stereotypic headache attacks from the age of 16. Each episode comprised a severe, constant, right-sided temporal pain that would usually last a few hours but could last up to a day. Mild nausea and photophobia were present, but there were never any autonomic features. He would have an attack every morning for a month. The attacks would then stop and he would be free of symptoms, often for a year or two. There was a strong family history of recurrent headaches, affecting his mother and two brothers. Previous MRI brain scan had been normal.

More complex admixtures of these two archetypes can sometimes be encountered. The following two cases exhibited features of both migraine and cluster headache during individual attacks.

CASE 222: SIMULTANEOUS MIGRAINE AND CLUSTER HEADACHE

A 35-year-old woman had suffered recurrent nondescript headaches every two months or so since childhood. Six years before consultation, and shortly after the birth of her first child, she began to have attacks of severe left-sided facial pain, with a visual aura of flashing lights followed by hemianopia in the left hemifield, together with nausea and photophobia. Attacks lasted several hours and occurred on a daily basis for some four or five weeks, before resolving completely. She was then free of symptoms for about two years. The second cluster of attacks, identical to the first, developed in the last trimester of her second pregnancy. This cluster lasted only two to three weeks, but she had another attack of similar duration two years later.

Just prior to consultation, she had been woken from sleep with an excruciating pain in the left occipital region, which radiated to the left face but resolved in one to two hours. Two days later, she had another attack but this time it was in the left periorbital region, radiating to the left occiput. She then had episodes of this headache every other day, some associated with nausea and vomiting and some preceded by the visual auras. In addition, she noticed that during attacks the left nostril would block up followed by a nasal discharge, and a left ptosis would develop.

Her mother had cluster headache and a maternal aunt had migraine. Examination revealed mild left ptosis and injection of the left conjunctiva.

The attacks became progressively more disabling, requiring hospital admission on several occasions. A number of treatments were used with variable success, including 100% oxygen therapy, injectable sumatriptan, high-dose steroids, and verapamil.

Periodicity in Cluster Headache

As noted above, the axiomatic feature of true cluster headache is its curious periodicity—the tendency of attacks to recur during cluster periods, often months or years apart. The duration of the cluster period can be quite variable, anything from seven days to a year, but is usually one to two months. Cluster periods are also seasonally related. Spring and autumn are particularly common times for cluster headache, as headache clinic personnel know only too well! Therefore, cluster headache may be driven not only by a diurnal rhythm but also a seasonal rhythm based on the length of daylight.

This circadian rhythm and circannual chronology is reflected in abnormal rhythms of cortisol, testosterone, growth hormone, and endorphins (reviewed in Ref. 38), strongly indicative of hypothalamic control.

Like migraine, cluster headache can be triggered by a variety of drugs such as alcohol and glyceryl trinitrate (GTN, see p. 68), but usually only during cluster periods. Positron emission tomography and blood-oxygen-level–dependent functional MRI studies have recently demonstrated specific ipsilateral posterior hypothalamic activation during attacks triggered by GTN during cluster periods. Activation was not observed when GTN was administered during cluster-free periods, providing further evidence that the hypothalamus might be the cluster headache generator (39,40). However, this same hypothalamic area is also activated in SUNCT/SUNA, another form of TAC; and activation of both the hypothalamus and the brainstem "migraine generator" region in the dorsal pons has been demonstrated recently in hemicrania continua, which has clinical features of both migraine and cluster headache (see below).

Paroxysmal Hemicrania

The symptoms of paroxysmal hemicrania (PH) are qualitatively identical to cluster headache, but the syndrome differs in a number of ways. PH is much less common than cluster headache, with prevalence of about 0.07%, and it is more common in women (the ratio is about 2.3:1). The attacks are shorter, lasting 2 to 30 minutes, and more frequent, usually occurring more than five times a day (range 2–40), and there is no nocturnal preponderance. During an attack, about half of patients prefer to sit or lie still, like migraineurs, whereas the remainder are restless and pace about, like the cluster headache patients. The majority of attacks are spontaneous, but some patients report that neck movements may trigger an attack. Only about 7% of patients find that alcohol is a trigger.

The key diagnostic feature of PH is that, unlike cluster headache, PH is exquisitely sensitive to indomethacin.

Like cluster, PH occurs in episodic and chronic forms. In fact, chronic PH was the first form to be described by Sjaastad and Dale in 1974 (41). Later it became clear that prolonged, pain-free remissions could occur between bouts in some patients, a syndrome now termed "episodic PH." PH is episodic in about 20% of cases and chronic in the remainder—the reverse of cluster headache—and most cases are chronic from onset. When episodic, the headache bouts usually last two weeks to five months, with remission periods ranging from 1 to 36 months. Unlike cluster headache, the bouts are not usually seasonally determined.

Chronic PH is defined under IHC-2 as attacks lasting for more than a year with less than one month of remission, and episodic PH as at least two attacks lasting seven days to a year, separated by remission of more than one month.

All patients with PH should have an MRI brain scan performed, because a high proportion of secondary cases has been reported.

PH can also occur in concert with trigeminal neuralgia (see below).

CASE 223: PAROXYSMAL HEMICRANIA

A 48-year-old woman presented with a new type of headache. For some three or four years, she had experienced occasional nondescript headaches that seemed to be related to work stress. These responded readily to simple analgesics. For a month prior to consultation, however, she had recurrent, stereotypic, exclusively right-sided headache attacks, initially once every other day. By the time of consultation, they were occurring three to four times daily. Without warning, she would develop a severe throbbing headache in the right temporal area, usually lasting half an hour. These headaches were not associated with nausea, photophobia, or phonophobia. On some occasions, an attack would occur during sleep and wake her, but there were no clear trigeminal autonomic symptoms. A diagnosis of PH was made and she was prescribed indomethacin 25 mg daily. She took the first dose with the next attack, and the headache resolved rapidly. She had no further attacks that day, and there were no further attacks while she continued this dose.

On inquiry two years later, there had been no recurrence although her previous nondescript headaches had become more frequent. They continued to respond to simple analgesics.

CASE 224: CHRONIC PAROXYSMAL HEMICRANIA

A 52-year-old woman was referred by her general practitioner because of headaches that had failed to respond to treatment with amitriptyline, carbamazepine, and pizo-tifen. She experienced exclusively left-sided headaches that were sharp and pene-trating, situated in and around the left eye and forehead. They would last 10 to 15 minutes and had occurred several times a day, most days, over a three-year period. When exacerbations occurred, they were extremely severe and would make her wince, and the scalp would feel tender. She would never get headache elsewhere. There was no lacrimation or nasal stuffiness, and her husband said that her eyelid did not droop during an attack. Between severe attacks, she felt otherwise perfectly well. Neurological examination and CT brain scan were both normal. She responded exceptionally well to indomethacin 25 mg once or twice a day.

However, an apparently selective response to indomethacin is not con-fined to PH and hemicrania continua, as the following case illustrates.

CASE 225: INDOMETHACIN RESPONSIVE HEADACHE

A 58-year-old woman began to suffer recurrent and disabling unilateral headaches following the onset of menopause. These were often very severe, sometimes throb-bing but not associated with nausea or visual disturbances. There was no response to a variety of analgesics and eventually she had a CDH, worsened by neck movements. On the presumption that the headaches resulted from "arthritis of the neck," her GP treated her with sustained-release indomethacin 75 mg, and this produced instant improvement. After two weeks of treatment, she stopped the drug and there was an immediate relapse. When indomethacin was reinstituted, the headache resolved rapidly once more. Eventually, she ran out of the drug, the headaches returned, and she was referred for evaluation. Ongoing treatment with indomethacin was recommended, and on review three months later, she was asymptomatic, on indomethacin 50 mg daily.

Hemicrania Continua

This rare syndrome appears to be an amalgam of chronic cluster headache and chronic PH, with the persistence of chronic migraine thrown in for good measure! In fact, it is a prime example of the principle of "overlap" in primary headache (see Chapter 6). Individual headache attacks are qualitatively similar to cluster and PH, but chronology and treatment responses differ. Like PH, hemicrania continua responds to indomethacin to the extent that this is considered part of the definition of the condition under IHC-2 (see also the "indotest," p. 312), although other types of nonsteroidal anti-inflammatory drugs can also sometimes be effective. Table 4 compares the features of chronic cluster headache, chronic PH, and hemicrania continua.

CASE 226
A 30-year-old woman presented with a 13-month history of unremitting unilateral headache that had started for no clear reason. It was right-sided and occurred daily for six months and then moved completely to the left side. The pain would vary in severity throughout the day, at times being described as severe. There were no autonomic features. She had a few MO attacks a few years previously but there

Table 4 Comparison of Chronic Cluster Headache, Chronic Paroxysmal Hemicrania, and Hemicrania Continua

	Chronic cluster headache	Chronic paroxysmal hemicrania	Hemicrania continua
Time course	< 1 mo remission per year	< 1 mo remission per year	Unremitting
Pain duration	15–180 mins	2–30 mins	20 mins-days, constant
Attack frequency	< 1–8 per day	5–40 per day	Persistent
Trigeminal autonomic symptoms	Yes	Often	Often
Indomethacin responsive	No	Yes	Yes

was no family history of migraine. No abnormality was found on examination and neck movements were full and pain free. She had tried carbamazepine, dothiepin, paracetamol, sumatriptan, and ibuprofen without success but had complete and almost immediate pain relief with indomethacin 25 mg three times daily, and remained headache-free when seen six months later.

SUNCT/SUNA and Trigeminal Neuralgia

Short-lasting Unilateral Neuralgiform headache attacks with Conjunctival injection and Tearing (SUNCT) is a very rare syndrome. The pain is strictly unilateral, abrupt in onset, of short duration (5 seconds to 4 minutes), and stabbing or burning in quality. During symptomatic periods, attacks can occur from 3 to 200 times per day, both during the day and at night, and may also cluster. The diagnosis demands that both conjunctival injection and tearing must both occur, but this is not invariable in otherwise typical cases and SUNCT is now increasingly considered part of the spectrum of Short-lasting Unilateral Neuralgiform headache attacks with Automatic Symptoms (SUNA).

In some respects, SUNCT/SUNA resembles trigeminal neuralgia and indeed is often mis-diagnosed as such. The chief distinguishing features are:

- SUNCT/SUNA involves the first division of the trigeminal nerve rather than the second or third divisions typically involved in trigeminal neuralgia, and the attacks are much more frequent.
- By definition, cranial autonomic symptoms are invariable in SUNCT/SUNA but are not a typical feature of trigeminal neuralgia.
- There is no clear history of triggering by tactile inputs, so characteristic of trigeminal neuralgia, in SUNCT/SUNA.

Paradoxically however, trigeminal autonomic symptoms can sometimes occur in association with what appears to be trigeminal neuralgia! The pathophysiological significance of the relationship, other than the common involvement of the trigeminal sensory pathways, is unclear, but it is conceivable that some forms of idiopathic trigeminal neuralgia are actually TACs.

Trigeminal neuralgia is a syndrome comprising severe, unilateral, *lancinating* facial pain, usually in the distribution of the second or third divisions of the trigeminal nerve (the first division is affected in less than 5% of cases), lasting seconds. The pain may be described as like an electric shock or a red-hot needle. As noted, an important characteristic is that the pain can often be triggered by inputs such as touching the face (washing, shaving etc.), chewing, cleaning teeth, or by cold wind. Rarely, it can be induced by inputs outside the trigeminal territory, such as stimulation of a limb, or by other sensory inputs such as loud noise, bright lights or strong odours. Sometimes the pain is so severe that it evokes spasm of the facial muscles (*tic doloreux*).

There is usually a refractory period following a paroxysm, during which a further attack cannot be triggered. However, this refractory period is said not to occur in cases secondary to structural pathology, such as multiple sclerosis or basilar aneurysm. There may also be a dull persistent facial pain between paroxysms.

Trigeminal neuralgia usually responds to anticonvulsants (such as carbamazepine, valproate, pregabalin etc.) and to various procedures to ablate pain fibres in the trigeminal ganglion, or to relieve vascular cross-compression of the affected trigeminal nerve (Janetta procedure). Unfortunately, by contrast, SUNCT/SUNA is notoriously refractory to treatment, although recently it has been reported that the syndrome may respond to intravenous lidocaine. This issue is discussed further in Chapter 7 (see p. 309).

CASE 227: SUNCT (WITHOUT THE T!)

A 51-year-old woman gave a 10-year history of head pains. Although history taking was a little challenging, she described one particular headache type that varied considerably in its frequency. At the first consultation, she described having had 10 or more attacks per hour, of pain lasting from a few seconds to a minute. It would start in the right occipital region and radiate to the right frontal region as a severe electric shock or stabbing sensation. There was no nausea, photophobia, or phonophobia and no aggravation of pain with movement. During the attacks, she would experience right-sided eye watering and right-sided ptosis without conjunctival injection, periorbital swelling, or rhinorrhea. Neck movements could trigger these attacks but light touch did not. The longest interval she had enjoyed without pain had been only a matter of hours over the ten years.

She had tried indomethacin 25 mg three times daily, which had helped for perhaps three days only. Carbamazepine did not affect the headache, but did reduce and almost eliminate the cranial autonomic symptoms. There was no family history of headache. She was a nonsmoker and did not drink alcohol. Examination was normal apart from marked right greater occipital nerve tenderness, and pain with eye watering could be triggered from that point.

SYMPTOMATIC MIGRAINE

We do not intend to discuss the many causes of secondary headache in this book, because our purpose is to examine the migraine mechanism and its manifestations. However, specific diseases and pathologies can occasionally cause the symptoms of migraine. Symptomatic migraine is defined under IHC-2 as "migraine-like headache secondary to other diseases." This may result from:

- Provocation of the migraine mechanism by a disease or disorder, for example, patients who develop platelet abnormalities
- Cerebral pathology in regions contiguous with or connected to the anatomical structures involved in the migraine mechanism (brain stem strokes, cerebral tumors, vascular malformations, etc.)
- Diseases involving intracranial or extracranial blood vessels, resulting in "vascular" headache (e.g., giant cell arteritis, arterial dissection, and cerebral venous thrombosis)

- Genetic disorders such as mitochondrial encephalopathy, lactic acidosis, and stroke-like episodes (MELAS) and cerebral autosomal dominant arteriopathy with subcortical infarcts and leukoencephalopathy (CADASIL) in which "migraine" is a constituent, as discussed in Chapter 4.

We will argue in Chapter 6 that the archetypical genetically determined "migraine" syndrome FHM should perhaps also be considered as a form of symptomatic migraine, because its pathogenesis and much of its symptomatology is different from typical primary headaches.

Platelet Disorders

In our experience, the most common cause of symptomatic migraine is platelet dysfunction. The early observations concerning the importance of platelets and serotonin in migraine pathogenesis were discussed in Chapter 1, and the possible involvement of platelets in migraineurs with right-to-left intracardiac shunts, migrainous infarction, and "migrainous TIAs" was considered in Chapter 4. In summary, the evidence is as follows:

- During a migraine attack, the concentration of serotonin in blood (platelets) falls. This phenomenon is apparently specific to migraine attacks and is not seen in other "stressful" conditions.
- Consequently, there is an increase in the urinary excretion of the serotonin metabolite 5-hydroxyindole acetic acid (5-HIAA) during a migraine attack.
- Intravenous infusion of serotonin relieves migraine headache, compatible with a deficiency of 5-HT activity at receptors involved in the headache mechanism, as discussed in Chapter 2.
- Migraineurs have lower levels of platelet (blood) 5-HT, reflecting reduced platelet 5-HT uptake kinetics into platelets, but have increased levels of platelet ADP and increased sensitivity to factors that precipitate the platelet-release mechanism.
- Platelets from migraineurs seem to exhibit a persistent state of increased activation and hyperaggregability when compared to that of nonmigraineurs. This does not affect the coagulability of the blood as measured in vitro, but platelet activation and increased aggregation might be important at a microvascular level in the cerebral circulation.

In Chapter 1, we noted that Damasio and Beck reported a number of patients who developed migraine in apparent conjunction with thrombocytopenia, and seemed especially likely to have migraine attacks at times when their platelets were reduced as a result of autoimmune destruction (42). We too have encountered patients whose migraine attacks seemed to be related to platelet abnormalities; but in our experience, the association has been particularly strong with essential thrombocythemia.

In the following cases, the normal upper limit for platelets is $440 \times 10^9/\text{L}$.

CASE 228: MIGRAINE AND ESSENTIAL THROMBOCYTHEMIA

A 55-year-old man was referred by hematologists with a three-year history of essential thrombocythemia, during which he had begun to experience stereotyped neurological events. These had first comprised a visual aura of "jagged lines" across the visual fields, which were particularly vivid if he closed his eyes. These attacks were later replaced by episodes of vertical splitting diplopia and ataxia that typically evolved over some five minutes. Just prior to consultation, he had three such attacks on consecutive days, and in one episode he also experienced paresthesiae affecting the mouth, tongue, and lips prior to the diplopia. None of these events were associated with headache or other migrainous symptoms, and he had no previous or family history of migraine. His platelet count was stable at around 748 to 791, and his MRI brain scan and MRA showed no abnormalities. He was treated with aspirin and had no further attacks.

CASE 229: MIGRAINE AND ESSENTIAL THROMBOCYTHEMIA

A 52-year-old man began to experience occipitofrontal headaches with associated nausea. Routine investigation revealed a persistent thrombocythemia, with platelet counts consistently in excess of 1000. He was treated successfully with anagrelide. The platelet count returned to normal, the headaches resolved completely, and the drug was discontinued. Some three years later, he suddenly developed a further attack of frontal headache and nausea. CT brain scan was normal but his platelet count was 1285. The anagrelide was restarted, together with aspirin. The platelet count gradually fell, but during this period he continued to have recurrent, nonspecific headaches with nausea. A year later, while his platelet count was still in excess of 700, he presented with a series of "transient ischemic attacks." At first, he suddenly had difficulty talking on his mobile phone. As this improved, he developed a pounding headache that persisted for two hours, followed by some right-sided weakness and paresthesiae. He recovered completely. Three days later, he awoke with a further severe pounding headache and nausea. CT brain scan was again normal, and he recovered fully after two days. But two days after recovery, he began to have episodic sensory disturbances in either hand or arm followed by a left-sided sensorimotor disturbance that lasted 15 minutes. Extracranial ultrasound studies were normal but MRI brain scan (Fig. 2) revealed widespread white matter lesions, considered "vascular" in origin. At this point, his platelet count was 1247. The dose of anagrelide was increased and his platelet count fell. On follow-up six months later, he indicated that the episodes of sensory disturbance had ceased and he had only very occasional non-specific headaches.

CASE 230: MIGRAINOUS INFARCTION IN FAMILIAL ESSENTIAL THROMBOCYTHEMIA

A 36-year-old man was screened because several members of his family had been found to have myeloproliferative disorders, notably thrombocythemia. He too was found to have thrombocythemia (platelet count 528), but at this point he was largely asymptomatic, although he did suffer recurrent "stress headaches," and his sister with the disorder had severe migraine attacks.

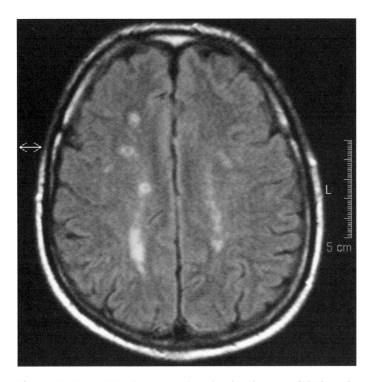

Figure 2 Case 229. Symptomatic migraine in essential thrombocythaemia. T2-weighted MRI brain scan showing extensive vascular white matter hyperintensities.

No treatment was instituted, but two years later he suddenly suffered a severe frontal headache, resulting in hospitalization. CT brain scan was normal. He was started on aspirin and anagrelide. The introduction of anagrelide coincided with a marked increase in the frequency and severity of the headaches (a recognized complication of the drug), and there was no improvement in the platelet count. He eventually developed CDH, with frequent episodes of typical MO. The CDH largely resolved when the anagrelide was withdrawn, but the migraine attacks continued and on some occasions were associated with visual auras. He continued to have frequent migraines, and two years later he suffered an episode of acute vertigo associated with severe headache, nausea, and vomiting during one of the attacks. MRI brain scan showed a left posterior cerebral infarct (Fig. 3), and he subsequently suffered recurrent episodes of migrainous vertigo. It was considered that the migraines and the strokes were the result of the continuing thrombocythemia and he was started on hydroxyurea. The platelet count gradually fell to normal and the migraine and migrainous vertigo attacks became much less frequent and severe.

CASE 231: AGGRAVATION OF MIGRAINE BY ESSENTIAL THROMBOCYTHEMIA

A 46-year-old woman was referred for management of her migraine attacks. She had a long history of mild and occasional MO, but she had recently begun to develop severe attacks with visual aura, and also acephalalgic visual and right hemisensory

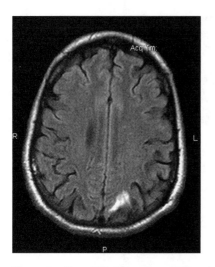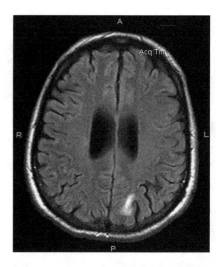

Figure 3   Case 230. Migrainous infarction due to symptomatic migraine in a patient with familial essential thrombocythaemia. MRI brain scan showing left posterior cerebral territory cortical infarction.

auras. Imaging and extracranial ultrasound studies were normal, but her platelet count was increased at 811. Investigations confirmed essential thrombocythemia. She was treated with alpha-interferon and aspirin, together with pizotifen 1.5 mg nocte. The platelet count returned to normal and the attacks of migraine headache and auras ceased completely for a protracted period. On inquiry 10 years later, her platelet count had remained normal but she had experienced further attacks of MA, although infrequently.

Extracranial Vascular Disease

It is well known that arterial dissection can cause severe headache. What is less well appreciated is that such headache can have the features of "migraine" (43). The cause of spontaneous dissection is unclear and is probably heterogeneous, but interestingly, an association with migraine has been reported recently (44). Headache with migrainous or vascular features can also occur in giant cell (cranial) arteritis. Could the observations concerning endothelin-1 and migraine pathogenesis noted in Chapter 2 be a unifying factor in these syndromes (see p. 169)?

Intracranial Vascular Disease

There are a number of reports of brainstem lesions, such as strokes, that have seemingly triggered migraine attacks because of their anatomical location (see p. 250), and we will describe a further instance of this in Chapter 6 (Case 254, see p. 273). Migraine-like headaches can also be a feature of intracranial vascular abnormalities in sites remote from the migraine generator, and it can be difficult to diagnose these if there is a previous history of primary headache.

Cerebral venous thrombosis seems to be the most common of these pathologies. This is being diagnosed more frequently because MRI imaging and MR venography has become commonplace. It is widely known that this condition is a cause of intracranial hypertension (benign intracranial hypertension, pseudotumor cerebri) and can also be an occasional complication of pregnancy, but it is now evident that it can also result from a range of relatively common coagulopathies such as Factor V Leiden deficiency, immunological disorders such as antiphospholipid syndrome, and in Behçet's disease. It can also be a consequence of altered cerebrospinal fluid dynamics in spontaneous and iatrogenic intracranial hypotension (post-lumbar puncture headache). The classical features of cerebral venous thrombosis are well known, but neuroimaging has recently shown that it can present with headache alone, both as a thunderclap headache and as "migraine" (45,46).

CASE 232: VENOUS SINUS THROMBOSIS

A 54-year-old woman awoke with a tingling sensation down the left side, several days prior to being seen. This was soon associated with a mild headache and nausea, which was improving by the time of consultation. She had suffered MA 20 years previously, and then MO a few times a year since then. Her mother, son, and daughter reported being migraine sufferers. Neurological examination was normal. Prolonged aura was suspected, but MRI brain scan showed a localized venous thrombosis involving the right parietal cortical vein and part of the superior sagittal sinus.

At review two months later, she was much improved. She had had two further migraine attacks. Repeat MRI imaging showed significant resolution of the thrombosis.

Symptoms suggestive of migraine can also be features of arteriovenous malformations (AVM) and other intracranial vascular abnormalities.

CASE 233: ARTERIOVENOUS MALFORMATION

A 27-year-old woman presented with a four-year history of intermittent, stereotyped symptoms. She would experience paresthesiae evolving over 10 minutes, beginning in the left hand and spreading up the arm to the face, the left side of tongue, and throat but sparing the leg. This would persist for another 10 minutes or so before gradually resolving. There was no associated weakness or headache with these events but she had a long previous history of recurrent, severe, throbbing headaches associated with visual blurring and sometimes numbness around the tongue but without associated nausea, vomiting, or photophobia. Sometimes, these headache attacks could be triggered by exposure to strong odors. Three years previously, one of these severe headaches had been associated with acute ataxia, and just prior to presentation, she had a further attack with ataxia, with a strange pulling feeling on the left side of her face. She then became confused and was found wandering around the house, evidently confused and talking incoherently. There was no previous or family history of note and examination showed no focal abnormalities. CT brain scan showed a large right-sided parietal AVM with associated hematoma.

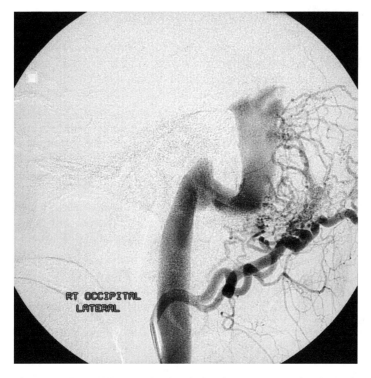

Figure 4 Case 234. Vascular headache due to Type 1 dural arteriovenous fistula. Selective right external carotid arteriogram.

CASE 234: DURAL AV FISTULA

A 37-year-old woman was referred with a two-month history of pain and tenderness in the right mastoid area. She had a long history of non-disabling MO occurring about three times monthly, and the new symptom had developed during an otherwise typical attack. However, on this occasion the discomfort persisted. It was worse on waking, and when severe she would feel nauseous. She subsequently developed pulsatile tinnitus localized to the right ear. On examination, there was a systolic bruit over the right mastoid. MRA and subsequent angiography confirmed a Type 1 dural AVM communicating with the sigmoid sinus (Fig. 4). The general view is that fistulas of this type do not require endovascular closure and often close spontaneously, and no specific treatment was instituted apart from occasional use of analgesics. On inquiry a year later, her headaches continued but were much less frequent or troublesome.

Structural Intracranial Disease

Headache with migrainous features or with symptoms of other primary headache syndromes can rarely result from structural intracranial disease. As we will discuss in Chapter 7, space-occupying lesions very rarely cause headache in isolation, and headache is almost never a primary manifestation of an infiltrating malignant parenchymal brain lesion. However, there are always traps for the unwary!

CASE 235: MENINGIOMA

A 49-year-old lady presented with a two-year history of typical MA. The stereotyped attacks would usually begin with a scintillating scotoma in the right hemifield that would migrate to the right and gradually resolve over about half an hour. The aura was followed by headache in the left parietal area, usually associated with nausea and some degree of visual blurring and photophobia. The episodes were infrequent, occurring perhaps once monthly, but more recently she had also had occasional headaches on the right side and particularly in the occipital area, without aura. These new headaches were rather nondescript in character but would last up to a day and were occurring about once weekly. However, they were not disabling and seemed to respond to ibuprofen. There was no previous personal or family history of headache.

She consulted her GP who considered the headaches to "vary from sinus/tension type to migraine". She was referred when the character of the headache seemed to change. One attack lasted three days and varied in site from occipital to frontal. In addition, she complained that for two months she had experienced increasing problems with her memory and concentration, and she had developed menorrhagia. On examination, she had a right upper quadrantianopia and very early papilloedema. An MRI brain scan revealed a very large left-sided tentorial meningioma (Fig. 5). Her symptoms were interpreted as being due to the irritative effects of the tumor adjacent to the occipital cortex triggering the migraine mechanism.

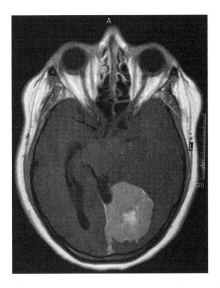 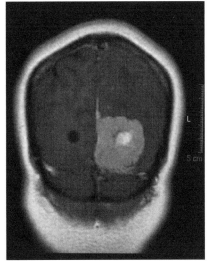

Figure 5 Case 235. Symptomatic migraine due to extra-axial tumor. T1-weighted MRI scans showing a large left-sided tentorial meningioma, with mass effect.

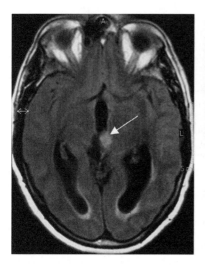 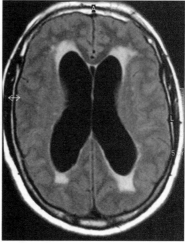

Figure 6 Case 236. Symptomatic migraine due to intraventicular lesion. FLAIR MRI brain scan. There is dilatation of the lateral and third ventricles with marked periventricular oedema. There is a 1.2 cm nodule in the left wall of the third ventricle causing displacement and distortion (*arrow*). The appearances suggest a thalamic hamartoma.

CASE 236: THIRD VENTRICULAR TUMOR

A 59-year-old man gave a history of two forms of stereotyped events over the previous year. The first comprised headaches in the frontal region that would develop insidiously and then resolve after a few minutes, to be followed by a bright halo of light in the right hemifield. This had a jagged edge and would migrate to the left over about five minutes before resolving. There was no associated nausea or vomiting. The other form comprised episodic dizziness and light-headedness precipitated by standing and relieved by sitting or lying. More recently, this symptom had worsened and he would seem mildly ataxic with the events. On occasions, the headache would follow such a dizzy spell, and at the end of the event, he would feel the need to micturate. On examination when asymptomatic, the only abnormality was mild papilloedema.

CT brain scan revealed mildly dilated lateral and third ventricles, whereas the fourth ventricle was normal. An MRI brain scan (Fig. 6) demonstrated obstructive hydrocephalus due to a tumor in the wall of the third ventricle close to the origin of the aqueduct. He became asymptomatic following third ventriculostomy. CSF studies for tumor markers and cytology were negative. The lesion was technically difficult to biopsy, and the decision was made to follow an expectant course. On follow-up over two years, he remained asymptomatic and there was no significant change in the lesion on serial imaging.

CASE 237: COLLOID CYST OF THE THIRD VENTRICLE

A 36-year-old man suddenly developed a headache one afternoon. The next morning on awakening, the headache was excruciating and he vomited, but struggled into work. The headache eventually subsided over a day or so, but then recurred, with nausea but no vomiting. This fluctuating pattern then continued. He also noted ''jagged lines'' across his visual fields from time to time during the attacks.

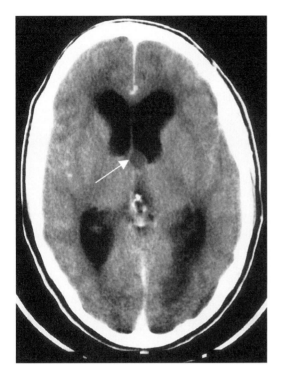

Figure 7 Case 237. Symptomatic migraine due to intraventicular lesion. Computed tomography brain scan, showing almost isodense colloid cyst at the foramen of Munro, and moderate hydrocephalus.

He had a previous history of typical MO dating from childhood, and there was a strong family history of migraine. In the previous two months, he had also woken some mornings with nondescript headaches that he had attributed to "hangover." Seven years previously, while abroad, he had awoken with a crushing headache with nausea and vomiting, and had been admitted to a local hospital. He could not recall precisely what had transpired but was told that he had "encephalitis."

Examination was entirely normal. A routine MRI scan was requested but in the interim, his condition deteriorated, and he was admitted as an emergency. CT brain scan demonstrated a colloid cyst of the third ventricle obstructing the foramen of Munro, with early hydrocephalus (Fig. 7). This was decompressed and marsupialized successfully by endoscopy. His acute symptoms resolved but he continued to have occasional migraine attacks, as before.

CASE 238: THALAMIC TUMOR CAUSING "STATUS MIGRAINOSUS"

A 27-year-old man presented with four-week history of persistent unilateral throbbing headache. The pain was localised to the left peri-orbital region, aggravated by movement, and associated with nausea and vomiting, photophobia and phonophobia. The patient was afebrile. There was no past history suggestive of migraine or any other headache syndrome and no family history of headaches. He was treated

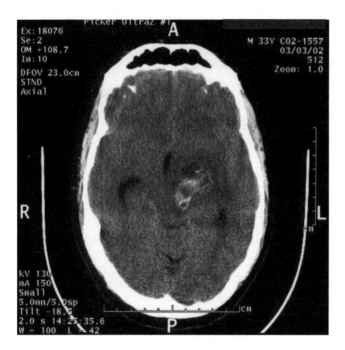

Figure 8 Case 238. Symptomatic migraine due to intra-axial tumor. Computed tomography brain scan showing left-sided hemorrhagic thalamic lesion.

with analgesics and anti-inflammatory drugs without benefit. The pain was so severe that his GP eventually gave him morphine, again without relief. He looked unwell and dehydrated. Examination was difficult because any movement of the head aggravated the pain, but there was no focal neurological abnormality and in particular, no evidence of papilloedema. The patient was admitted as an emergency for intravenous fluids and bed rest, and was started on sumatriptan 6 mg subcutaneously. He made a dramatic recovery within two hours. The headache settled almost completely and he asked to be discharged home.

The clinical presentation and the rapid response to sumatriptan suggested that the likely diagnosis was status migrainosus but CT brain scan showed a left-sided thalamic tumor, with minor hemorrhage extending down to the third ventricle in the region of the periventricular gray matter (Fig. 8).

In this instance, the typical migraine without aura symptoms presumably resulted from activation of key structures involved in the migraine mechanism, such as the periaqueductal gray matter. This association was first reported over 20 years ago in relation to deep brain stimulation in that area (see p. 244).

Migraine in Genetic Disorders

Familial hemiplegic migraine (FHM) is considered the prime exemplar of migraine due to a single gene abnormality. Although this disorder is cited as evidence of the likely primacy of genetic factors in migraine pathogenesis, the condition is so unusual by comparison to migraine in general that we will argue in Chapter 6 that it would be more appropriate to consider it as a form of symptomatic migraine, along with other genetic diseases in which migraine can be a feature. These include CADASIL and MELAS. A common feature of the migraine syndrome of all these genetic disorders is the high prevalence of aura symptoms, sometimes "atypical," suggesting major cortical involvement in pathogenesis.

Cerebral Autosomal Dominant Arteriopathy with Subcortical Infarcts and Leukoencephalopathy

CADASIL is an autosomal dominant disease characterized by strokes or stroke-like episodes, dementia and neuropsychiatric syndromes. Migraine, almost always with aura, is a cardinal symptom. Indeed, it may be the only manifestation and typically develops at least a decade before the onset of clinical strokes (47). The disease is caused by mutations in the *notch 3* gene at 19p13 (a "hot spot" for migraine genes, as noted in Chapter 2). *Notch 3* is expressed exclusively in the smooth muscle cells of small- and medium-sized blood vessels, and defective function of the gene appears to affect vasoreactivity, leading to progressive multifocal ischemia (48). We also noted in Chapter 4 that the prevalence of patent foramen ovale seems even higher in this condition than in idiopathic MA.

The disease causes characteristic accumulations of granular osmiophilic material within the basement membrane surrounding pericytes and smooth muscle cells of blood vessels, a disease-specific feature that can be seen readily on skin biopsy (49). The type and distribution of MRI scan abnormalities may be strongly suggestive of the diagnosis, even in asymptomatic individuals. These lesions include white matter infarcts and more confluent ischemic changes, seen as high signal intensities on T2-weighted images, that tend to be particularly prominent in the subcortical white matter of the frontal and temporal lobes, sparing the inferior surfaces and the occipital cortex. Lesions are also common in the deep gray nuclei of the basal ganglia and in the brain stem (50,51).

CADASIL is probably underdiagnosed. White matter lesions have a wide differential including multiple sclerosis, small vessel ischemia, and vasculitis. Knowledge of the typical distribution of such lesions in different conditions is important (52). The diagnosis may be suspected on the basis of clinical features and MRI scan findings but skin biopsy findings are diagnostic, although lymphocyte DNA analysis is increasingly available.

CASE 239: CEREBRAL AUTOSOMAL DOMINANT ARTERIOPATHY WITH SUBCORTICAL INFARCTS AND LEUKOENCEPHALOPATHY
A 33-year-old man was referred for advice on the management of his migraine with aura, which he had suffered for 10 years. His attacks would begin with moderate

(A)

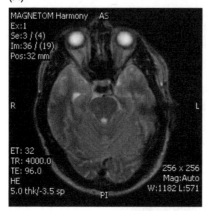

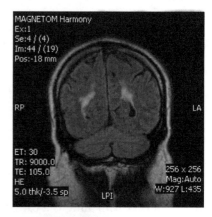

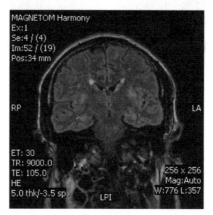

(B)

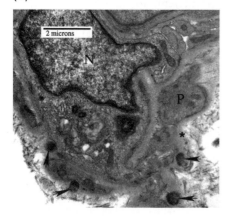

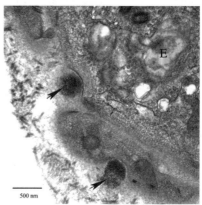

Figure 9   (*Caption on facing page*)

dysphasia followed by tingling in one or other hand that would slowly progress up the arm. These symptoms lasted less than an hour. As they eased, he would develop a very severe bifrontal headache with nausea, photo and phonophobia, and he would retreat to a quiet, darkened room. These attacks had occurred only once or twice a year, but just before referral, he had experienced a cluster of attacks for five consecutive days. His mother, sister and maternal uncle all suffered from "bad migraine" and he was aware that his mother at least had similar aura symptoms. His mother and maternal aunt had also suffered strokes at any early age. MRI brain scan showed extensive periventricular hyperintensities with some anterior temporal involvement (Fig. 9A) and skin biopsy showed the characteristic granular, electron dense osmiophilic deposits diagnostic of CADASIL (Fig. 9B)

Mitochondrial Encephalopathy, Lactic Acidosis, and Stroke-Like Episodes

As discussed in Chapter 4, strokes and stroke-like episodes may be complications of the migraine mechanism, particularly in young people. MELAS is a mitochondrial disease, most commonly due to a mitochondrial DNA (mtDNA) point mutation in the mitochondrial leucine transfer RNA gene. A full discussion of this complex disease is beyond the scope of this book, but a syndrome of migraine-like headache attacks, seizures, and strokes that do not conform to single vascular territories, particularly in the posterior circulation, are classical manifestations. MRI findings, lactic acidosis, and typical changes of mitochondrial disease on muscle biopsy are usually diagnostic, and the culpable mutation can usually be identified by mtDNA analysis. Occasionally, migraine can be the presenting feature (53).

CASE 240: MELAS
A 24-year-old woman presented to a local hospital with malaise, drowsiness, headache, nausea, and vomiting. She had a mild degree of mental handicap dating from childhood and had suffered seizures between age seven and nine, treated with carbamazepine. She was known to have polycystic ovary disease, and two years previously, had developed insulin-dependent diabetes. She had also suffered occasional episodes of headache with nausea and vomiting throughout her life.

Figure 9 (*Continued from previous page*) Case 239. Symptomatic migraine in CADASIL. (**A**) MRI brain scan in a patient with CADASIL. T2-weighted images showing confluent hyperintensities in the frontal and anterior temporal regions. The ischemia tends to spare the inferior surfaces of the brain. (**B**) Electronmicroscopy of skin biopsy. Three of 24 dermal blood vessels showed granular, electron-dense, osmiophilic deposits closely associated with the basal lamina of capillary and arteriolar pericytes. These are diagnostic of the condition. The electron micrographs show the electron-dense deposits (*arrows*) in the basal lamina (*). *Note*: N, nucleus; E, cytoplasm of endothelial cell; P, pericyte. *Abbreviations*: CADASIL, cerebral autosomal dominant arteriopathy with subcortical infarcts and leukoencephalopathy; MRI, magnetic resonance imaging.

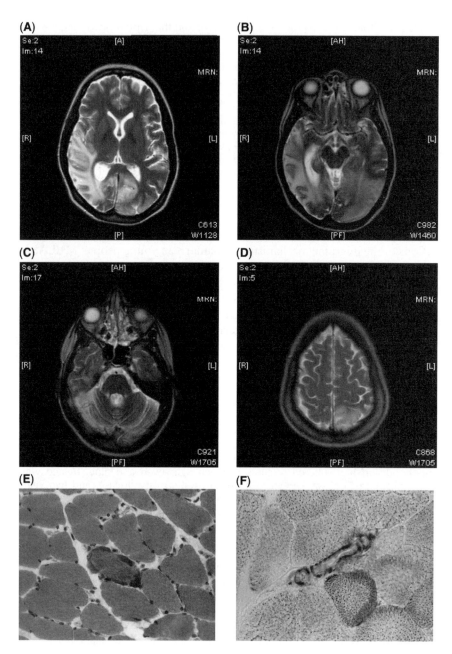

Figure 10   (*Caption on facing page*)

Figure 10 (*Continued from previous page*) Case 240. Symptomatic migraine in mitochondrial encephalopathy, lactic acidosis, and stroke-like episodes (MELAS). Magnetic resonance (MR) images. (**A**) At first presentation, when the patient had left hemifield neglect, MRI brain scan showed high signal abnormality compatible with infarction in the distribution of both the right posterior and middle cerebral arteries. (**B**) She subsequently developed bilateral cortical blindness. The MRI now showed additional infarction in the left posterior cerebral territory. (**C**) and (**D**) Subsequent scans demonstrated further extension of the infarction into the left thalamus, temporo-occipital and parietal regions. [MRA (not shown) demonstrated normal proximal intracranial vessels, but the right calcarine branch had become occluded.] (**E**) Muscle biopsy findings. H & E section from vastus lateralis biopsy, showing subsarcolemmal accumulations of abnormal mitochondria. These would appear red on Gomori trichrome staining—the classical "ragged red" fibers of mitochondrial myopathy. (*See color insert.*) (**F**) Succinate dehydrogenase (SDH) stain. The abnormal mitochondrial accumulations in the walls of endomysial blood vessels are characteristic of MELAS. (*See color insert.*)

On examination, she was hirsute and small in stature. It became apparent that she had visuospatial neglect to the left. CT and subsequently MRI brain scans revealed low density with mass effect compatible with acute infarction in the right temporal and occipital lobes (Fig. 10A).

She was investigated and treated as a "young stroke" patient, but no specific cause was established by the time she had recovered sufficiently to be discharged.

Two months later, she had a further acute illness comprising progressive headache, confusion, and fluctuating visual disturbances, followed a day later by headache, nausea, vomiting, dysphasia, and total loss of vision due to cortical blindness. MRI brain scan now showed infarction in the left occipital lobe in addition. At this point, she was found to have significantly raised lactate levels in blood and CSF. A muscle biopsy revealed typical features of mitochondrial disease (Fig. 10B) and she was subsequently shown to have the common A3243 tRNA Leu mtDNA mutation in blood, urinary epithelial cells, and muscle.

In this chapter, we have considered the attempts made to introduce a conceptual framework for the diagnosis of primary headache syndromes. This has proved invaluable for headache research and, in particular, for defining patients likely to respond to one form of treatment rather than to another. However, it must always be borne in mind that the diagnosis of primary headache is by definition, one of exclusion. In the next chapter, we will consider the issue of whether these primary syndromes are truly distinct entities or different manifestations of a single process.

REFERENCES

1. Headache Classification Subcommittee of the International Headache Society. The International Classification of Headache Disorders 2nd ed. 2004. Cephalalgia 2004; 24(suppl 1):1–160.

2. Eriksen MK, Thomsen LL, Olesen J. Sensitivity and specificity of the new international diagnostic criteria for migraine with aura. J Neurol Neurosurg Psychiatr 2005; 76:212–217.

3. Bahra A, May A, Goadsby PJ. Cluster headache: a prospective study with diagnostic implications. Neurology 2000; 58:354–361.

4. Kunkle EC, Pfeiffer JB Jr, Wilhoit WM, et al. Recurrent brief headache in 'cluster' pattern. Trans Am Neurol Assoc 1952; 85:75–79.

5. Isler H. Episodic cluster headache from a textbook of 1745: Van Swieten's classic description. Cephalalgia 1993; 13:172–174.

6. Sjaastad O. So called "tension headache:" a term in need of revision? Curr Med Res Opin 1980; 6:41–54.

7. Olesen J. IHS Classification: present and future. Cephalalgia 1993; 13(suppl 12): 94.

8. Friedman A. Ad Hoc Committee on the Classification of Headache of the National Institutes for Health. J Am Med Assoc 1962; 179:717–718.

9. Vahlquist B. Migraine in children. Int Arch Allergy Appl Immunol 1955; 7: 348–355.

10. Blau JN. Towards a definition of migraine headache. Lancet 1984; i:444–445.

11. Lance JW. Mechanisms and Management of Headache. 4th ed. London: Butterworth Scientific, 1982:122.

12. Lance JW, Zagami AS. Ophthalmoplegic migraine: a recurrent demyelinating neuropathy? Cephalalgia 2001; 21(2):84–89.

13. Maranhao-Filho PA, Martins-Ferreira H, Vincent MB, et al. Sumatriptan blocks spreading depression in isolated chick retina. Cephalalgia 1997; 17: 822–825.

14. Pandit JC, Fritsche P. Permanent monocular blindness and ocular migraine. J R Soc Med 1997; 90:691–692.

15. Killer HE, Forrer A, Flammer J. Retinal vasospasm during an attack of migraine. Retina 2003; 23:253–254.

16. Hedges TR, Lackman RD. Isolated ophthalmic migraine in the differential diagnosis of cerebro-ocular ischaemia. Stroke 1976; 7:379–381.

17. Linn FH, Wijdicks EF, van der Graaf Y, et al Prospective study of sentinel headache in aneurysmal subarachnoid haemorrhage. Lancet 1994; 344: 590–593.

18. Wijdicks EFM, Kerkhoff H, van Gijn J. Long-term follow-up of 71 patients with thunderclap headache mimicking subarachnoid haemorrhage. Lancet 1988; ii:68–70.

19. Hughes PJ, Davies PTG. Exertional Headaches. Clin Sports Med 1990; 2: 37–40.

20. Dalessio DJ. Effort migraine. Headache 1974; 14:53.

21. Wang KC, Fuh JL, Lirng JF, et al. Headache profiles in patients with a dilated cyst of the cavum septi pellucidi. Cephalalgia 2004; 24:867–874.

22. Nightingale S, Williams B. Hindbrain hernia headache. Lancet 1987; I:731–734.

23. Evers S, Lance JW. Primary headache attributed to sexual activity. In: Olesen J, Goadsby PJ, Ramadan, et al. eds. The Headaches. 3rd ed. Philadelphia: Lippincott Williams and Wilkins, 2005:841–845.

24. Fisher CM. Painful states: a neurological commentary. Clin Neurosurg 1984; 31: 32–53.
25. Day JW, Raskin NH. Thunderclap headache: symptom of unruptured cerebral aneurysm. Lancet 1986; ii:1247–1248.
26. Valenca MM, Valenca LPAA, Bordini CA, et al. Cerebral vasospasm and headache during sexual intercourse and masturbatory orgasms. Headache 2004; 44:244–248.
27. Jackson M, Lennox G, Jaspan T, et al. Migraine angiitis precipitated by sex headache and leading to watershed infarction. Cephalalgia 1993; 13:427–430.
28. Odell-Smith R. Ice cream headache. In: Vinken PJ, Bruyn GW, eds. Handbook of Clinical Neurology. Amsterdam: Elsevier, 1968, Vol. 5:188–191.
29. Negoro K, Morimatsu M, Ikuta N, et al. Benign hot bath-related headache. Headache 2000; 40:173–175.
30. Mak W, Tsang KL, Tsoi TH, et al. Bath-related headache. Cephalalgia 2005; 25:191–198.
31. Raskin NH. The hypnic headache syndrome. Headache 1988; 28:534–536.
32. Dodick DW, Mosek AC, Campbell JK. The hypnic ("alarm clock") headache syndrome. Cephalalgia 1998; 18:152–156.
33. Dodick DW. Polysomnography in hypnic headache syndrome. Headache 2000; 40:748–752.
34. Pearce JM. Exploding head syndrome. Lancet 1988; 2(8605):270–271.
35. Raskin NH, Schwartz RK. Ice pick-like pain. Neurology 1980; 21:203–205.
36. Selby G, Lance JW. Observations on 500 cases of migraine and allied vascular headache. J Neurol Neurosurg Psychiat 1960; 23:23–32.
37. Dodick D, Pascual J. Primary stabbing, cough, exertional and thunderclap headaches. In: Olesen J, Goadsby PJ, Ramadan, et al. eds. The Headaches. 3rd ed. Philadelphia: Lippincott Williams and Wilkins, 2005:831–839.
38. Cluster Headache and Related Conditions. In: Olesen J, Goadsby PJ, eds. Oxford: OUP, 1999.
39. May A, Bahra A, Buchel C, et al. Hypothalamic activation in cluster headache attacks. Lancet 1998; 352:275–278.
40. Sprenger T, Boecker H, Tolle TR, et al. Specific activation during a spontaneous cluster headache attack. Neurology 2004; 62:517.
41. Sjaastad O, Dale I. Evidence for a new(?) treatable headache entity. Headache 1974; 14:105–108.
42. Damasio H, Beck D. Migraine, thrombocytopenia and serotonin metabolism. Lancet 1978; I:240–242.
43. Silverman IE, Wityk RJ. Transient migraine-like symptoms with internal carotid artery dissection. Clin Neurol Neurosurg 1998; 100:116–120.
44. Pezzini A, Granella F, Grassi M, et al. History of migraine and the risk of spontaneous cervical artery dissection. Cephalalgia 2005; 25:575–580.
45. De Bruijn SF, Stam J, Kappelle LJ. Thunderclap headache as first symptom of cerebral venous sinus thrombosis. CVST Study Group. Lancet 1996; 348:1623–1625.
46. Slooter AJ, Ramos LM, Kappelle LJ. Migraine-like headache as the presenting symptom of cerebral venous sinus thrombosis. J Neurol 2002; 249:775–776.

47. Vahedi K, Chabriat H, Levy C, et al. Migraine with aura and brain magnetic resonance imaging abnormalities in patients with CADASIL. Arch Neurol 2004; 61:1237–1240.

48. Lacombe P, Oligo C, Domenga V, et al. Impaired cerebral vasoreactivity in a transgenic mouse model of cerebral autosomal dominant arteriopathy with subcortical infarcts and leucoencephalopathy arteriopathy. Stroke 2005; 36:1053–1058.

49. Brulin P, Godfraind C, Leteurtre E, et al. Morphometric analysis of ultrastructural vascular changes in CADASIL: analysis of 50 skin biopsy specimens and pathogenic implications. Acta Neuropathol (Berlin) 2002; 104:241–248.

50. Yousry TA, Seelos K, Mayer M, et al. Characteristic MR lesion pattern and correlation of T1 and T2 lesion volume with neurologic and neuropsychological findings in cerebral autosomal dominant arteriopathy with subcortical infarcts and leucoencephalopathy (CADASIL). Am J Neuroradiol 1999; 20:91–100.

51. Coulthard A, Blank SC, Bushby K, et al. Distribution of cranial MRI abnormalities in patients with symptomatic and subclinical CADASIL. Br J Radiol 2000; 73:256–265.

52. Porter A, Gladstone JP, Dodick DW. Migraine and white matter hyperintensities. Curr Pain Headache Rep 2005; 9:289–229.

53. Ohno K, Isotani E, Hirakawa K. MELAS presenting as a migraine complicated by stroke: case report. Neuroradiology 1997; 39:781–784.

6

Conceptualizing Primary Headache

> A tendency on the part of the nervous centres to the irregular accumulation and discharge of nerve-force to disruptive and uncoordinated action...and the concentration of this tendency in particular localities, or about particular foci will mainly determine the character of the neurosis in question.
> —*Edward Liveing (1873)*

> So common that it is become a proverb as a sign of a more rare and admirable thing that his head did never ake.
> —*Thomas Willis (1668)*

INTRODUCTION

In this book, we have traced the origins of migraine, considered the complex processes underlying the migraine mechanism, and have described the multitude of neurological symptoms, both benign and serious, that can be manifestations of the process. We have also described the many primary headache "variants" that can be encountered, with illustrative case histories from our practices. These observations lead us to propose two very simple principles, which in a sense echo the sentiments of the quotations from Liveing and Willis.

- All primary headache is migraine.
- Everyone has migraine.

In other words, we suggest that *all* the various defined primary headache syndromes are manifestations of a single fundamental process that is inherent in all of us. Such an extreme, even heretical, view can hardly pass unchallenged. Is it a *reductio ad absurdum* or a plausible hypothesis?

259

HOW MANY FORMS OF PRIMARY HEADACHE ARE THERE?

As we noted in Chapter 1, Arateus in the first century A.D. taught that there were but three forms of headache: *heterocrania* (later the Galenic hemicrania, which gradually evolved to "migraine"), *cephalalgia* (briefer, more frequent, but less severe headaches), and *cephalea* (more protracted but milder headaches). One might argue that these relate broadly to today's "big three" problem headaches: migraine; episodic tension-type headache, including "cervicogenic headache" and "sinus" headache; and chronic daily headache, often referred to as "chronic tension headache." By contrast, the present classification of primary headache is much more complex. ICH-2 includes about 40 defined primary headache syndromes (Appendix 1). While it can be argued that this approach is useful, even essential for headache research, are these disorders all really separate entities? Which view approximates more closely to the truth—the simplicity of the ancients or our modern complexity?

Primary Headaches: To Lump or to Split?

The question of whether the various primary headaches represent unique pathophysiologies or simply heterogeneous manifestations of a common mechanism has been debated for decades. The delineation of "migraine" as a distinctive syndrome comprising aura and headache phases was a crucial step. The studies by Wolff and colleagues, discussed in Chapter 1, seemed to confirm the view that migraine was fundamentally a vascular disorder, with aura reflecting intracranial vasoconstriction and headache being due to vasodilatation. As a result, any recurrent and reasonably protracted primary headache that lacked symptoms perceived to be of "vascular" origin were considered not to be migrainous and were described variously as "tension" or "stress" headaches, "muscle contraction" headaches, "sinus" headaches, and so forth, without evidence of such pathogenesis.

The alternative view, that primary headaches represent a continuum, is not new (1,2), although our concept extends the scope of the spectrum beyond "migraine" and "tension headache" to include all primary headaches.

Cady et al. (2) argued persuasively that migraine and tension headache share many characteristics. Either form can be triggered by similar factors; both can have premonitory and aura symptoms, and may be unilateral, focal, or holocranial; and both may be associated with combinations of nausea and photo- or phonophobia. There is also good evidence that either form will respond to triptans if treated sufficiently quickly, before central sensitization has developed (2). As noted previously, there is no particular symptom or symptoms that can reliably distinguish one form of primary headache from another (Table 1).

It is interesting to compare the position of headache, arguably the most common human malady, with that of muscle diseases, which are relatively rare. Prior to 1830, all forms of muscle wasting were thought to be secondary

Table 1 Incidence of Particular Symptoms in Different IHC-2-Classified Primary Headache Syndromes

Headache type	Unilateral (%)	Severe (%)	Nausea or vomiting (%)	Aura (%)	Autonomic (%)	Stabbing (%)
Migraine	61	84	87	20	5	42
Cluster headache	100	100	53	5	100	?
Hemicrania continua	100	73	53	10	73	26
Chronic paroxysmal hemicrania	98	?	14	?	100	?
Chronic tension-type	20	1	53	?	?	?
Episodic tension-type	18	60	?	?	?	?

Source: Young WB, Peres MFP, Rozen TD. Modular headache theory. Cephalagia 2001; 21:842–849.

to the disease of the spinal cord or nerves. The realization that skeletal muscle could be the site of primary disease resulted in the evolution of entirely new fields of clinical and basic sciences. We now recognize dozens of different forms of muscle disease, each defined by unique genetic, immunological, or pathological characteristics. This relatively new science has taught us that:

- Conditions that are phenotypically similar may be caused by wildly different molecular pathologies,
- Very different pathologies and phenotypes can result from identical molecular abnormalities, and
- Very similar phenotypes can result from different genetic abnormalities.

The number of recognized forms of both primary headache and muscle disease has increased over the years. While this is fully justified in the case of muscle disease, because the entities can be clearly differentiated on molecular grounds, the integrity of the different primary headache diagnoses lies far from this ideal. It is now difficult to be entirely confident of a primary muscle disease diagnosis on the basis of clinical assessment alone. Laboratory investigations are paramount. By contrast, a primary headache diagnosis is essentially unverifiable. Just because different types of headaches behave differently or respond to different treatments—even on a habitual basis—it does not necessarily mean that different processes cause them.

As we discuss next, the characteristics of one form of primary headache can overlap with another or the symptoms can transform completely to an alternative headache form. The symptoms may straddle an intermediate position between one headache diagnosis and another or several forms of primary headache can sometimes occur concurrently.

Evidence for Phenotypic Continuity in Primary Headache

Overlaps: We often encounter patients whose symptoms straddle the boundaries of two or even more ICH-2 primary headache forms, and we have described many patients who illustrate this principle throughout this book. We refer to these as *primary headache overlaps*. In its simplest and most common manifestation, this concept applies to the archetypical syndromes of migraine with aura (MA) and migraine without aura (MO). For example, we know that most migraineurs who habitually experience MO will occasionally experience aura in one form or another (not necessarily "typical" aura), and will sometimes have aura without associated headache. Conversely, migraineurs who typically experience MA will often have headaches without aura. While it is possible that the tendency to experience MA rather than MO is genetically determined, twin studies have not clearly demonstrated that the genes underlying these two phenotypes are different (see Chapter 2), and the factors that determine whether an attack will be associated with aura are unclear. Indeed, as we have discussed, there is reasonable evidence that the processes underlying the aura and headache phases of migraine are probably independent.

This principle is particularly well illustrated by the syndrome of hemicrania continua. As discussed in Chapter 5, this is clinically an amalgam of migraine and cluster headache, but is characterized by a rapid and dramatic response to indomethacin in most instances. In keeping with this, recent neuroimaging studies in this condition have shown concurrent activation of both the "migraine generator" sites in the brainstem and also the posterior hypothalamus, as seen in other trigeminal autonomic cephalgias (TACs) (3). Interestingly, like posttraumatic migraine, this syndrome can also be triggered by head injury (4).

Transformation: Some patients also experience *transformation* of their habitual stereotyped primary headache symptoms into another primary headache phenotype at some point in their lives. Perhaps the commonest example of this is the "maturation" of childhood migraine syndromes to more typical phenotypes in adulthood. As we discussed in Chapter 1, Edward Liveing believed that migraine was an exemplar of the "neuroses" (conditions not apparently resulting from defined pathology), and as the quotation from "Megrim" above infers, he noted that one form of "neurosis" could apparently transform into another. Although the interchangeable conditions that he cited included diseases that we now recognize not to have a neurological basis (such as asthma and gout), we might reasonably apply the general notion of "transformations" to the primary headaches themselves. The following cases are illustrative of transformation.

CASE 241: TENSION-TYPE HEADACHE EVOLVING TO MIGRAINE WITHOUT AURA, TO MIGRAINE WITH AURA (ALL WITH CLUSTER PERIODICITY), THEN TO TYPICAL CLUSTER HEADACHE, AND THEN TO SUNCT/SUNA VARIANT

A 42-year-old man developed new onset, recurrent, dull, nonspecific holocranial headaches. These comprised a "tight" feeling over the head, occasionally associated with slight dizziness and nausea. At times he would feel faint during these episodes, and even attended an emergency room on a couple of occasions with presyncopal symptoms. He was under a lot of pressure at work and at home. A diagnosis of tension-type headache was made. These attacks eventually resolved spontaneously. Two years later, he suddenly developed a more intrusive headache problem. These new attacks would begin with nausea followed by severe and exclusively right-sided headache, occasionally throbbing in character, with photophobia and nausea. He could gain some relief by using a cold compress over the affected temple. Again, he would sometimes experience faintness during the attacks. Biochemistry, including screening for pheochromocytoma, was normal and computed tomography (CT) brain scan demonstrated only an innocent arachnoid cyst in the left Sylvian fissure. The following year he presented with similar attacks, but with headache affecting the left side. Occasionally an aura of flashing colored lights and visual blurring would precede these attacks. A diagnosis of MA was made and he was treated with pizotifen and sumatriptan. As with the first headache problem, these attacks resolved completely.

Three years later, he suddenly began to experience a completely new type of headache problem. These attacks would commonly (80% of the time) wake him from sleep (at any time of the night) but could also occur during the day. They comprised severe pain on one side of the face, particularly behind the eye, with ipsilateral epiphora, nasal blockage and swelling, and drooping of the eyelid, together with severe nausea. There was no conjunctival injection. Each attack would last between 25 and 45 minutes and would recur five to nine times per day. The attacks came in clusters: mild attacks on a daily basis for five to eight weeks on one side of the head, then more severe attacks on the other side for a similar period, and then a third series on the first side again. Over the next six years, he suffered six clusters of this type (four of the left and two on the right), each lasting about four to six months, followed by cluster-free periods of 9 to 12 months. This syndrome was diagnosed as cluster headache. Individual attacks responded to subcutaneous sumatriptan, and he was also treated at various times with methysergide, 100% oxygen, and steroids, with variable benefit.

A third pattern of headaches then emerged. Although these headaches had many features of the cluster headache attacks, they occurred almost exclusively during the day and were associated with severe recurrent stabbing pains in the affected eye and lower face, in the manner of trigeminal neuralgia. It was felt that these attacks were more suggestive of SUNCT/SUNA syndrome, although they would occur only up to 10 times daily. They were not particularly responsive to subcutaneous sumatriptan. He was plagued with regular attacks of this type over the next year, but suddenly they stopped spontaneously, and on follow-up, he reported experiencing only occasional twinges of facial pain.

CASE 242: THUNDERCLAP COITAL CEPHALALGIA EVOLVING TO CHRONIC DAILY HEADACHE

A 42-year-old woman developed "the worst headache ever" at climax during sexual intercourse. The pain was located in the right parietal area, and she likened it to a blow to the head. There was no associated nausea, photophobia, meningism, or alteration in consciousness, and although she was very alarmed by the attack, she simply took some analgesics, and the headache gradually receded. Over the next few weeks, however, she began to have recurrent spontaneous headaches of a similar type, associated with scalp tenderness. These would last about an hour, but became progressively more protracted as she began to use increasing amounts of analgesics—which were ineffective. She was eventually admitted with a four-week history of unremitting daily headache. Neuroimaging was normal. The headache persisted despite eliminating the analgesics. Coincidentally, she subsequently underwent an elective laparoscopic bilateral salpingo-oophorectomy. On recovery from the anesthetic, the headache had vanished and never returned.

Many years earlier, she had suffered attacks of MO, which seemed to have been provoked by drinking strong coffee, and stopped when this trigger was avoided.

CASE 243: MIGRAINE WITH AURA EVOLVING TO EPISODIC CLUSTER HEADACHE

A 35-year-old man suffered MA as a teenager. He would get attacks every six months or so and they would last about two days. He could not recall the exact location of the headache. His last attack was at the age of 19. At the age of 29, he started to suffer from episodic cluster headache. He would get attacks every eight months or so, and in the month-long cluster period, he would experience severe left-sided headache lasting about 30 minutes associated with running of the eye ipsilateral to headache. Attacks typically occurred at 2:00 A.M. and 10:00 A.M.

CASE 244: MIGRAINE WITHOUT AURA TRANSFORMS TO MENSTRUAL MIGRAINE, THEN CHRONIC MIGRAINE WITH COITAL CEPHALALGIA

A 34-year-old woman gave a history of headache attacks dating back to childhood. After menarche, these were exclusively related to menstruation. The attacks consisted of a constant frontal and bitemporal headache with photophobia and would usually last about a day. They stopped completely after her first pregnancy and did not start again until a year prior to referral. She described a particularly severe new headache attack in which, on waking, she had developed marked rotatory vertigo and a severe occipitonuchal headache that then persisted for many months to a variable degree. During this period of chronic migraine, she suffered a typical attack of coital cephalalgia superimposed on the background headache She described a severe preorgasmic exacerbation of the ongoing headache in the occipitonuchal area, and then about two minutes after climax, paresthesiae in the left arm that continued for about an hour. Nausea was prominent throughout the attack, which gradually subsided over some two days. She had two further identical coital cephalalgia attacks in the next few weeks. Her mother was a migraineur.

CASE 245: CHILDHOOD MIGRAINE SYNDROME EVOLVING TO MIGRAINE WITHOUT AURA, THEN CHRONIC DAILY HEADACHE WITH IDIOPATHIC STABBING HEADACHES

A 63-year-old woman was referred with a new headache syndrome. She had experienced migraine-related symptoms since childhood, and had a family history of the condition. The first symptom was reflex syncope following trauma, and then she had recurrent vertigo and syncope. This evolved into recurrent but infrequent episodes of MO for many years. These became increasingly frequent after menopause until she had developed chronic daily headache. She then developed a new headache pattern. On a weekly basis, she would wake in the early hours with an excruciating, thumping headache and nausea. In addition, she began to get attacks of sudden stabbing headaches, "like a red-hot needle" shooting through the head causing her to wince. She might experience two or three such stabs per day, two or three times weekly.

CASE 246: MIGRAINE TRANSFORMS TO "CLUSTER HEADACHE"

A 76-year-old woman presented with recurrence of episodic headache. She had first suffered occasional headaches at about the age of 16. These attacks were nearly always left sided, with photophobia, nausea, and vomiting but without aura. They would last several hours. They ceased completely following the birth of her first child. However, some 20 years prior to consultation, at around the menopause, she began to be troubled again. However, these later attacks were different both in terms of symptoms and in terms of chronology. They would occur about three times weekly and were highly stereotyped. They would wake her from sleep at around 3 am and were invariably left sided. During each event, she would experience ipsilateral nasal blockage and sometimes discharge, and during one particularly severe attack, she developed ipsilateral ptosis. The attacks were not associated with nausea or vomiting, and she would typically pace the floor during the attack. A grandson suffered from similar attacks, but there was no other family history.

CASE 247: MIGRAINE TRANSFORMS TO HEMICRANIA CONTINUA

A 32-year-old man presented with a change in his habitual headache pattern. He had suffered typical MO attacks about three times a year from the age of 11. The headache was always right sided, associated with nausea and photophobia, and usually lasted one to two days. He was later prescribed sumatriptan, which settled the headache rapidly.

In the two years before consultation, he began to experience a new pattern of symptoms. Again these were exclusively right sided but generally more severe than the migraine headaches, and, in particular, were associated with ipsilateral conjunctival injection, epiphora, clear discharge from the nostril, and swelling of the eyelids. He also felt that the right cheek was numb. There was little response to sumatriptan, and none to various analgesics and over-the-counter anti-inflammatory drugs. These attacks became progressively more frequent and severe. He consulted his general practitioner, who referred him to an ENT department, with the comment that the condition was "plainly a sinus infection." He was admitted for intravenous administration of antibiotics, which were eventually stopped when the CT scan of his sinuses showed no abnormality. A local neurologist diagnosed cluster headache and recommended a course of prednisolone, starting at 60 mg daily. This seemed to bring the attack under control temporarily, but the headache and recurrent trigeminal autonomic symptoms returned. He was treated with verapamil without benefit and eventually referred to the Headache Clinic. He was diagnosed with hemicrania continua and obtained immediate relief with indomethacin 25 mg three times daily. Unfortunately, he developed dyspepsia and had to stop the drug. The headache returned but he responded to indomethacin again, with omeprazole cover. The indomethacin was maintained for some three months. Five months later he remained headache free.

CASE 248: MIGRAINE WITHOUT AURA AND REFLEX CEPHALALGIA TRANSFORMS TO IDIOPATHIC STABBING HEADACHES

A 36-year-old man developed recurrent unilateral headaches in his early 30s. These would nearly always affect the right side of the head, and had a throbbing quality consistent with MO, and occured once or twice weekly. Over the year prior to referral, there had been a dramatic change in the quality of the attacks. He now experienced very severe, sharp stabbing pains in the same territory as his previous headaches. Each stab would last 20 to 30 seconds, and would make him wince. The stabs would occur irregularly and without warning several times in a day, on two or three days of each week. On one occasion in the past, he recalled that he had experienced an isolated episode of very severe head pain when someone had poured ice-cold water on his head.

Intermediate Forms: We have already mentioned overlap headache cases, in which symptoms include elements of two or more primary headache types. One also encounters cases with features that are strongly suggestive of a particular primary headache diagnosis but do not strictly fulfill the IHC-2 criteria for that condition. For example, the following patient had attacks that in essence were primary stabbing headaches, except that their duration was atypical.

CASE 249: ATYPICAL PRIMARY STABBING HEADACHE
A 35-year-old year man presented with three attacks of very severe left parietal head pain. On the first occasion, the pain was so severe that he thought he had been shot! It lasted about 30 seconds. The second and most severe attack occurred while he was driving a truck at work. On this occasion, there was a premonition of a build up of pressure in the left side of the head, which became rather numb. The pain became intense and somewhat pulsatile, and he thinks he lost consciousness for about 30 seconds. On recovery, the headache vanished and there were no other sequelae, although he felt frightened. The third attack occurred a few weeks before he was seen in clinic and lasted for only a very short period. On that occasion there was no loss of consciousness. Examination and neuroimaging were normal.

In the following example, the patient had symptoms in individual attacks that were very similar to paroxysmal hemicrania, but the tendency of the attacks to alternate from one side of the head to the other, to occur in clusters, and not to respond to indomethacin, was atypical.

CASE 250: EPISODIC ALTERNATING PAROXYSMAL HEMICRANIA
A 38-year-old woman had suffered recurrent headaches over the previous six years. The attacks occurred in clusters. The first cluster lasted for eight months; the second, two years later, lasted three months and recurred for a similar period the following year. In each of the succeeding two years she had clusters lasting eight months. Between clusters she had no significant headaches. The pain was either right or left sided, never bilateral, and would last 2 to 10 minutes (she had been instructed to time them accurately). She would get 2 to 50 episodes each day. There were no other symptoms, and, in particular, no trigeminal autonomic symptoms. Neurological examination and magnetic resonance imaging (MRI) brain scan were normal. Treatment that was unsuccessful included indomethacin (up to 200 mg/day) and sodium valproate, but she gained almost complete and sustained relief with gabapentin 600 mg t.d.s.

In the next case, the symptoms are again suggestive of paroxysmal hemicrania, but the duration of attack was too brief to conform to the accepted definition of this condition, and yet too protracted to be idiopathic stabbing headache. We presume the head injury was the trigger.

CASE 251: POST-TRAUMATIC HEADACHE WITH CHARACTERISTICS INTERMEDIATE BETWEEN PAROXYSMAL HEMICRANIA AND STABBING HEADACHE

A 36-year-old woman accidentally injured her face. The injury was superficial, but she developed a nosebleed and bilateral periorbital hematoma. There was no change in consciousness, and she did not seek medical attention. Shortly after this, she began to experience recurrent stereotyped headache attacks. She would have severe pain starting around the right eye and spreading to the right parietal and occipital area, lasting 20 seconds at a time, usually two or three times a day, with a maximum of six times, daily. Skull X ray was normal, and the symptoms responded rapidly and completely to indomethacin.

Multiple Primary Headaches: The final category that illustrates the continuity of primary headache phenotypes includes patients who seem to be experiencing two or more different primary headache phenotypes at different times over the same period. For example, primary stabbing headache may be associated with tension-type headache, cluster headache, cervicogenic headache, and in up to two-thirds of patients with hemicrania continua during painful exacerbations (5). The following cases are typical.

CASE 252: COITAL CEPHALALGIA AND STABBING HEADACHES

A 39-year-old woman recalled having occasional episodes of relatively mild pain in the right temple exclusively during sexual intercourse some two years previously. This had occurred on only a few occasions before resolving completely. She then remained headache free until six months before presentation with a new headache syndrome. She had first developed a constant "muzzy" feeling on the right side of her head, and then four months later, started to note two different types of headache. The most severe form had occurred on 30 to 40 occasions. This was a pain behind the right eye and around and behind the ear and temple that evolved over seconds and would then last an hour or two before gradually waning. It had never occurred on the left side. Some form of activity always triggered this pain. It came on every time she had sexual intercourse, as orgasm was approaching. If she did not desist, the pain would become severe and was associated with mild nausea and photophobia. If she lifted weights in the gym, she might feel the same type of pain developing and would have to stop, but the pain never occurred when she coughed, sneezed or, bent over. The second type of headache comprised sharp, brief, stabbing pains perhaps twice a day, again in the right but never the left temple. There was no other past or family history of note. She drank very little alcohol, but had noticed only recently that alcohol could make the headaches worse. Neurological examination and MRI brain scan were normal.

CASE 253: POST-TRAUMATIC MIGRAINE AND STABBING HEADACHES

A 24-year-old woman accidentally fell down some stairs and hit her head on the right side. She lost consciousness briefly and suffered mild postconcussion symptoms, including headache at the site of injury. This evolved into a chronic daily headache, with intermittent throbbing qualities and photophobia. Two weeks later, she began to experience stabbing headaches, again in the area of the injury. She described severe, lancinating pains occurring every five seconds or so throughout the day on the background chronic headache. Pressure over the affected area seemed to help. This headache syndrome gradually eased over several months, with the stabbing headache becoming infrequent.

A New Perspective on Primary Headaches

We suggest that the primary headache syndromes represent coherences of symptoms defined essentially by headache intensity, frequency, duration and the prevalence of trigeminal autonomic reflex activity (Fig. 1). Any patient's primary headache syndrome can be positioned within the continuum. Some headache sufferers will have symptoms that habitually conform to the strict criteria of the IHC-2 definitions, but some will fall outside these confines, and others will move from one coherence to another from time to time.

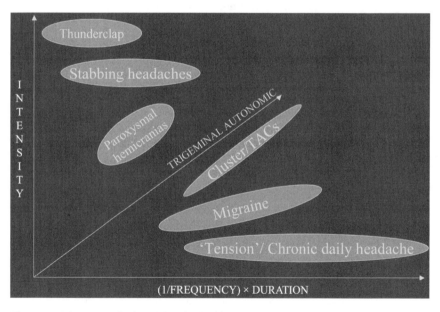

Figure 1 Ideogram of primary headache syndromes viewed as a continuum defined by parameters of headache intensity on the *Y*-axis, inverse frequency and duration on the *X*-axis, and the extent to which manifestations of the trigeminal autonomic reflex are found on the *Z*-axis. Some of the ICHD-2-defined phenotypes are shown, representing coherent aggregations of these defining features. Any patient's primary headache could be depicted on the graph. Thus, thunderclap headache is shown as a very brief but high-intensity pain, while at the other extreme, chronic daily headache is of low intensity, but low frequency or "high/long" duration. Neither have trigeminal autonomic symptoms, unlike trigeminal autonomic cephalgias, and occasionally migraine, which also have *Z*-axis dimensions. *Abbreviation*: TACs, trigeminal autonomic cephalgias.

We further suggest that the primary paroxysmal headaches represent *migraine fragments* within this continuum. Thus, thunderclap headache, idiopathic stabbing headaches, and paroxysmal hemicrania are much more common among migraineurs and those with a family history of migraine. Broadening the argument further, primary "tension-type" headache is typically experienced in the occipitonuchal area, spreading to involve the vertex and parietal regions in a symmetrical fashion, usually without nausea and photophobia. Yet there are many patients who have this quality of headache but find that sometimes it is unilateral, throbbing in quality, and responds to triptans; but the symptoms do not meet the IHC-2 criteria for migraine. It is likely, therefore, that most instances of "tension-type" headache are also migrainous.

Is Headache Quantal?

We noted in Chapter 2 that some authorities believe that migraine has to "run its course." That is, once the migraine mechanism has been triggered, its progress, as judged by the persistence and severity of symptoms, is predetermined unless some intervention terminates it. Thus, *the product of headache severity and the reciprocal of frequency or duration might be a constant for a particular individual but would vary between individuals.* Simply stopping the headache may not be sufficient because the processes underlying the migraine mechanism may still be active. The symptoms can recur, referred to as "rebound," requiring further intervention. However, too frequent use of rescue medication can actually result in prolongation of the attack and the problem of medication overuse headache.

Are Cluster Headache and Other TACs Really Different from Migraine?

A recurring dilemma germane to our argument is the extent to which "cluster headache" is pathophysiologically distinguishable from migraine. In Chapter 5, we documented numerous examples of patients with headaches that seemed to have elements of both migraine and cluster/TAC. It can be argued that in many respects, the similarities between the *symptoms* of migraine and cluster headache are more striking than their differences. Thus, nausea, vomiting, and aura typical of "migraine" are well described in "cluster headache" (6), while symptoms and signs due to activation of the trigeminal autonomic reflex can sometimes be encountered in migraine attacks. Conversely, occasional patients with otherwise typical cluster headache behavior have attacks without autonomic symptomatology. It is certainly true that patients with migraine tend to lie still in quiet dark rooms while cluster patients are typically restless and agitated during attacks, but these features are not the exclusive province of either form of headache.

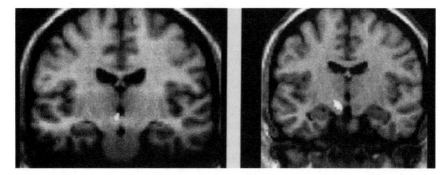

Figure 2   (*See color insert*) Positron emission tomography study showing the activation of the posterior hypothalamus in a patient during a spontaneous attack of cluster headache. Similar activation can also be seen in other forms of TAC. *Source*: With Permission from May A, Bahra A, Buchel C, et al. Hypothalamic activation in cluster headache attacks. Lancet 1998; 352:275–278.

Arguably the most important difference between migraine and cluster headache is not the symptoms but the *periodicity* of cluster attacks, which has been linked to the hypothalamic dysfunction evident from neuroendocrine studies (see Chapter 5). The neuroimaging evidence supports this. Migraine is associated with brainstem and/or cortical activation, while cluster and SUNCT show specific posterior hypothalamic activation (Fig. 2) (7,8). Moreover, the SUNCT syndrome can be a manifestation of pituitary tumors (9). On the other hand, migraine attacks can also cluster in time, and patients with cluster headache can also have typical MA and MO attacks. For example, in the study by Bahra discussed in Chapter 2, a patient with habitual cluster headache developed MO following glyceryl trinitrate (GTN) infusion, with typical brainstem activation on positron emission tomography (PET) (10).

In summary, we believe that rather than being distinct disorders caused by different and specific genetic factors and neurochemical events, the primary headache syndromes are all driven by the same process—the migraine mechanism. We also suggest that, in typical primary headaches, it is the *threshold for activation* of this mechanism rather than the particular primary headache syndrome that is genetically determined. We would suggest, therefore, that the group of rare and unusual genetic disorders that can feature prominent migraine symptoms, particularly aura, such as familial hemiplegic migraine (FHM), cerebral autosomal dominant arteriopathy with subcortical infarcts, and leukoencephalopathy (CADASIL), and migraine associated with mitochondrial disease, should be considered as forms of symptomatic migraine (Chapter 5).

Of course, it is entirely possible that further advances in molecular biology will demonstrate that cluster headache and other forms of TAC— and indeed each and every form of primary headache as defined by

IHC-2—actually are distinct entities, in which case our conjecture will be no better (but no worse) than the many theses that have preceded it!

Reflexes, Modules, and Chaos

How does the migraine mechanism work? In Chapter 2, we discussed the components of the process and noted that the structures involved are integral to normal human brain function. So how do these elements interact to produce primary headaches, and what provokes them to do so? If the migraine mechanism drives all primary headaches, why are there so many different forms, and what determines the habitual syndrome in a particular headache patient? If each syndrome is indeed genetically determined and distinct, this would explain it; but the existence in clinical practice of so many examples of "overlaps," "transformations," and "intermediate forms" of primary headache seems counterintuitive to that argument.

Migraine as a Reflex

As we discussed in Chapter 2, the migraine mechanism can involve up to four distinct phases:

- Premonitory symptoms or prodrome
- Aura
- Headache phase, in which headache severity tends to evolve from mild, to moderate to severe, and may become increasingly lateralized and throbbing in quality, and may be associated with trigeminal autonomic symptoms
- Recovery phase, including resolution of the headache and sometimes recapitulation of premonitory symptoms (*postdrome*)

We could view these phases as components in a complex reflex, comprising a number of simpler reflexes modulated by the antinociceptive pathways. As with all reflexes, the output (symptoms) would be stereotyped— representing the habitual headache pattern—and many sensory inputs would be capable of triggering that reflex. However, factors such as stress and hormones could alter the sensitivity of the reflex pathways and this might at times lead to changes in the activation pattern, resulting in different headache symptoms.

In Chapter 2, we suggested that the symptoms resulting from the activation of the migraine mechanism—primary headaches—might serve a biological purpose in resetting sensory thresholds. The reflex mechanism would be engaged when the nervous system encountered a change in environment (i.e., sensory inputs, internal or externally generated) that exceeded its adaptive capabilities. In support of this concept, it is interesting to note that the *neurological* symptoms associated with "migraine"—auras—tend to be the converse of the aura symptoms of epilepsy: migraine symptoms tend to be "posterior and sensory," and epileptic symptoms are generally "anterior and motor" (Table 2).

Table 2 Comparison of Aura Characteristics in Migraine and Epilepsy

Aura	Migraine	Epilepsy
Visual	++++	+
Somesthetic	+++	+
Dysphasic	++	++
Olfactory	+	+++
Motor	+/−	++++
Epigastric	+/−	++++

All the inputs to the migraine mechanism, centrally from the cortex, thalamus, hypothalamus, and limbic areas, and peripherally from the primary sensory organs, the neck, and vestibular system, converge on the trigeminocervical complex. Activation of this key region results in central sensitization and progressive sensory neuronal windup. This sensitization might account for the initial mild-to-moderate headache, vague neck stiffness, and pericranial muscle tenderness that may be encountered in the early part of some primary headache attacks. If further windup and sensitization occur, the trigeminovascular system might be engaged, resulting in neurogenic inflammation, with resulting "vascular" components to the headache, and further central sensitization by antidromic stimulation via the trigeminal nerve. More aggressive provocation still might result in stimulation of the trigeminal autonomic system, with the development of "cluster headache" symptoms. The duration and severity of any phase could vary and the process could abort at any stage. The clinical phenotype would then be a reflection on the extent of engagement of the different parts of the reflex. For example, if there is no premonitory or aura phase and the headache resolves during the "mild-to-moderate" intensity stage, the attack might be diagnosed as a "tension-type headache." There could also be prolonged activation of this stage, interpreted as "chronic tension headache." Different components of the trigeminocervical system might be sensitized, giving rise to more focal pain, interpreted as "sinus" headache, "cervicogenic" headache, "facial migraine," and so forth.

This concept presupposes a hierarchy of activation sensitivities. Elements are recruited in a linear order, depending on the extent of the provocation. While in some cases these phases would indeed occur in sequence, premonitory and aura phases are experienced in only a minority of typical migraine attacks [much less in our experience than the 70% quoted in some studies (11)], and trigeminal autonomic symptoms are uncommon. On the other hand, the evidence from the GTN activation studies discussed in Chapter 2 does suggest that at least the typical visual aura is relatively difficult to provoke, suggesting a "high activation threshold." Perhaps this is why auras occur less frequently than migraine headache.

Modular Theory

This "linear, threshold-dependent reflex" explanation of the migraine mechanism seems too elementary to explain phenomena such as acephalalgic migraine and other situations in which events occur "out of order." For example, aura can develop during the headache phase (see p. 115). Bill Young and colleagues in Philadelphia (12) proposed that primary headache symptoms were a function of the activation of particular networks of nerve cells and their associated vasculature, which together function as "modules." This concept is in effect an extension into pathophysiology of the regional activation that occurs in normal brain functioning as revealed by functional neuroimaging. During a primary headache attack, several such modules would be activated and the types of modules activated would determine the resulting syndrome. For example, throbbing headache is envisaged as representing the activation of the module comprising the trigeminovascular system, while nausea would result from the activation of the module including the nucleus tractus solitarius. Individual aura phenomena would represent the activation of different cortical modules, either individually or sequentially. As with the reflex concept, the authors suggested that the thresholds for activation of individual modules also vary, again resulting in a hierarchy of headache-related symptoms. As the trigger or input to the migraine mechanism becomes greater, the likelihood of modules with greater activation thresholds being recruited would increase. Differential rates of inhibition from higher pain-control centers may be another factor involved.

The authors suggested that the stereotypy and repetitive nature of most primary headaches is the result of *anatomical and functional links* forged between symptom modules by repeated activation. Some links would be forged more commonly than others; so the elements involved in "migraine" and "tension-type headache" would be the commonest. For example, the strong association between "throbbing headache" and "nausea" might relate to the anatomical proximity of the trigeminal nucleus caudalis and the nucleus tractus solitarius. The following case illustrates this principle to some extent.

CASE 254: STATUS MIGRAINOSUS AND INTRACTABLE VOMITING FOLLOWING BRAINSTEM STROKE

A 77-year-old man with no notable previous history of headache was admitted to a local hospital following the acute onset of vertigo and ataxia, with severe nausea, vomiting, and headache. He had experienced a brief episode of vertigo with diplopia a month earlier but had not sought medical attention. He had a history of mild hypertension on treatment, but no other notable personal or family history. On examination, he was complaining of headache with marked photophobia. He was severely ataxic and unable to stand, dysarthric, and showed bilateral cerebellar signs, much more marked on the left than the right, together with nystagmus on left lateral gaze. A diagnosis of posterior circulation infarction was made. However, initial CT brain scan and screening for sources of thromboembolism were negative. He was transferred to the neurosciences center for further evaluation when he was still suffering continuous headache, nausea, vomiting, and photophobia six weeks after presentation!

MRI brain scan showed multiple infarcts confined to the posterior circulation territory, with a particularly notable lesion in the region of the left vestibular nucleus. Extracranial ultrasound showed an occluded left vertebral artery, and CT angiogram revealed generalized hypoplasia of the posterior circulation, while the anterior circulation and indeed the rest of the brain was entirely normal for age. He was also found to have developed a generalized autonomic failure, with severe postural hypotension, absent sinus arrhythmia and Valsalva response, and loss of pressor response to isometric exercise and performance of mental arithmetic.

The vomiting having shown no response to dopamine receptor blockers (phenothiazines) and only minimal response to odansetron (a $5HT_3$ inhibitor), he was treated with topiramate and steroids. The headache quickly resolved and the vomiting stopped. On review following three months rehabilitation, he was well but remained mildly ataxic. No postural hypotension could be detected.

There was a remarkable concordance between the position of the most prominent infarct in this patient and the area of activation in migraine demonstrated by PET in the recent study by Shazia Afridi, mentioned previously (see p. 98) (Fig. 3). We hypothesized that this infarct provoked status migrainosus and might also have been involved in the genesis of the autonomic failure, being close to autonomic nuclei such as the nucleus tractus solitarius and nucleus ambiguus.

We would note that there would be intrinsic flexibility in this modular system. Modules typically activated in one form of primary headache could be recruited in a different combination to "create" another "classical" primary headache type. Additional or substitute modules could be activated on some occasions, resulting in overlaps or intermediate forms, or the activation links could change dramatically for some reason, resulting in transformations.

Young and colleagues concluded, at the time, that the activation sites demonstrated by functional neuroimaging might represent some of their "modules," but thus far, the number of such sites has actually proved very restricted. In particular, as we noted in Chapter 2, activation of the trigeminocervical complex has not yet been demonstrated by functional neuroimaging.

Migraine and Chaos

The concepts discussed so far are based on linear dynamics, in which the components of the migraine mechanism—the neural networks of the cortex and brainstem—are normally maintained in a state of homeostatic equilibrium. Perturbations such as environmental and endogenous inputs are essentially eliminated by feedback mechanisms. In such systems, an understanding of the individual components allows an understanding of the system as a whole. However, David Kernick has recently pointed out that complex biological systems, such as those underlying the neural networks that drive migraine and epilepsy, almost certainly do not operate in this way. He has

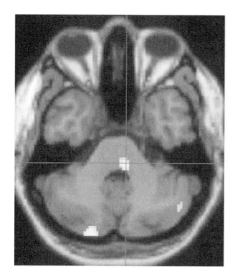
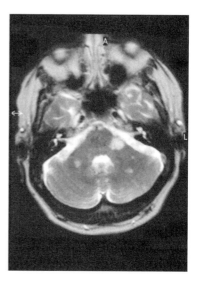

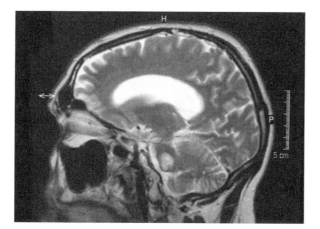

Figure 3 Comparison of the location of brainstem activation in glyceryl trinitrate–triggered migraine in the patient reported by Afridi et al. (see p. 274, *left panel*) and the posterior circulation lesions in Case 254 (*right and lower panels*).

suggested that such behavior might be better described and understood using nonlinear dynamics, the basis of *chaos theory* (13).

In nonlinear systems, there is rarely a simple relationship between cause and effect. Small inputs can lead to large system changes, whereas large inputs may have little impact. The concept of a butterfly fluttering its wings in one part of the world causing a hurricane in another is often quoted, and one can see that Edward Liveing had also grasped this idea from this quotation:

> Megrim... A primary and often hereditary... disposition of the
> nervous system itself... to the irregular accumulation and discharge of the
> nerve-force... a gradually increasing instability to equilibrium in the nervous
> parts: when this reaches a certain point, the balance of forces is liable to be
> upset and the train of paroxysmal phenomena determined by causes in
> themselves totally inadequate to produce such effects—just as a mere scratch
> will shiver to dust a mass of unannealed glass.
>
> — Edward Liveing (1873)

Individual neurons either fire or do not fire depending on the integrated output of excitatory or inhibitory synapses. The complex interactions of the myriads of neurons that together comprise a functional network determine that the overall output cannot be predicted. No one element is in control or has an "overview" of the system, and the information about the system is encoded in a distributed manner involving the interaction of elements at a local level without external direction or the presence of internal control. This property is known as *emergence* and gives such systems the flexibility to adapt and self-organize in response to external challenge. Emergence is a pattern of system behavior that could not have been predicted by an analysis of its component parts. However, such "chaotic" behavior does show patterns that are predictable over time. "Chaotic attractors" operating in various dimensions of time and space determine these patterns, and the number of these attractors determines the complexity of the system. The emergent patterns at elemental level, known as fractals, are mirrored by the system as a whole.

Chaotic behavior is a signature of healthy physiology. For example, the electrocardiogram and electroencephalogram (EEG) show chaotic behavior. Things "go wrong" when the behavior becomes less complex due to pathological or pathophysiological processes that result in periodicity or repetitive activity. For example, aging and sleep result in less complex chaotic EEG activity, and system behavior becomes most simplified in pathological periodic states such as cardiac dysrhythmias and status epilepticus. It has also been reported that the EEG in nocturnal migraine demonstrates a simplification of normal chaotic behavior (14).

Kernick suggests that in health, interrelated neural systems operate within a narrow range of attractor dimensionality, i.e., their complexity is coherent. In migraineurs, the midbrain networks that integrate sensory inputs cannot always accommodate the necessary dimensional range. If certain conditions arise, the gap between the attractor dimensions of sensory integration and cortical control networks becomes too great, resulting in a loss of synchronization and a global transition to a significantly lower dimensional state—a feature of dysfunctional physiological systems, in this context, the migraine phenomenon. This provokes a behavioral response that, in turn, reduces the level of sensory input, restoring the sensory-integrating network to a compatible attractor dimension and resolution of the attack.

This model would explain why migraine is rare at the extremes of age when cortical dimensions are lower and there is less possibility of dimensional incoherence between neural subsystems.

WHAT NEXT?

At present, research continues to focus on understanding the elements of the migraine mechanism, such as the processes underlying aura and the various components of the headache phase. Many questions remain unanswered. For example, can auras other than visual be demonstrated by functional neuroimaging, and will it be possible to demonstrate activation of the trigeminocervical complex, which appears so central to our current understanding of the migraine mechanism? Some parts of the puzzle are falling into place. The confirmation using PET, of the explanation of lateralization of the headache in typical migraine based on the paradigm outlined in Chapter 2, is encouraging. With regard to our hypothesis that all primary headache is migraine, the provocation of "migraine" with typical brainstem activation in a patient with habitual cluster headache, the demonstration that both cluster headache and SUNCT show identical activation sites in the posterior hypothalamus, and that hemicrania continua shows activation characteristics of both migraine and TACs, has been important.

We would like to speculate still further. In Chapter 3, we discussed recent observations that suggest that migrainous vertigo is almost certainly generated in the brainstem. Because vertigo, in this instance, is a migraine aura, we suggested that this might be caused by spreading depression in the brainstem, by analogy to cortical spreading depression. Could it be, therefore, that the brainstem activation typically seen on neuroimaging during migraine attacks reflects this process? The recent demonstration of activation of both the brainstem and occipital cortex during a GTN-triggered attack of migraine with aura (see p. 98) would support this proposition.

Although it is possible that all forms of primary headache might be driven by a common mechanism, it is clear from clinical experience that the different headache syndromes that result respond better to some interventions than others, and that treatments have to be tailored to individual need. This will be the subject of our final chapter.

REFERENCES

1. Featherstone HJ. Migraine and muscle contraction headaches: a continuum. Headache 1985; 25:194–198.
2. Cady R, Schreiber C, Farmer K, Sheftell F. Primary headaches: a convergence hypothesis. Headache 2002; 42:204–216.

3. Matharu MS, Goadsby PJ. Functional brain imaging in hemicrania continua: implications for nosology and pathophysiology. Curr Pain Headache Rep 2005; 9:281–288.
4. Lay CL, Newman LC. Post traumatic hemicrania continua. Headache 1999; 39:275–279.
5. Dodick D, Pascual J. Primary stabbing cough, exertional and thunderclap headaches. In: Olesen J, Goadsby PJ, Ramadan NM, et al. eds. The Headaches. 3rd ed. Philadelphia: Lippincott Williams and Wilkins, 832.
6. Bahra A, May A, Goadsby PJ. Cluster headache: a prospective clinical study with diagnostic implications. Neurology 2002; 58:354–361.
7. May A, Bahra A, Büchel C, et al. Hypothalamic activation in cluster headache attacks. Lancet 1998; 352:275–278.
8. May A, Bahra A, Buchel C, et al. Functional magnetic resonance imaging in spontaneous attacks of SUNCT: Short-lasting neuralgiform headache with conjunctival injection and tearing. Ann Neurol 1999; 46:791–794.
9. Massiou H, Launay JM, Levy C, et al. SUNCT syndrome in two patients with prolactinomas and bromocriptine-induced attacks. Neurology 2002; 58: 1698–1699.
10. Bahra A, Matharu MS, Buchel C, et al. Brainstem activation specific to migraine headache. Lancet 2001; 357(9261):1016–1017.
11. Giffin NJ, Ruggiero L, Lipton RB, et al. Premonitory symptoms in migraine. An electronic diary study. Neurology 2003; 60:935–940.
12. Young WB, Peres MFP, Rozen TD. Modular headache theory. Cephalalgia 2001; 21:842–849.
13. Kernick D. Migraine—new perspectives from chaos theory. Cephalalgia 2005; 25:561–566.
14. Strenge H, Fritzer G, Gőder R, et al. Non linear electroencephalogram dynamics in patients with spontaneous nocturnal migraine attacks. Neurosci Lett 2001; 390:105–108.

7

Management of Migraine

This contumacious and rebellious disease ... deaf to the charms of every
Medicine.

—*Thomas Willis (1672)*

INTRODUCTION

There can be few more rewarding experiences in clinical medicine than
correctly diagnosing and successfully treating a patient with a severe, recurrent and disabling headache problem, particularly when that patient may have
followed previously the all too common "circuit of diagnostic destitution"—
optician, dentist, ENT surgeon, physical therapist, and so forth—without
benefit. On the other hand, there are few more frustrating experiences for a
physician than to be faced with a patient who has headache "all day every
day" that is refractory to each and every intervention. There is nothing to
see or measure, no "tests" to help to understand the basis of the problem.

In this chapter, we will review briefly the history of headache treatments,
examine the burden of headache in the community, and then review current
recommendations for the treatment of the various primary headache syndromes, concluding with a look toward future prospects. Given that we have
advanced the thesis that all primary headaches are "migraine," we will use this
term generically to denote "primary headache" where appropriate.

HISTORICAL BACKGROUND

Ancient Remedies

In Chapter 1, we noted that in prehistoric times, medical treatments were
based largely on magic and exhortations to supernatural forces. This was

also evident in the medicine of the ancient Egyptian civilization, although more rational treatments also evolved based on clinical observation (1). Measures to treat headache often included compresses of various forms, presumably because it was common experience that pressure over the painful area could sometimes help the pain. The Greeks and Romans too, considered their gods important in causing and curing disease, but emphasis was placed on imbalances in bodily "humors" and "vapors," and treatments often involved bleeding and purging.

Civilization moved east after the fall of the Roman Empire. In Persia, one method used to treat headache involved the embedding of cloves of garlic under the skin of the temples to cause suppuration (2)! Even as late as the 13th century, topical headache treatments tended to be the rule. In Italy, sufferers often had a poultice of opium and vinegar placed upon their heads, and the Incas would incise the scalp and drip coca juice into the incision, the cocaine presumably acting as a local anesthetic (3).

In the 17th and 18th centuries, surgical division and ligation of the superficial temporal artery became a popular treatment. Thomas Willis treated his eminent patient Lady Conway (see p. 18) with mercurials, venesection, and an arteriotomy, while William Harvey suggested she should have "opening of the skull." She went to France for the procedure, but the physicians baulked at this and elected to perform "opening of the jugular!"

Gradually, internal medicines became more popular. Coffee was introduced to Oxford in the mid-17th century, and Thomas Willis used caffeine and also the leaves of the feverfew plant (*Tanacetum*) or chrysanthemum (*Parthenium*) to treat headache. Feverfew continues to have its adherents as a migraine treatment and it does appear to be effective (4).

The 19th century saw an increasing emphasis on conservatism in headache treatment, a move away from interventions toward evaluation of sufferers' lifestyles as possible causes. William Gowers wrote (5)

> If any error in mode of life or defect in general health can be traced, the removal of this is the first and most essential step in treatment.

The Evolution of Acute and Prophylactic Treatments

Gowers was one of the first physicians to separate headache treatments into episodic (for acute headaches) and prophylactic measures. He advocated bromide as a prophylaxis, often as part of the famous Gowers' mixture (Fig. 1 and see p. 21) (5), and Indian hemp (marijuana), sedative doses of chloral, or a hypodermic injection of morphia as acute treatments. William Osler favored particularly *cannabis indica*. However, the potency of cannabis preparations was too variable, and individual responses to orally ingested cannabis seemed erratic and unpredictable. Hemp products are insoluble in water and so, with the invention of the hypodermic syringe in the 1850s, which allowed water-soluble drugs to be injected for fast pain

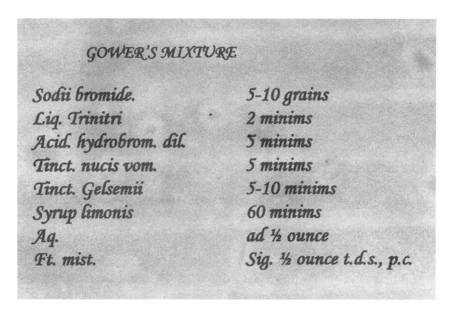

Figure 1 Gowers' mixture. Several modifications of this original formula were produced, including the Charing Cross Hospital formula, which omitted the glyceryl trinitrate!

relief, the use of cannabis for analgesia slowly declined. Osler also noted that antipyrin and phenacetin (the forerunners of acetylsalicyclic acid and acetaminophen) could be effective if given early in the attack.

The early 20th century saw the publication of *Die Migräne* by Flatau (6). This was the most comprehensive book on migraine treatment up to that time but some of the suggested remedies were brutal and sometimes dangerous, and included subcutaneous arsenic injections and treatment with silver nitrate, quinine, nicotine, stramamonium, and other poisons.

Ergot and Its Derivatives

In Chapter 1, we recounted in detail how the rye fungus ergot came to be used to treat migraine headache. *Dihydroergotamine* (DHE) was synthesized by Stoll and Hofmann in 1943 and first used to treat migraine in 1945, by Horton and colleagues (7). A nasal spray version of this drug was approved for use as late as 1997 and was available briefly, as "Migranal" in the United Kingdom, but was withdrawn for commercial reasons. It remains available in the United States.

Serotonin, Its Receptors, and the Development of Triptans

As knowledge of serotonin grew in the 1950s and 1960s, its potential as a key compound in migraine pathophysiology became increasingly appreciated.

The vascular theory of migraine was favored at the time and soon there was an explosion of work on serotonin and platelets in migraine. As discussed in Chapter 1, the triggering of migraine by the administration of reserpine (which releases serotonin from nerve terminals) and the efficacy of methysergide in migraine prophylaxis, first reported in 1959 (8), all helped to provide circumstantial evidence that serotonin played a key role in migraine pathogenesis. Those who supported a neural basis for migraine could nevertheless be consoled with the concept that perhaps platelets were a model for serotonergic neurones!

Over time, more and more types of receptors for serotonin were discovered and their classification became worthy of international meetings of experts (9,10). By about 1980, it seemed reasonable to say that serotonin agonists stopped migraine and serotonin antagonists seemed useful migraine prophylactics. The Holy Grail was to develop a more specific serotonin agonist than ergotamine—one that was more effective and better tolerated, and did not significantly constrict the coronary arteries.

The pharmaceutical giant Glaxo (now part of GlaxoSmithKline) started a development program, led by Pat Humphrey, to discover such a drug (11). We noted in Chapter 1 that the vasoconstrictor activity of serotonin in the cerebral vasculature could not be accounted for in terms of the "two serotonin receptor" model of the time. Humphrey and his colleagues studied numerous modifications of the serotonin molecule in a dog saphenous vein system, a supposed model of the carotid vasculature, and eventually discovered a compound that acted specifically on these vessels. The initial hypothesis was that this compound, GR43175, acted on "shunts" between arteries and veins. This was indeed the basis for Heyck's theory of migraine pathogenesis (see p. 33), but, there is no evidence that such shunts exist in the human cerebral circulation. Nevertheless, the compound proved to be a potent and highly selective $5-HT_{1b}$ and $5-HT_{1d}$ (5-HT, 5-hydroxytryptamine) agonist with selective vasoconstrictor effects in the cerebral circulation. It soon looked a promising acute migraine treatment and Professor Paul Turner, then chairman of the British Pharmacopoeia Sub-committee on Drug Names, invited Humphrey to London to find a name for the compound. Because it worked by mimicking some of the actions of 5-HT, the suffix "triptan" was used to reflect the action on "tryptamine receptors," while "suma" was chosen as a specific prefix for the 5-sulphonamide group of its chemical structure (11). *Sumatriptan*, a new and revolutionary treatment for acute migraine headache was born. Much experimental work followed, using this compound as a tool to better understand the migraine mechanism.

The latter part of the 20th century saw a mushrooming in the number of new migraine treatments. Imigran, the trade name for sumatriptan in the United Kingdom, was available by 1991 and was soon followed by six other triptans. The clinical trial data for these new treatments was of high quality and better than anything that had been produced previously.

New measurement scales for symptoms had been devised and cost effectiveness and quality of treatments were discussed for the first time.

Other Acute Interventions

Along with the development of the triptans, there appeared a number of other drug formulations specifically for migraine. The problem of gastric stasis, and subsequent poor drug absorption during acute attacks, was addressed by a number of companies by using soluble analgesics such as paracetamol or nonsteroidal anti-inflammatory drugs (NSAIDs) such as aspirin, in combination with soluble antiemetics such as metoclopramide. Some of these were only available on prescription but others were available "over the counter" (OTC) to a population of sufferers keen to find better treatments for their attacks. In the United Kingdom, it is likely that triptans will become available OTC in the near future. We will consider this further later.

Development of Prophylactics

By comparison, migraine prophylactic drugs have been relatively slow to develop. Many drugs have been reported to have prophylactic effects in migraine, but for the most part, trials have been inadequate, or the results inconsistent. After methysergide, propranolol, pizotifen, and clonidine were reported to be useful, but clonidine was eventually shown to be ineffective (12). In the United Kingdom, other drugs such as sodium valproate and calcium antagonists are used off-licence, as prophylactics although flunarizine was never licensed here. In 2005, Topamax (topiramate) became the first new migraine prophylactic drug to be licensed in the United Kingdom for many years following large scale trials (13,14). Other anticonvulsants such as lamotrigine have also been found to be helpful (15), and levetiracitam is currently under trial in the United Kingdom.

THE BURDEN OF HEADACHE

The Global Perspective

Having discussed the development of headache treatments, this is perhaps an appropriate point to address the burden of headache in a global context.

In an average week, more than 80% of the normal population experiences one or more troublesome somatic symptoms. The most common of these are headache and fatigue (16). One of our primary contentions is that "everyone has migraine." If this is true, the potential headache burden is obviously enormous. Some large epidemiological studies of headache in the general population report prevalences approaching 100% if the question is posed appropriately: "do you ever have headache?" rather than "do you suffer from headache?" (17).

The prevalence of migraine across the world, is similar (Fig. 2). In Chapter 3, we noted that the prevalence of migraine aura was notably higher in physicians than in the general public, because doctors are more likely to recognize the basis of such symptoms. In another study (18), neurologists (who should know) recorded their one-year and lifetime prevalences of migraine. Of 220 respondents, the respective figures for male neurologists were 34.7% and 46.6%. For male headache specialists (who *really* should know) the figures were 59.3% and 71.9%. The corresponding figures for female neurologists were 58.1% and 62.8% and for female headache specialists, 74.1% and 81.5%. A subsequent study of neurologists showed very similar results (19).

Is this a selection bias or is migraine often unrecognized when experienced by people who are not able to diagnose it in themselves? We would suggest the latter. Headache disorders are certainly under-recognized, underdiagnosed, and undertreated (20). Migraine has the potential to cause significant handicap to sufferers, their families, and society in general. Table 1 shows the World Health Organization (WHO) list of diseases that cause suffering worldwide, and lists migraine as a major cause of disability—in fact above diabetes.

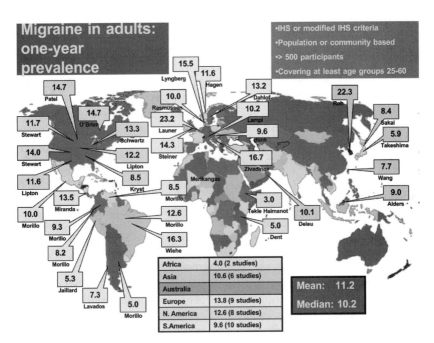

Figure 2 The Scale of the Problem. The 1-year prevalence rates of migraine in population-based studies using IHS criteria (or modified criteria). *Source*: With permission from the Global Campaign to Reduce the Burden of Headache Worldwide, a collaboration between World Health Organization, World Headache Alliance, International Headache Society and European Headache Federation.

Table 1 The Migraine Burden Compared with Other Disease Burdens in the World[a]

Both sexes, all ages	% Total
1. Unipolar depressive disorders	11.9
2. Hearing loss, adult onset	4.6
3. Iron-deficiency anemia	4.5
4. Chronic obstructive pulmonary disease	3.3
5. Alcohol use disorders	3.1
6. Osteoarthritis	3.0
7. Schizophrenia	2.8
8. Falls	2.8
9. Bipolar affective disorders	2.5
10. Asthma	2.1
11. Congenital abnormalities	2.1
12. Perinatal conditions	2.0
13. Alzheimer's and other dementias	2.0
14. Cataracts	1.9
15. Road traffic accidents	1.8
16. Protein-energy malnutrition	1.7
17. Cerebrovascular disease	1.7
18. HIV/AIDS	1.5
19. Migraine	1.4
20. Diabetes mellitus	1.4

[a]See Appendix 2 for World Health Organization Website and Reference.
Source: Adapted from World Health Organization Report 2001.

Headache Services and Organizations

The International Headache Society (IHS) was founded in 1981 and embraces the national headache societies of 41 countries. Other organizations having a global interest include the headache section of the World Federation of Neurology, the WHO, and the World Headache Alliance, while on a continental scale there is the European Headache Federation, the American Association for the Study of Headache, and the Australian Headache Society.

In the United Kingdom, the premier specialist organization for headache is the British Association for the Study of Headache (BASH). Other interested U.K. organizations include the Migraine in Primary Care Advisors (MIPCA) and the patient organizations the Migraine Trust, the Migraine Action Association, and the Organization for the Understanding of Cluster Headache (OUCH), which together constitute Headache UK. Website information is given in Appendix 2. There is a wealth of information on these websites for all involved in headache management as well as for headache sufferers, including useful downloads such as headache diaries and patient information leaflets.

Headache Politics

The medical services for headache naturally vary from country to country. Each has differing priorities and varying numbers of neurologists, headache specialists, and other medical and nursing staff who might deal with headache. In the United Kingdom, the provision of the National Health Service (NHS) has meant a "top down" prioritization of services in which patients have relatively little say in setting priorities other than by lobbying their Member of Parliament or forming patient organizations that can shout more loudly than individuals! In a private or insurance-funded system, patients with common conditions such as migraine dictate the provision of services to some extent—a "bottom up" approach. The United States accordingly has a large number of headache clinics, the United Kingdom relatively few.

Headache in the United Kingdom

Migraine (as defined by the IHS) affects about 15% of the British population. A British study (21) found the median attack frequency to be 12 per year, with 54% of migraineurs reporting at least one attack per month (approaching the accepted threshold for needing prophylactic treatment), while 13% had more than one attack weekly (certainly in prophylactic treatment territory). Thus, each day it is estimated that migraineurs suffer about 190,000 migraine attacks, and as a result almost 100,000 people are absent from work or school. The socioeconomic cost of this illness through lost productivity is immense, estimated at about £1.5 billion (US $2.5 billion) a year in the United Kingdom alone (21). The NHS spends a mere fraction of this cost on headache treatments, which if used correctly can significantly alleviate the problem for most sufferers. The conclusion is inescapable. The total costs of migraine to society, including treatment costs, would be reduced if more resources were directed to managing more sufferers more effectively. But how and where should these resources be allocated?

We think it would be fair to say that most general practitioners (GPs) (and a good proportion of neurologists) in the United Kingdom have no particular interest in headache. Part of the problem may lie (at least for the authors' generation of doctors) in the fact that as medical students we had little or no formal teaching in this area. As a result, for many headache patients seeking medical help, advice is inexpert. As noted above, the "treatment trail" often starts with a visit to the local optician if the headache is frontal; an osteopath, physical therapist, rheumatologist, or orthopedic surgeon if it is cervico-occipital, or perhaps a dentist if it is facial pain, sometimes resulting in inappropriate teeth extractions. "Sinus" headache, particularly, is vastly overdiagnosed in primary care, and treatments such as inhalations, topical nasal mucosal vasoconstrictors, antibiotics, and even sinus drainage procedures may be being used indiscriminately. Real sinusitis is a severe disease (see below) and the mere presence of headache in the region of the "sinuses," or even opacification of a sinus on an X-ray or scan, does not establish the diagnosis.

While some patients may benefit from advice from these sources, it seems that many do not, other than by excluding other diseases. The correct treatment, if ever received, is delayed. By contrast, epidemiological surveys show that rescue medications such as OTC analgesics, if used excessively, can actually make the problem worse, by causing another major problem—medication overuse headache (MOH). Some 1% of the entire Norwegian population have chronic daily headache (CDH) caused by long-term, inappropriate, over-frequent use of analgesics and other rescue medications (22)!

What can be done to improve the situation? Currently the NHS priority lies in identifying and dealing with "serious" causes of headache; but these are rare. Hopkins and Ziegler (23) reported that, in one year, among a U.K. population of 100,000,

- 79,000 to 83,000 had a headache,
- 24,000 had suffered a headache in the previous fortnight sufficient to require an analgesic,
- 9100 had at least one "very severe" of "almost unbearable" headache,
- 1600 had consulted their family doctor, and
- 272 referrals were made to the hospital for investigation,

but only 10 brain tumors were found, of which only two were benign and treatable by current intervention.

Paradoxically there is no special provision for primary headache, which is extremely common. Yet it requires no special facilities. What is needed is time to listen to the patient, genuine professional interest in the condition, the appropriate knowledge and clinical skills, and the freedom to prescribe appropriately and to follow-up patients to ensure they are using their medication correctly and effectively. Undoubtedly, nurses can play an important role in this area, as they do already in other common conditions managed principally in the community or on an outpatient basis, such as asthma, diabetes, epilepsy, and Parkinsonism.

Like primary care, neurology clinics suffer resource limitations. Conflicting pressures from other conditions considered of greater clinical priority limit what the migraineur can be offered. Specialist headache clinics in the United Kingdom see only the tip of the migraine iceberg. In addition, perhaps inevitably, these clinics are also populated with the most recalcitrant and difficult cases, often suffering the consequences of protracted inappropriate treatments. Here too, specialist nurses in headache can play a pivotal role, but at present there are very few such nurses in secondary care in the United Kingdom.

Primary care groups offer the ideal opportunity for reforming headache services to the public, with only quite a small number of interested GPs with a specialist interest needed in each Primary Care Trust (PCT) to develop and maintain the requisite specialist skills. This new ideal world of headache services would see formal links established between PCT-based headache clinics in primary and intermediary care, and local secondary care and regionally based specialist headache clinics, whose number should be increased to provide this support. Only the most difficult cases would need to be referred to a neurology department, including the small number needing special investigations.

Reducing the Burden of Headache

It is likely that better education of health professionals, and indeed the public, and greater understanding of headache in general, will lead to a reduction in its social and economic impact. For example, there is evidence that triptans reduce lost work time from migraine (24), and efforts are being made in the United Kingdom currently, to allow for these medications to be available "OTC," as well as by prescription.

BASH aims to improve the recognition and treatment of headache in Britain at all levels. Members of BASH Council, the governing body, have over time included many of the recognized U.K. headache specialists from primary and secondary care, mostly neurologists but including several GPs, a pediatrician, a physician with a specialist interest in homeopathic medicine, and a nurse specialist. BASH covers most aspects of headache that need guidance at a national level and has published recommendations on the organization of headache services. Details of all BASH activities, including its updated guidelines (in pdf format), a set of PowerPoint slides for teaching purposes, membership application, and other information can be found at its Web site (see Appendix 2).

MANAGING THE HEADACHE PATIENT

We will now discuss the management of individual primary headache syndromes. As stated in the Preface, this book is not primarily concerned with the evaluation and treatment of headache in general, for which there are many excellent reference works available, but we will start with some general points.

First, we have proposed that all primary headaches are driven by the migraine mechanism and that we are all potentially vulnerable to its manifestations, chiefly headache. For the vast majority of people, "ordinary headaches," whether interpreted as "tension-type" headaches related to work stress or excessive concentration, "sinus" headaches, or whatever, are an occasional and trivial nuisance that is either ignored or swatted away with a couple of painkillers. Professional help is neither needed nor required. At the other extreme, recurrent attacks of IHS-defined migraine or trigeminal autonomic cephalalgia (TAC) can be devastating and incapacitating, resulting in severe handicap and even a state of persistent fear and apprehension, requiring expert and ongoing medical help and support.

Second, while all primary headaches might stem from a common mechanism, the syndromes that result vary considerably. As we described in Chapter 5, IHC-2 divides primary headaches into four broad categories: *migraine, tension-type headache*, the *TACs*, and *other primary headaches*. Experience has taught that some syndromes respond best to certain interventions, so in the absence of a "universal headache panacea," accurate diagnosis of primary headache types, as defined by IHS criteria, is crucial for meaningful clinical trials and thus effective treatments.

What Does the Headache Patient Want?

As a rule, the medical profession overemphasizes the use of headache treatments and underestimates the patient's need to understand better the nature and basis of their headache syndrome. Packard (25) found that patients attending a headache clinic were, contrary to their doctors' expectations, more likely to be interested in finding the *cause* of their headache rather than a symptomatic treatment. Diagnosis is important, particularly if the definition of a headache syndrome leads to a specific treatment.

"Cluster headache" and "migraine" are useful terms that patients usually find easy to understand in relation to treatment and management plans. In our experience, the term "tension-type headache", particularly chronic tension-type headache, is less useful because patients (as well as doctors) often have difficulty understanding what it really is. Patients with "chronic tension headache" often find it difficult to understand why painkillers do not resolve their headache and also why doctors sometimes suggest treatment with tricyclic antidepressant drugs for this disorder. Their correct use in such patients is often a challenge in terms of compliance and dose escalation.

It is helpful to consider the patients' own concepts of the origin of their headache, and for patients to understand the limitations of the treatments available. We have found it useful in management, particularly of chronic headache, to check that patients are confident that causation has been fully addressed and that they are assured of the benign nature of their condition before addressing the question of symptomatic treatment. Patients concerned as to the cause of their headaches, and who believe that the doctor must find the cause of headache before treating it, do not readily accept symptomatic remedies (26).

Lipton and Stewart set out to explore what patients wanted from migraine therapy (27). They identified 688 individuals with migraine and asked them, over the phone, using a computer-assisted interview, about their migraine and its treatment. The key information obtained from this study group, which had a mean age of 43 years, was that:

- About a 30% had never consulted a doctor.
- About 50% did not think their headache was "that bad," while the other 50% had a treatment that worked for them.
- 40% did not think that doctors had any useful remedies.
- About 30% thought that seeing a doctor was too expensive (this being the United States!).
- About 20% had seen doctors previously but had not done so in the past year, largely because treatments were working or their headaches had improved.
- 50% thought that their doctor could not help them or was not interested in headache.
- 70% of patients were "not very satisfied" with their treatments, generally due to lack of efficacy of treatment rather than due to side effects.
- Most people thought satisfactory pain relief should be within one hour and more than half thought it should be within 30 minutes.

The responses to questions about what patients wanted from their doctors produced a constellation of answers, all of which demonstrated that patients see their relationship with their doctor as a partnership. They wanted questions answered and to be educated about controlling their migraines.

"Red Flag" Headaches

It goes without saying that the first responsibility of a doctor faced with a patient complaining of headache is to exclude a serious underlying cause. Whether one works in general practice, a neurology clinic, or the emergency room, serious causes of headache are uncommon and a good working knowledge of the primary headache syndromes keeps the physician alert to symptoms that might indicate serious underlying pathology.

All doctors should be aware of the following two (rather self-evident) facts:

- Headache *in isolation* is most unlikely due to a brain tumor or serious intracranial abnormality.
- The worse the headache, the more times it has occurred, and the longer it has been present, the less likely it is to be due to such abnormalities.

"Red flags" in the history lead to a focused physical examination and appropriate investigations. It can be helpful to ask at the outset, the question, "How many different types of headache do you suffer from?" The history for each type can then be taken in turn. In general, when a headache is the *only* symptom, it is unlikely that a definable pathological cause will be discovered. Serious headaches generally present acutely or subacutely, although cranial arteritis, for example, may grumble on for months before the diagnosis is made, and exertional cephalalgias due to structural posterior fossa abnormalities may have caused symptoms for years.

We would highlight the following as "red flags" in the history.

Severe Headache "Out of the Blue"—"Thunderclap" Headache

This means intracranial hemorrhage—usually subarachnoid hemorrhage (SAH)—until proven otherwise. In typical SAH, the headache is severe (usually the worst ever headache, like being hit over the head with a bat), lasts several hours at least, and is usually associated with vomiting, neck stiffness (on flexion/extension rather than on lateral rotation, which is more often due to cervical spondylosis), and almost always some degree of impairment of consciousness, at least transiently. Computed tomography (CT) scanning should be undertaken immediately. If performed more than 12 hours after the ictus, the scan is unlikely to show subarachnoid blood. Conversely, if the scan does not show blood, lumbar puncture must be undertaken but should be delayed 12 hours, because it can take this long for xanthochromia to develop. The "sentinel headache" of SAH (28) may raise little suspicion of impending catastrophe, as the following case illustrates.

CASE 255: SENTINEL HEADACHE—MISSED SUBARACHNOID HEMORRHAGE

A 28-year-old man suddenly developed a generalized headache, not related to sexual intercourse, whilst in bed with his girlfriend. Their was no nausea or vomiting and it seemed to pass off over about an hour. His girlfriend was concerned but the patient brushed the problem aside and simply went to sleep. The next morning, he still had a mild nonspecific headache and his girlfriend insisted he attend the hospital. No abnormalities were found on examination. The CT brain image was scrutinized on the scanner monitor. It seemed to show no abnormalities and because the patient seemed fully recovered, he was discharged. However, when a neuroradiologist saw the hard copies of the image some hours later, it was clear that the man had suffered a SAH (Fig. 3). The Police eventually found the patient and he had an angiogram that day, which demonstrated a right posterior communicating artery aneurysm. This was clipped successfully shortly afterwards.

As we noted in Chapter 5, the great majority of "thunderclap headaches" prove to be benign and are probably migraine variants. Unless there is alteration of consciousness or some more alarming or protracted consequences, many patients actually ignore this type of headache, especially

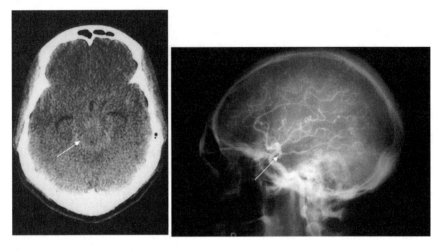

Figure 3   Case 255. (*Left panel*) CT brain scan shows a thin veneer of blood in the peripontine cistern (*arrow*), with mild dilatation of the temporal horns of the lateral ventricles. (*Right panel*) Carotid angiogram shows a right posterior communicating artery aneurysm (*arrow*).

when associated with sexual intercourse! If attacks occur repeatedly, they are also of course unlikely to be due to hemorrhage.

Headache Brought on by Maneuvers that Alter Intracranial Pressure

Again, as discussed in Chapter 5, some headaches are precipitated exclusively by Valsalva maneuvers (e.g., cough headache) and some are brought on by exertion—generally termed "exertional cephalalgia." The latter needs to be distinguished from exertion-triggered migraine, in which the headache develops some time after the exercise (29).

As discussed in Chapter 5, Valsalva headaches may be caused by posterior fossa pathology such as a Chiari malformation, by tumors or intraventricular lesions, or by venous sinus thrombosis. It is therefore particularly important to look for evidence of brainstem dysfunction (unsteadiness, double vision, downbeat nystagmus, etc.). Scanning is mandatory, but most Valsalva and exertional headaches are benign and typically remit spontaneously over some weeks or months.

Conversely, *spontaneous intracranial hypotension* can start explosively as a thunderclap headache, but is then characterized by severe headache induced by upright posture and relieved by lying flat (as with post–lumbar puncture headache). The investigation and management of this headache is reviewed in Ref. (30).

Patients over the Age of 50 Years Presenting with
a New Headache

Giant cell ("cranial" or "temporal") arteritis must always be considered, but migraine variants and headache related to cervical spondylosis will be much more common. Occasionally Paget's disease of the skull, skull metastases, and occult meningiomas (see p. 294) may present with headache.

Progressively Worsening Headaches

Headache of progressively increasing frequency and severity is naturally of grave concern to patients, and often their doctors, and must always be carefully evaluated. But a serious cause will seldom be found; brain tumors almost never present with daily headache alone. While progressive morning headache with nausea and/or vomiting should always alert the clinician to the possibility of a space-occupying lesion, migraine is the most common cause of these symptoms.

SCANNING

Does a patient with a troublesome headache need a brain scan? In some parts of the world, all headache patients are scanned routinely but the pickup rate for culpable pathology is extremely low and this practice is wasteful of resources. Most patients simply need a clear and adequate explanation of their problem. It is often a matter of telling the patient what they have not got, rather than being able to tell them exactly what they do have!

Many headache patients are referred for specialist opinion "to exclude an intracranial lesion." Such patients will often have had "bad" headaches for a long time, and they will sometimes say they know of a friend or relative who had had such headaches and was found to have a "brain tumor" or "a clot on the brain"—a scenario that by contrast is a rare experience for most physicians. Certainly, some such patients will be helped by a "therapeutic brain scan." However, we have had patients who still believe they have a brain tumor even when the scan is normal! It is also worth bearing in mind that magnetic resonance imaging (MRI) brain scans, particularly, are very likely to disclose lesions that are irrelevant to the patient's problem. For example, in one study (31), 29% of 3085 normal asymptomatic Japanese subjects were found to have abnormal MRI—18.8% had white matter high signal lesions (14.8% deep cortical, 4% periventricular), 8.3% had infarctions (8.1% lacunar basal ganglia infarcts, the remainder cortical), and there were a significant number of unsuspected instances of hemorrhages, arteriovenous malformations, cavernomas, low-grade malignant or benign brain tumors, pineal cysts, and hydrocephalus.

But be warned! Requesting a "therapeutic" scan can sometimes reveal the unexpected, as the following two cases illustrate.

CASE 256
A 46-year-old woman complained of a six-month history of persistent frontal headache. There were no other symptoms and examination was completely normal. She said she was certain that she had a brain tumor. She had experienced a similar headache in her teens and had been convinced at the time that she had a tumor but was reassured by a normal skull X-ray. Five years before presentation, she had developed bowel symptoms and associated cancer phobia, which responded to counselling.

A CT brain scan was arranged to reassure her. Unfortunately, this did actually reveal a very long-standing left anterior parafalcine meningioma (Fig. 4). However, on receiving the news over telephone, she was relieved to be told that although she did indeed have a tumor, it was not the cause of her headache!

CASE 257
A 43-year-old man developed a "flu" that led to a chest infection associated with severe bouts of coughing. The repeated coughing resulted in persistent headache in the right supraorbital region, radiating over the right frontoparietal area. The pain tended to occur in waves, often present on wakening and worsened by coughing and straining. He denied associated nausea, vomiting, or visual disturbances, but at the onset of headache there had been a small amount of bloody nasal discharge from

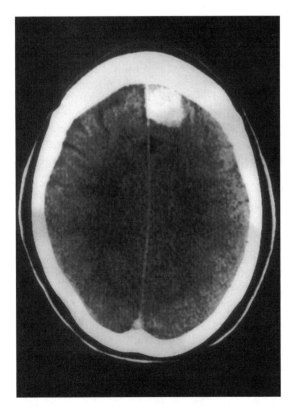

Figure 4 Case 256. CT brain scan. Incidental left anterior parafalcine meningioma.

(A)   (B)

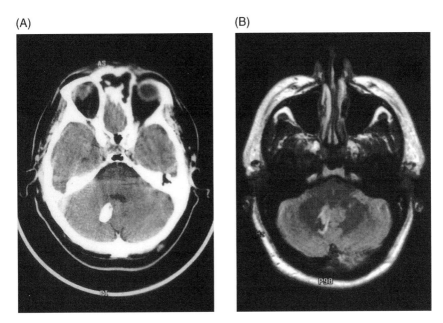

Figure 5 Case 257. (**A**) CT brain scan showing right-sided cerebellar hematoma, close to the fourth ventricle. (**B**) MRI brain scan, showing residual hemosiderin in the hematoma cavity. The underlying lesion was probably a cavernoma.

the right nostril. There was no previous history of significant headache but his sister suffered from migraine. He had been treating his headache with a sinus preparation from the chemist.

Neurological examination was completely normal. A diagnosis of mild sinusitis was suspected and an X-ray of his sinuses revealed "some clouding of the right frontal sinus, but no fluid levels."

Two weeks later the patient's wife wrote in reporting that her husband's MRI brain scan had shown an intracerebral hemorrhage! (Fig. 5). He had seen another neurologist for a second opinion when his headaches had not settled. A subsequent angiogram showed no abnormality. The hematoma was removed but the headache attacks continued as before, and it was concluded that he was actually suffering from migraine.

MYTHS, CONTROVERSIES, AND FALLACIES

Common misconceptions concerning the causes of headache abound among the general public, and indeed many doctors. The relationship to hypertension, eyestrain, the sinuses, and the neck are the main areas of concern.

Headache and Hypertension

The relationship between headache and hypertension has been debated for years and is considered established by many headache sufferers, and indeed many doctors. However, there is in fact no good evidence that headache is caused by "high blood pressure." The problem is that there is a high prevalence of both headache and hypertension. Patients complain of headache, seek medical help, and are found to have an elevated blood pressure—*quod erat demonstrandum.* So many people are taking antihypertensives that it would now be difficult to examine the relationship, but population surveys undertaken when blood pressure surveillance was less assiduous provide useful data. A U.S. Health Examination Survey of Adults (32) conducted between 1960 and 1962 found that headaches that occurred "every few days" or bothered subjects "quite a bit" were reported by 22.8% of people with a systolic pressure less than 140 mmHg, 23.2% of people with a systolic pressure of 140 to 159 mmHg and 24.4% of people with a systolic pressure greater than 160 mmHg. This trend was not statistically significant. In another study [reviewed in Ref. (32)] of 200 consecutive patients, all of who had a diastolic pressure of 120 mmHg or above, 44% admitted to headache, but the blood pressure did not distinguish those with and without headaches. The factor that reliably predicted headache was whether or not the patients were aware of their hypertension! Of 96 patients who were aware, 74% complained of headache; but of 104 who were unaware of their hypertension, only 16% complained of headache, despite an average diastolic pressure of 135 mmHg. This trend was also seen in 18 individuals with malignant hypertension. It was concluded that while a true "hypertensive headache" might exist in patients with significant hypertensive retinopathy and in malignant hypertension, this is exceptional (32). Overall, there is no evidence that hypertension alone causes headache, unless the blood pressure is very high, or perhaps rises very quickly.

Eye Strain and Headache

Headache due to refractive errors does seem to exist. The IHC-2 criteria for diagnosis are:

- Mild headaches in the frontal region and in the eyes themselves.
- Pain absent on awakening and aggravated by prolonged visual tasks at the distance or angle where vision is impaired.
- Uncorrected refractive error, e.g., hyperopia, astigmatism, presbyopia, or wearing of incorrect glasses.
- Close temporal relation between headache and refractive error.
- Headache disappears within seven days after correction of refractive error.

The public considers eyestrain to be a common cause of recurrent headaches and the great majority of patients referred to our clinics have consulted their optician previously about the problem. Many will have had glasses prescribed or had their prescriptions changed, possibly unnecessarily.

However, in our experience, it is very uncommon for headache to be cured by correcting an unrecognized refractive error.

"Sinus" Headache

As mentioned above, "sinus" as a cause of headache does seem to be greatly overdiagnosed. *Chronic sinusitis is not validated as a cause of headache or facial pain unless it relapses to an acute infective stage.* The use of antibiotics should be based on fulfilment of the IHC-2 criteria for the disease.

- Frontal headache accompanied by pain in one or more regions of the face, ears, or teeth.
- Clinical, nasal endoscopic, CT and/or MRI imaging and/or laboratory evidence of acute or acute-on-chronic rhinosinusitis.
- Headache and facial pain develop simultaneously with onset of acute exacerbation of rhinosinusitis.
- Headache and/or facial pain resolve within seven days after remission or successful treatment of acute or acute-on-chronic rhinosinusitis.

The Neck and Headache

In Chapter 2, we saw that cervical and trigeminal sensory inputs overlap in the trigeminocervical complex (TCC), allowing pain to be referred from one area to the other. Headaches may therefore arise from disorders in the neck, but the definition and management of cervicogenic headache is controversial. The general public, rightly or wrongly, commonly blames the neck for headache. The IHC-2 diagnostic criteria, listed below, are rigorous. *Cervicogenic headache* can be diagnosed if pain is referred from a source in the neck and perceived in one or more regions of the head and/or face, together with:

- Clinical, laboratory, and/or imaging evidence of a disorder or lesion within the cervical spine or soft tissues of the neck known to be, or generally accepted as, a valid cause of headache.
- Evidence that the pain can be attributed to the neck or lesion, based on at least one of the following:
  a. Demonstration of clinical signs that implicate a source of pain in the neck.
  b. Abolition of headache following diagnostic blockade of a cervical structure or its nerve supply compared to placebo or other adequate controls.
  c. Resolution within three months after successful treatment of the causative disorder or lesion.

Whilst we would not argue with the outline above, few neck conditions have actually been validated as a cause of headache and there are no reliable clinical signs.

We described earlier, a patient whose migraine attacks were actually precipitated by neck manipulation (Case 11, p. 76). Colleagues have provided some further examples.

CASE 258: MA TRIGGERED BY NECK MOVEMENT

A 17-year-old girl described two headache types. The first started when she was 11 years old. This was usually a frontal headache that built up over an hour, was throbbing in nature and associated with nausea but no photo- or phonophobia, and often associated with periods of stress. The frequency varied from at most two to three times a week to just one episode in the previous six months, before consultation. The second headache type had started about a year previously, in association with learning to drive. This headache was exclusively triggered by turning her head to the left 90°, to look behind when reversing. A few seconds later she would see little sparkling lights in both visual fields for about five minutes followed by a few dark spots, each lasting a few seconds. The total phenomenon would last several minutes, but was followed about 30 minutes later by a severe migrainous headache that would last up to two hours. She had never lost consciousness during these episodes. Neurological examination was normal. She had a normal MR brain scan, MR cerebral angiogram, and trimodal evoked potentials.

CASE 259: MO TRIGGERED BY NECK MOVEMENT

A 50-year-old man had suffered with typical migraine without aura (MO) for some 25 years. For the last six years he had experienced four or five attacks per year. Over this period, he realized that neck movements could set off a typical attack. If he looked to the left, but not to the right, he would get, within 30 to 90 seconds, blurring of vision for a few minutes followed by a "closing in" of his visual fields. At worst he "would not be able to see a Transit van five feet away." His vision would recover within 40 minutes and he would then experience dizziness, nausea, and headache, with tiredness and yawning. The headache could last several days and was worsened by activity. Neurological examination, CT brain scan, and carotid Doppler studies were normal. Attempted migraine prophylaxis with amitriptyline, propranolol, sodium valproate, and pizotifen was unsuccessful, and acupuncture and chiropractic treatment were similarly ineffective.

THE BRITISH ASSOCIATION FOR THE STUDY OF HEADACHE MIGRAINE MANAGEMENT (BASH) GUIDELINES

> Patients will inevitably take their medication in whatever fashion suits them.
> —*Hippocrates*

A small proportion (but a very large number) of people are badly afflicted by primary headaches and need treatment. The following is an outline of the BASH recommendations for treating migraine. The full article, which includes the evidence base for the recommendations, is available at www. bash.org (not to be confused with www.bashh.org, which is the British Association for Sexual Health and HIV, which provides details of "genitourinary medicine clinics and guidelines, and sexually transmitted infection foundation courses!")—and is updated at least annually. It is not produced in hard copy because new treatments appear and are reviewed regularly. The guidelines also cover headache relapses, "long duration" migraine, slowly developing migraine, migraine in children, and also nondrug therapies, including physical and psychological therapies, homeopathy, and alternative remedies.

British Association for the Study of Headache Management Principles

There are four elements to good migraine management:

- Correct and timely diagnosis
- Explanation and reassurance
- Identification of predisposing factors and triggers
- Appropriate intervention (drug or non-drug)

Asking the patient to keep a dairy of the headaches over a few weeks may be helpful in determining the pattern and severity of attacks, and to identify any trigger factors. As noted above, patients may experience more than one type of headache and separate histories are necessary for each.

We would suggest that particular attention is paid to the timing of onset of nausea and/or vomiting. If this occurs early in the attack, it may well compromise the efficacy of standard oral medications, requiring consideration of an antiemetic or the use of parenteral (rectal, nasal, or subcutaneous) preparations.

The Acute Treatment Ladder

The Guidelines propose a treatment ladder that begins with drugs that are the cheapest and safest, while having proven efficacy. An important principle is that *any treatment should be tried for at least three attacks before being abandoned*, because no treatment can be expected to work for every attack. Patients who can recognize attacks of different sorts or severity may use different steps on the treatment ladder accordingly. Acute treatment should not be taken regularly on more than two days a week, to avoid the potential development of MOH.

Step One: Simple Oral Analgesic With or Without Antiemetic

(1a) Aspirin (600–900 mg) or ibuprofen (400–600 mg) in buffered soluble or oro-dispersible formulations, best taken early in the attack. There is little evidence base that paracetamol alone is helpful, although it is widely used. *Codeine and dihydrocodeine should be avoided*, because opiate-based drugs are often implicated in MOH.

(1b) Aspirin or an NSAID combined with an antiemetic, ideally a prokinetic antiemetic to prevent gastric emptying. Domperidone is particularly useful. It is a peripheral dopamine D2-receptor antagonist that does not readily cross the blood–brain barrier and therefore exhibits a very low incidence of central nervous system side effects. It improves gastric motility by inhibiting fundic receptive relaxation and enhancing antral contractions. It also acts on the D2 receptors in the area postrema, providing antiemetic activity (see below). It is quite widely used in the United Kingdom but was discontinued in the United States due to cardiovascular events. Prochlorperazine (3 mg buccal tablet), although not prokinetic, is also useful and available without prescription.

Step Two: Parenteral Analgesic With or Without Antiemetic

For example, diclofenac 100 mg suppositories for pain, domperidone 30 mg suppository for nausea. In an emergency, intramuscular chlorpromazine and diclofenac are recommended. We also use subcutaneous sumatriptan in this situation, but there have been no direct comparisons with first-line treatments.

Step Three: Specific Antimigraine Drugs

Triptans have a range of efficacy and duration of action, and also vary in cost. There are unpredictable individual variations in response to triptans, so patients may wish to try different preparations to find the one that suits them best. It can also be helpful to use some validated instrument, such as the Migraine Disability Assessment Program or the Headache Impact Test 6 (see Appendix 2), to determine whether prescription of a triptan is justified. Above all these drugs are very convenient to use.

Triptans have no effect on aura. They appear to be most effective if taken early in the headache phase when the pain is still mild but may be helpful at any time in the attack. Triptans currently available in the UK are shown in Figure 6.

A good response to a triptan would be resolution of all attack symptoms within an hour, and a satisfactory response would be amelioration of symptoms to the extent that the sufferer was able to conduct all required activities despite ongoing minor symptoms.

Headache relapse occurs in 20% to 50% of patients who initially respond to treatment with a triptan. A further dose may be needed within 24 hours but too frequent use can, as with all interventions, lead to MOH. We have had some success by sequential use of "short-acting" triptans (e.g., zolmatriptan and rizatriptan) and "long-acting" triptans (such as naratriptan and frovatriptan) in individual attacks. Ergotamine preparations may also be useful for patients with repeated relapses as they have a long duration of action.

Triptan Side Effects

Triptan side effects may include tingling, numbness, warm/hot sensations, and sensation of pressure or tightness in different parts of the body, including chest and neck. Chest pain, dizziness and sedation, sometimes claimed to

Name	Trade name	Normal Adult Dose	Melt/ orally dispersible	Nasal Spray	S.C	Therapeutic Gain at 2 hrs	Headache Recurrence
Sumatriptan	Imigran	50mg 100mg	Radis 50mg/ 100mg	20mg	6mg	29% 33% 30% 51%	20-40% overall
Zolmitriptan	Zomig	2.5mg 5mg	2.5mg 5mg	5mg		34%	31% overall
Naratriptan	Naramig	2.5mg				21%[a]	27%
Rizatriptan	Maxalt	10mg	10mg			36%	35%
Eletriptan	Relpax	40mg				36%	31%
Almotriptan	Almogran	12.5mg				27%	
Frovatriptan	Migard	2.5mg				20%	17.5% overall

Figure 6 Some comparisons of the seven different triptans available in the United Kingdom. The normal adult dosages are shown. Only two of the many parameters of efficacy are shown—therapeutic gain (mean of absolute and placebo subtracted headache relief) and headache recurrence (initial therapeutic success followed by an increase in headache to moderate or severe within 24 hours). [a]Primary end point was relief at four hours. *Source*: Adapted from Therapeutic Class Summaries. 5-HT$_1$ agonists ("triptans") for migraine in adults. http://www.ukmi.nhs.uk/Med_info/NewProd.asp.

be side effects, are often actually part of the migraine attack—they may not occur if the drug is taken at other times.

If step three fails,

- Review the diagnosis.
- Review compliance.
- Review the manner of use of medication.
- Exclude MOH.

Step Four: Consider Combination of Steps One and Three or Steps Two and Three

Prophylaxis

Prophylaxis is considered when migraine attacks are insufficiently controlled by trigger avoidance and optimal acute therapy, and to reduce the risk of MOH. As a general rule, we might advise prophylaxis if disabling attacks continue to occur more than three times monthly. The evidence base for efficacy is good for beta-blockers, valproate, and topiramate and, adequate for amitriptyline, but poor for other drugs. Prophylactics *must be titrated slowly* up to an effective dose in order to avoid side effects. Drugs that are effective should be continued for four to six months. Withdrawal by tapering the dose should then be considered.

First-Line Prophylactic Drugs

- *Beta-blockers*, unless contraindicated. Any history of asthma must be documented and considered before prescribing these drugs. Atenolol 25 to 100 mg b.i.d., metoprolol (50–100 mg b.i.d.), and propranolol sustained release (80–320 mg) are widely used.
- *Amitriptyline* 10 to 150 mg one to two hours before bedtime, is first-line therapy when migraine coexists with troublesome "tension-type" headaches, other chronic pain conditions, disturbed sleep, or depression. Many experts think that depression in this context needs specific treatment, however.

Beta-blockers and amitriptyline can both have significant side effects, notably fatigue and parasomnia.

As the neurogenic basis for the migraine mechanism has been slowly elucidated (see Chapter 2), there is increasing interest in the role of anticonvulsants in migraine prophylaxis. Sodium valproate and topiramate have been clearly shown to be effective prophylactic agents. Trial data for other antiepileptic drugs is very limited. Lamotrigine may find a place in the treatment of aura and in SUNCT, and levetiracitam is currently under investigation in the UK.

Second-Line Prophylactic Drugs

- Sodium valproate 300 to 1000 mg twice daily
- Topiramate 25 mg daily to start, increasing to 50 mg twice daily

Third-Line Prophylactic Drugs

- Gabapentin 300 mg daily to 800 mg three times daily
- Methysergide 1 to 2 mg three times daily
- Beta-blockers in combination with amitriptyline

Other Drugs Used in Prophylaxis But with Limited or Uncertain Efficacy, including

- Pizotifen 1.5 to 3 mg daily
- Verapamil slow release 120 to 240 mg twice daily

On the international scene, the calcium antagonist flunarizine is widely used in migraine prophylaxis (33), but because it is not readily available in the United Kingdom we shall not comment on it further.

A number of "non-orthodox" drug therapies have been subjected to limited clinical trial. Magnesium, riboflavin, and coenzyme Q may prove to be of benefit but further studies are needed because of the relatively small number of patients recruited into trials thus far (34).

Antiemetics in Migraine

In Chapter 2, we reviewed the anatomy and physiology of the vomiting center and the chemoreceptor trigger zone (area postrema). It was noted that acetylcholine and histamine were key transmitters in the vomiting center while the area postrema was subject to dopaminergic and serotoninergic influences. Not surprisingly, antagonists to all these transmitters can suppress the vomiting mechanism to some degree and are widely used. Intriguingly, antiemetics used alone may have antimigraine actions. While metoclopramide (35,36) and domperidone (37) in combination with aspirin, were found to have efficacy comparable to triptans, and demonstrated superior control of nausea, metoclopramide and domperidone alone also appeared effective (38,39), although it is not clear if the benefit relates to central nervous system effects or prokinetic actions (40).

One interesting study looked at the roles of migraine and olfaction in nausea and vomiting in pregnancy, by comparing normal women and women with anosmia. Nausea and vomiting were found to be very rare in pregnant anosmic women, but the prevalence of nausea and vomiting was significantly greater in pregnant women who were migraineurs compared to non–migraine sufferers, and a third of mothers who suffered hyperemesis were also migraine sufferers (41). This could imply that nausea and vomiting in pregnancy might be yet another manifestation of the migraine mechanism.

There are two further situations in which migraine treatment can be problematic—menstrual migraine and migraine during pregnancy and lactation.

Menstrual Migraine

Menstrual migraine is defined as migraine occurring within 48 hours of the onset of menstruation in at least two out of three menstrual cycles and at no other time. A migraine diary is needed for accurate diagnosis. IHC-2 defines menstrual migraine as a form of MO, but we have seen cases with aura. The attacks are often prolonged and rather difficult to treat. Because they seem to be related to falling estrogen levels, at least in some women, exogenous estrogen given throughout the menstrual period may be helpful. This can be in the form of estrogen patches or gel (42). Taking the combined oral contraceptive pill continuously for nine weeks rather than three ("tricy-cling"), followed by the usual seven-day pill-free interval, results in 5 rather than 13 withdrawal bleeds per year (and thus fewer menstrual migraines) and is an alternative approach. In some women, regular administration of progesterone can be effective.

Treating Migraine in Pregnancy and Lactation

About 80% of migraineurs who become pregnant find that their migraine improves, particularly during the second and third trimesters (43). This may well result from stabilization of estrogen levels, and women with menstrual migraine are most likely to notice an improvement. Although sudden worsening may occur immediately postpartum, the benefit usually continues while breast-feeding and until the return of menstruation.

Rest and relaxation are important, and as few drugs as possible should be used at the lowest effective dose, using those with least potential to cause harm. Paracetamol is often used, despite formal proof of efficacy, and aspirin seems safe in the first and second trimesters but should be avoided near term because it inhibits platelet aggregation, increases the risk of hemorrhage, and is associated with premature closure of the fetal ductus arteriosus. It is also excreted in breast milk and could cause Reye's syndrome in the newborn infant. Codeine is not generally recommended in the management of migraine in the United Kingdom, but occasional use in combined analgesics is unlikely to cause harm. The antiemetics that have been used widely in pregnancy and lactation without apparent harm include buclizine, chlorpromazine and prochlorperazine, but domperidone and metoclopramide can also be used.

Triptans are not currently recommended. Safety in pregnancy has not been established, although data from inadvertent use of sumatriptan in pregnancy is reassuring (44). Ergot preparations are contraindicated because these can precipitate premature labour (ergot has been used to procure abortions since the Middle Ages).

Occasionally, the use of prophylactic drugs is unavoidable. Of the beta-blockers, the adverse effects of propranolol have been most studied, in connection with the treatment of hypertension in pregnancy (45). There appears to be about a 25% risk of intrauterine growth retardation. It is assumed that this is a class effect and experts therefore advocate the use of the lowest effective dose. Pizotifen safety data in pregnancy are limited, but there are no reports of adverse outcomes during pregnancy or lactation. Amitriptyline is probably safe, but sodium valproate and topiramate are contraindicated.

THE PLACEBO RESPONSE AND ALTERNATIVE MEDICINE IN PRIMARY HEADACHE

Many troublesome headaches resolve of their own accord and reassurance of their benign nature may be all that a patient needs. We can all recall instances of patients referred by their GP because of worrisome headaches, who, when seen weeks later, sheepishly admit that the symptoms have got better!

It has been said of placebo treatments that "their undoubted effectiveness in some disorders, along with their obvious safety and lack of side effects, makes them in some way ideal treatment" (46). In the triptan trials in acute migraine, a placebo response rate of about 30% was commonly seen. It is also clear that placebos can and do have side effects, and the

Table 2 A Summary of the Considered Efficacy of Some Alternative Therapies Used in the Treatment of Migraine and Tension-Type Headache

Headache type	Alternative therapy	Effective?	Comments
Migraine	Feverfew	Yes	Conflicting results, but recent big study showed efficacy (4)
	Biofeedback	Yes	Time intensive. No adverse effects
	Homeopathy	No	No adverse effects
	Spinal manipulation, e.g., chiropractic	No	But can help nausea of various forms
	Acupuncture	No	No adverse side effects
Tension-type headache	Biofeedback	Probably	No adverse side effects
	Hypnotherapy	Possibly	Control for placebo effects not possible
	Relaxation	Probably	Free of adverse effects!

Source: Ernst EP. The Desktop Guide to Complementary and Alternative Medicine. An Evidence-Based Approach. Amsterdam: Elsevier, 2001.

placebo effect does not help everyone. There can be difficulties and ethical problems if placebo is being used in headache management. Is the doctor being deceitful knowing the treatment is a placebo while the patient is obviously benefiting but does not know? These and many other issues regarding this difficult area of placebo treatment have been addressed recently (47).

Patients often ask about the effectiveness of various alternative medicines. The comments in Table 2 are based on the conclusions of *The Desktop Guide to Complementary and Alternative Medicine* (48), although we appreciate that some will not agree with these views.

Homeopathy and Migraine Treatment

Homeopathy is nontoxic and safe. Drug costs should be low. Efficacy has been hard to demonstrate objectively in clinical trials. Nevertheless, it is still used by some headache experts (49).

Acupuncture and Migraine Treatment

Alecrim-Andrade and colleagues evaluated the effectiveness of acupuncture in migraine prophylaxis (50). Twenty-eight migraineurs (MA and MO) were randomized to real or sham-acupuncture (placebo) groups. Sham acupuncture in this trial consisted of a very superficial insertion of the needle in the acupuncture points. By the third and final month of treatment, 28.6% of patients in the standard acupuncture group and 42.3% in the sham-acupuncture group had a 50% or more reduction in migraine-attack frequency compared with the run-in period. Standard acupuncture treatment was thus no different from placebo in preventing migraine and indeed the sham-treated group responded significantly better!

TREATMENT OF OTHER PRIMARY HEADACHES

Episodic "Tension-Type" Headache

Patients with this type of headache do not usually seek medical advice but may use OTC remedies such as simple analgesics and NSAIDs. The cause of their headache is often apparent, such as too much studying, a busy day at the office, or other stresses, but the mechanism or mechanisms are speculative.

Chronic Daily Headache: Chronic Migraine and Chronic "Tension-Type" Headache

As discussed in Chapter 5, there are a number of causes of CDH (see Chapter 5, Table 3). The treatment is obviously directed to the underlying cause if it can be identified, but such cases are very rare in practice. MOH is the most important differential (see below). Excluding this, it is likely that chronic migraine accounts for the majority of cases and our approach here is to use migraine prophylactics and acute migraine treatments as required, and to avoid opium-based drugs.

    Chronic tension-type headache probably also includes a number of secondary headache causes such as cervical degenerative diseases and psychological disorders. In contrast to acute tension-type headache, chronic tension-type headache responds poorly or not at all to simple analgesics and NSAIDs. The standard intervention is with tricyclic antidepressants. We have found that it is important to tell patients that these drugs are being used for their pain relieving properties and not because the problem is "all in the mind." If the patient has tried one before (and patients seen in secondary care often have), it is usually amitriptyline at small doses. If it was ineffective but tolerated well, we would restart it at bedtime and build the dose up in small steps (by 10 mg or possibly 25 mg increments) every few days until it is effective, or has to be discontinued because of side effects, or because the maximum of 150 mg nocte has been reached. If this was not effective, we would use an alternative tricyclic antidepressant (Table 3).

    The management of MOH, a common form of CDH, is discussed later in this chapter.

Cluster Headache and Other Trigeminal-Autonomic Cephalalgias

There are no more unpleasant primary headache syndromes than the TACs. The pain is devastating. The diagnosis is usually easy to the tutored eye, but unfortunately is generally often delayed by six or more years (OUCH Web site, see Appendix 2).

Table 3 Tricyclic Antidepressants and Related Drugs Available in the United Kingdom

	Dose range
Sedating tricyclics	
Amitriptyline	10–150 mg
Clomipramine	10–150 mg
Dosulepin (dothiepin)	25–225 mg
Doxepin	10–300 mg
Maprotiline	25–150 mg
Mianserin	30–90 mg
Trazodone	100–600 mg
Trimipramine	50–300 mg
Less-sedating tricyclics	
Amoxapine	100–150 mg
Imipramine	10–300 mg
Lofepramine	140–210 mg
Nortriptyline	10–150 mg

The pathophysiology of cluster headache has been reviewed (51). Other TACs, particularly paroxysmal hemicrania, must be differentiated, sometimes by a trial of indomethacin (see below), and there are a few case reports of secondary cluster headache, for example, in association with pituitary lesions, parasellar meningiomas, lesions in the region of the third ventricle, and so forth, so neuroimaging should certainly be considered (52).

The relatively brief duration of pain (20–30 minutes) means it is actually unlikely to respond to oral medication, which usually takes half hour to kick in, although many patients attribute the resolution of the attack to such an intervention. However, effective treatment is available and its institution can be a very rewarding experience for the physician.

Management is based largely on clinical experience and anecdote, as relatively few randomized controlled trials have been published. In general, the treatment of cluster headache differs from that of migraine but there are some similarities. The trigger factors so typical of some migraine attacks are lacking in cluster headache, although vasodilators such as alcohol and nitrates should be avoided. The fastest relief for acute attacks is brought about by oxygen inhalation, and subcutaneous or nasal preparations of triptans or DHE (not currently available in the United Kingdom). Intranasal lignocaine (lidocaine) has also proved helpful (53).

Acute Treatments

- Oxygen (100%) given via a non-rebreathing mask (e.g., continuous positive airway pressure) at a flow rate of 7 to 10 L/min. This is effective in about 70% of patients and often within five minutes (54).

> In most countries, small portable oxygen cylinders are available. In the United Kingdom, the correct valve and the masks can be obtained through OUCH.

- Subcutaneous sumatriptan is also a remarkably effective treatment. It may produce benefit within five to seven minutes after administration (55). The current injectors are easy to use and dummies are available from the manufacturer to demonstrate to patients how they should be used.
- DHE is available in some countries in injectable and intranasal forms.
- Non-parenteral analgesics and narcotics have little or no place in the treatment of cluster headache.

Prophylactic Treatments

Preventive treatment is directed at shortening the bouts of episodic cluster and controlling the frequency of the attacks in both the episodic and chronic forms of the disorder. Most patients require preventive treatment at some time in the cluster period. Medications that are generally regarded as effective in preventive treatment include verapamil, lithium carbonate, methysergide, corticosteroids, valproic acid, ergotamine, and sometimes indomethacin. Medication should be started early in the cluster period, continued until the patient has been headache free for two weeks, and then tapered. The choice of drug will depend on previous drug responses and side effects, whether the condition is acute or chronic cluster (expected length of treatment), contraindications to drug usage, frequency and timing of attacks, and the age and lifestyle of the patient.

- Verapamil is considered by many as the drug of first choice for episodic and chronic cluster headache. However, high doses (960 mg/ day or even more) are often needed and it takes a little while to titrate to that dose.
- Corticosteroids-prednisolone 60 mg/day, tapering over two weeks, or dexamethasone 4 mg twice daily two weeks, then 4 mg/day for one week, are effective (56).
- Methysergide is effective in about 65% of patients with episodic cluster headache, although its efficacy in chronic cluster headache has been questioned (57). Doses up to 12 mg/day are often needed. Prolonged periods of treatment have been associated with fibrotic reactions such as retroperitoneal fibrosis, so it is generally only used in episodic cluster headache, particularly where bouts do not last more than a few months.

The efficacy of lithium in episodic and chronic cluster headache was first reported by Ekbom in 1993, and to date, a total of 28 clinical trials comprising 468 patients have been published. Lithium was found to be effective in chronic cluster headache in 236 (78%) of 304 patients in 25 trials. It also works against episodic cluster headache although to a lesser degree, an overall remission rate of 63% having been obtained in a total of 164 patients treated (58).

In-depth coverage of the management of cluster headache can be found in Ref. 59 and we will discuss surgical treatments for cluster headache later in this chapter.

SUNCT/SUNA

This is a particularly taxing group of conditions to treat and until recently was generally considered refractory to intervention. However, clinical experimental studies by Peter Goadsby and colleagues at the National Hospital have shown convincingly, that attacks can be aborted, often for protracted periods, by drugs that block neuronal sodium channels (60). Thus, in a group of 43 short-lasting unilateral neuralgiform pain with conjunctival injection and tearing (SUNCT) patients and nine severe unilateral neuralgiform headache attacks with cranial autonomic symptoms (SUNA) patients, none responded to 100% oxygen or intramuscular indomethacin, but all responded to 100 mg of intravenous lignocaine. From a practical point of view, good responses were also obtained with lamotrigine (400 mg daily), topiramate (in SUNCT but apparently not in SUNA, although only one patient was studied) 400 mg daily, and gabapentin (3600 mg daily).

Other Paroxysmal Headaches

Thunderclap Headache and Exertional and Reflex Cephalalgias

Many of the headaches in this group, fully discussed in Chapter 5, are "one-off" (e.g., primary thunderclap headache) or situation dependent (e.g., exertional and reflex cephalalgias), and are either self-limiting or can be avoided. No intervention is required beyond excluding definable causes. They usually resolve spontaneously in due course although they may be replaced by other primary headache.

Paroxysmal Hemicrania

The treatment of *paroxysmal hemicrania* is prophylactic, with indomethacin the treatment of choice. It may stop attacks after a couple of doses and usually produces resolution within one or two days with typical maintenance doses of 25 to 100 mg/day. Where indomethacin is not tolerated, treatment can be difficult but calcium channel antagonists, acetazolamide and corticosteroids seem to have some effect.

Hemicrania Continua

This, like paroxysmal hemicrania, is an indomethacin-responsive headache and is treated with a similar regime.

Hypnic Headache

Like cluster headache, hypnic headache may respond to lithium. The dose is taken at bedtime and often a small dose (200 mg) is sufficient to stop attacks. Other treatments recommended are verapamil, indomethacin, flunarizine, and caffeine (two cups of caffeinated coffee in the late evening has been reported to be effective). Treatment of this condition has been reviewed in Ref. 61.

"DIFFICULT" HEADACHES

Medication Overuse Headache

It has long been recognized that excessive use of analgesics and other drugs used to treat headache may in fact worsen the problem. Repetitive use of "rescue medications," particularly those containing opiate derivatives such as codeine, or anti-inflammatory drugs, results in headache becoming progressively more frequent, until it occurs "all day, every day" to some degree. When the rescue medications are withdrawn, the headache improves, often considerably so, confirming a diagnosis of MOH.

The medical community in general—doctors, nurses, pharmacists, and pharmaceutical companies—has been extremely slow in spreading awareness of what is a preventable problem. Indeed the problem is growing. Most patients when told that their painkillers or other headache medications are actually contributing to the problem find it difficult to comprehend; others have their suspicions realized. Despite the size of this global problem, there has been virtually no experimental work into the mechanisms of MOH, and what we know about it comes from clinical series describing such patients and their treatments. Although it is a secondary headache, MOH must be considered in all patients with difficult, frequent primary headache.

The problem has been reviewed recently (62). Initial reports on MOH came from Switzerland after the Second World War. The excessive use of the analgesic phenacetin led to chronic headache (and renal disease) in over 30% of female workers in some factories. Soon afterwards, the first descriptions of headaches due to the abuse of ergotamine appeared. About a year after the introduction of sumatriptan, reports appeared confirming that it too could cause this problem.

MOH is not just confined to Europe and North America. Population-based studies show that chronic headache has a prevalence between 2% and

5%, with a prevalence of MOH around 1% to 2%, and these prevalence figures also apply to China, for example. Specialist headache clinics report that 5% to 10% of their patients have MOH.

The diagnosis is dependent, like all headache problems, on a good clinical history and a careful and sympathetic assessment of the patient's drug history. Often patients are ashamed or reluctant to divulge their frequent use of rescue medications. Taking the patient through a typical day, asking whether their headache responded to a drug and when they then took the next dose, often brings the problem to light more readily than by simply asking how many painkillers they take in a week.

MOH is likely to occur in patients taking more than 12 triptan tablets per month, analgesics on more than 15 days a month, or combination of analgesics on more than 10 days a month. The IHC-2 diagnostic criteria for MOH are:

- Daily or nearly daily occurrence.
- The headache problem has taken many months to develop.
- Headaches vary in type, location, and intensity from time to time.
- They are invariably refractory to prophylactic treatments.
- Withdrawal symptoms occur when patients are taken off medication.
- Headache improves spontaneously a few days after analgesia is withdrawn.

Although all drugs may cause MOH, some do so more readily than others and patients will often be found to be taking several rescue medications in excess at the same time. Triptans seem to produce this problem most quickly (two years on average), but improvement is generally speedy once the drug is withdrawn. The timeline is more protracted for ergotamine (two to three years), with analgesics taking the longest to produce MOH (about five years), with a proportionally longer recovery period after withdrawal. Even when the different prevalence of migraine between men and women is accounted for, MOH is slightly more common in women.

Strangely, not all recurrent primary headache syndromes are prone to this problem. Perhaps surprisingly, it has not been reported in cluster headache sufferers, despite drug overuse.

DIAGNOSTIC THERAPEUTIC TRIALS

The syndromic diagnosis of a primary headache is usually simple but sometimes the phenotype is unclear or the headache fails to respond to intervention in the expected manner. In these circumstances, it may be helpful to study *under observation*, the patient's response to a range of treatments. These might include trials of parenteral triptans, 100% oxygen, intravenous lignocaine, and a range of anticonvulsants. In addition, responses to parenteral indomethacin and aspirin can be informative.

The "Indotest"

We have mentioned how a positive response to indomethacin is part of the diagnostic criteria for paroxysmal hemicrania and hemicrania continua. It can be helpful to observe the response to this drug in a controlled trial in patients whose symptoms could include elements of this spectrum of disorders. Intramuscular indomethacin 50 mg is given after recording baseline attacks in a headache diary. The test is considered positive if there is absolute relief lasting four hours at least. An intramuscular placebo is given 24 hours before or after the active drug for comparison. Contraindications to this test include asthma, NSAID intolerance, and renal impairment.

Intravenous Aspirin

There are a number of protocols available for "detoxification" in MOH. Intravenous aspirin can be a useful drug to help withdrawal from medication in inpatients. Intravenous aspirin 1 g is given over five minutes and can be repeated after four hours, to a maximum of 3 g/day. This regime has also been used to treat refractory attacks of migraine and status migrainosus.

SURGICAL TREATMENTS

A number of surgical treatments are available for cluster headache. These include:

- Glycerol injection (or other procedures used in the treatment of trigeminal neuralgia) into the trigeminal ganglion.
- Complete trigeminal nerve section.
- Deep brain stimulation.
- Occipital nerve injection.
- Occipital nerve stimulation.

Procedures to the Trigeminal Nerve

CASE 260: TRIGEMINAL NERVE SECTION IN CHRONIC CLUSTER HEADACHE

A 42-year-old man, with no previous or family history of headache, developed increasingly severe attacks of pain beginning at the angle of the left jaw and then spreading into the left side of his head and face. Initially it was thought that he might have dental disease, and over the years most of the teeth had been removed from the left side of his upper and lower jaws, without benefit. At the outset, the attacks occurred about twice a month. Each lasted about half an hour and could occur at any time of the day or night. During the attacks he would invariably develop epiphora, nasal blockage, reddening of the eye, and ptosis ipsilateral to headache.

He would typically also feel hot and clammy, agitated, and sometimes breathless, but there was no nausea or vomiting.

A diagnosis of chronic cluster headache was eventually made. Over the next four years, he continued to have attacks varying in frequency from once every two days to three times daily, and he was never free of attacks for more than a week. For most of this time he was taking between 12 and 16 Solpadeine (paracetamol, codeine, and caffeine) tablets a day. Other treatments included verapamil up to 120 mg q.i.d., sodium valproate to 2.2 g daily, pizotifen, ergotamine tartrate, and carbamazepine. Sumatriptan caused side effects and had no therapeutic benefit, but lithium produced almost immediate relief and he had no attacks for six months. The attacks then returned despite lithium, and he was treated with methysergide up to 2 mg t.d.s. The attacks were then less severe but just as frequent. He also tried naratriptan and zolmatriptan, with some benefit from the latter.

Six years after presentation, he had a glycerol injection around the right Gasserian ganglion, and following this he was pain free for six weeks. When the attacks returned, he became suicidal. He was now getting two to six attacks a day, half of these waking him at night. A complete section of the right trigeminal nerve in the posterior fossa resulted in immediate and complete freedom from attacks. On follow-up some five years later, he remained asymptomatic. Although he had right facial numbness, he had not experienced any problems with his cornea and had experienced surprisingly little problem with chewing, with only minimal objective weakness of the jaw muscles.

Deep Brain Stimulation

The techniques for deep brain stimulation that are now being employed around the world for the treatment of Parkinson's disease are also being used to treat some cases of intractable headache (63). There is growing literature on the use of deep brain stimulation for the treatment of intractable chronic cluster headache (64).

CASE 261: INTRACTABLE CHRONIC CLUSTER HEADACHE TREATED BY DEEP BRAIN STIMULATION

A 56-year-old man gave a history of typical episodic cluster headache with recurrences in September or October every year, over the previous 11 years. Over the last three years however, he had developed secondary chronic cluster headache. He had tried prophylaxis with carbamazepine, methysergide (up to 9 mg/day), ergot, verapamil (up to 960 mg/day), and amitriptyline without significant benefit and, at the time of referral, the attacks were partially controlled by injections of sumatriptan and high-dose prednisolone. Using standard coregistration CT and MRI stereotaxis, a deep brain stimulator was placed in the region of the ipsilateral hypothalamus (Fig. 7). The mere insertion of the electrode resulted in complete abolition of the attacks, and no further cluster attacks occurred in the twelve months following surgery.

Occipital Nerve Stimulation

The term "occipital neuralgia" is used widely and loosely to refer to any pain felt in the occipital region. The term implies pain stemming from an occipital nerve but there is no compelling evidence for such a disorder, or for entrapment of the greater occipital nerve where it pierces the trapezius.

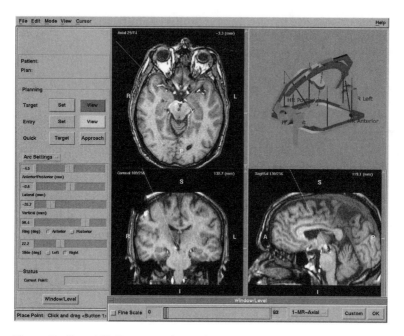

Figure 7 Case 261. Postoperative sagittal MRI brain image showing the placement of the deep brain stimulating electrode. Following placement the patient's cluster headache remitted. T-1 weighted axial MRI scan (2 mm, thickness, zero spacing) to confirm correct electrode placement. *Source*: Courtesy of Professor Tipu Aziz, Oxford University, UK.

There is predictably no consensus on the definition or diagnostic criteria for this condition. The reader wanting to delve into these murky waters is referred to an excellent chapter in Ref. (65). Nevertheless, as noted above, there is good evidence that sensory inputs from the cervical region can aggravate the migraine mechanism and reducing this sensory traffic might be a useful intervention. "Injection of the greater occipital nerve" by local anesthetics and steroids is a time-honored treatment for "occipital neuralgia" and continues to be a useful treatment in our hands. More recently, chronic occipital nerve stimulation has been used to good effect, for the treatment of intractable chronic migraine (66).

Botulinum Toxin Injection

The mechanism by which this form of treatment might work is less clear than that for occipital nerve stimulation. The role of muscle spasm in the generation of headache, as we have seen, is unclear. The toxin is taken up by nociceptive neurons and could lead to an attenuation of peripheral neuropeptide release and possibly less pain. The efficacy of this treatment has yet to be shown conclusively (34).

HEADACHE TREATMENT—WHERE ARE WE NOW?

> It is astonishing how successful we have been in treating headache without really knowing what pain is or being able to define accurately how drugs can relieve it.
>> —*Arnold Friedman* [One of the greatest headache physicians of the twentieth century (3).]

Before considering possible future directions for the treatment of primary headache, we must consider the extent to which the fact that different primary headache syndromes seem to demand different treatments challenges our concept that "all primary headache is migraine." The evidence is not compelling! Effective treatments for migraine were introduced over time despite what proved to be an erroneous concept of how migraine is caused. In turn, ideas of causation have been influenced by what treatments seem to be effective. Although tryptans are clearly very effective in the treatment of the "migraine" phenotype, there are reports of triptans helping the pain of "tension-type" headache in migraineurs, cluster headache, temporal arteritis, ergotamine withdrawal, and SAH. By way of analogy, cough headache may respond to methysergide (67) and, as noted, a range of headache phenotypes respond to indomethacin (68). Although it is clear that not all primary headaches respond to any currently available single drug, it is also true that not all "IHC-2 migraine" patients respond to a triptan. Trials show that, at best, the response to any oral triptan in migraine is only about 70%. Failure to respond to a triptan does not, however, negate the view that a particular headache is fundamentally migrainous and some patients will respond to one triptan and not another (69).

Thus, it is not justifiable to base ideas of headache causation on response to treatment: indeed, conversely, a generally or consistently beneficial response to a particular class of drug across different headache phenotypes lends some support for a unitary concept.

HEADACHE TREATMENT—THE FUTURE

There is no doubt that the introduction of sumatriptan for the treatment of acute migraine attacks was a major advance, and there is now a useful range of triptans to choose from. However, some 20% to 30% of primary headache attacks do not respond adequately to triptans, and rebound headache and triptan-related side effects are significant problems for some patients. In addition, although topiramate was licenced for migraine prophylaxis in 2005, following the largest controlled trials ever conducted of a migraine prophylactic, the currently available prophylactics are not dramatically successful. There is a need for new migraine treatments.

We reviewed the key processes underlying the migraine mechanism in Chapter 2. Overall, the key to primary headache generation seems to be *activation of the TCC*. It is helpful to consider possible interventions as being "upstream" or "downstream" of this process.

Downstream Targets

One conceptual approach to stopping a migraine attack would be to *reduce sensitization of the primary trigeminal afferents involved in the activation of the trigeminovascular system*. At present, drugs used to treat acute migraine attacks, and indeed most prophylactics, appear to work mainly on such "downstream" targets. Thus, simple analgesics, NSAIDs, triptans, β-blockers, pizotifen, calcium antagonists, methysergide, and so on, mainly affect peripheral nociceptors, serotonin receptors, blood vessels, and processes involved in neurogenic inflammation, although triptans also act centrally.

We noted in Chapter 2 (p. 62), that there are several lines of evidence that suggest that inhibition of neurogenic vasodilatation and plasma protein extravasation (consequences of activation of the trigeminovascular system) alone is unlikely to be fully effective in the treatment of migraine headache. However, drugs that inhibit neurogenic inflammation are certainly reasonably effective for many people, and might be all that is required. In Chapter 2 we also noted that the powerful vasodilator calcitonin gene–related peptide (CGRP) was released during neurogenic vasodilatation and that CGRP infusions can cause a migraine-like headache. CGRP receptor antagonists would be likely to show antimigraine actions, in both acute attacks and prophylaxis, and trials of such drugs are planned (70).

Further engineering of the triptans is also a possibility. The effective molecules to date are mainly 5-HT_{1b} and 5-HT_{1d} receptor agonists, but they have some unwanted peripheral vascular effects. Trials are taking place in France, of oral donitriptan mesilate. This drug may exert greater intrinsic activity at $5\text{-HT}_{1b/1d}$ receptors than naratriptan, rizatriptan, and zolmatriptan. A marketing application is expected in 2007. Without-water quick-dissolving tablets of naratriptan and of sumatriptan are in development and a needle-free injection of sumatriptan is in the pipeline. There is also expectation that 5-HT_{1F} receptor agonists would be effective in migraine without having systemic vascular complications.

Triptans have been shown to hyperpolarize trigeminal ganglion cells by increasing the Ca^{2+}-activated K^+ current, and they also block nitric oxide synthesis. As we discussed in Chapter 2, nitric oxide may well play a pivotal role in the migraine mechanism, and specific nitric oxide–synthase inhibitors could prove to be powerful antimigraine drugs. GR79236, an adenosine A1–receptor antagonist, inhibited CGRP release in animals and aborted headache in man, and trials of such agents are already planned (70,71).

Upstream Targets

The ideal "universal primary headache treatment" would be one that markedly reduced the nociceptive output of the TCC without adverse effects.

Inhibition of trigeminal nociceptive transmission to second-order neurons, the associated process leading to sensitization and allodynia, is an attractive therapeutic possibility. Glutamate is a major excitatory neurotransmitter, playing a key role in nociception. Ionotropic receptor channel blockers such as MK-801 acting on the N-methyl-D-asparate (NMDA) receptor, and GYKI-52466 acting at the 2-amino-3-(3-hydroxy-5-methylisoxazol-4-yl) propanoic acid (AMPA) receptor, have been shown to inhibit trigeminovascular nociception in the TCC, and it is likely that glutamate receptor antagonists would have antimigraine actions A mixed AMPA/kainite receptor antagonist, LY-293558, was shown to be effective and well tolerated in acute migraine (70,71).

More information on the different calcium channel types for neurotransmitter release at central trigeminal synapses might also lead to effective and selective migraine treatments. Ziconotide was shown to block, specifically, the $Ca_v2.2$ neuronal channel (see p. 80). This drug proved too toxic for use in man but drugs with such action might be of interest. Another strategy to reduce central sensitization would be the desensitization of vanilloid VR1 receptors by the continuous application of VR1 agonists (70).

Treatment of Aura

As we noted above, the precise relationship between cortical spreading depression (CSD) and the other parts of the migraine mechanism is not clear and may vary with circumstance. However, it is entirely possible that inhibition of CSD might abort migraine attacks. Unfortunately, thus far we have made little progress in this direction. This is a problem because for a significant minority of patients aura is the most troublesome or indeed the only manifestation of the migraine mechanism.

The influence of drugs on the initiation and propagation of CSD has been studied in the chick retina model but no clear picture has emerged. Some effective prophylactic drugs such as topiramate can inhibit CSD in this model (72) but β-blockers do not. Tonabersat, a benzopyrene with anticonvulsant properties, blocked K^+-induced CSD in the feline brain, and NMDA receptors also seem to be involved in CSD (70). This may explain the observation that ketamine relieved aura in patients with familial hemiplegic migraine (73).

In practical terms, it was recently shown in a controlled clinical trial that lamotrigine to a dose of 300 mg daily reduced the frequency and duration of aura, and that 75% of the patients who responded also enjoyed a reduction in the frequency of their migraine attacks (15).

CLOSURE OF PATENT FORAMEN OVALE

In Chapter 4, we touched on the issue of migraine and its apparent association with structural cardiac abnormalities, particularly patent foramen ovale (PFO). We noted that the prevalence of PFO was significantly greater in patients with active migraine (especially migraine with aura) compared to nonmigraineurs and that closure of PFOs seemed to reduce the frequency of migraine attacks. A number of groups have since reported their experience with this procedure. As shown in Table 4, the trend was universally supportive of the original claim: closure of PFO appears to dramatically reduce the frequency of migraine attacks in both MA and MO (74–79). The reported adverse event rates for the procedure were very low.

These studies were uncontrolled and mostly retrospective, involved only relatively small numbers of patients, and had rather short periods of follow-up. Mindful of the very high placebo response rate in migraine, as discussed earlier, a formal placebo-controlled trial was urgently needed.

The Migraine Intervention with STARFlex® Septal Technology (MIST I) Trial

The MIST I trial was an international, prospective, randomized, double blind, placebo-controlled (sham operation) study, involving 432 patients with

Table 4 Resolution or Reduction in Migraine Attack Rates Following Closure of PFO

Authors (Ref.)	No. of patients with migraine	Follow-up	Migraine resolution n (%)	Migraine resolution or improvement n (%)
Wilmshurst et al. (76)	16 MA	"Long term"	7 MA (43.8%)	15 MA (93.8%)
	5 MO		3 MO (60.0%)	3 MO (60.0%)
Sztajzel et al. (77)	15 MA	13 mo	7 (46.7%)	No data provided
Morandi et al. (78)	17 MA	6 mo	5 MA (29.4%)	15 (88.2%)
Post et al. (79)	12 MA	≥6 mo	9 MA (75%)	No data provided
	14 MO		8 MO (57.1%)	
Reisman et al. (80)	38 MA	9 mo	21 MA (54%)	26 MA (68%)
	12 MO		7 MO (62%)	8 MO (67%)
	50 MA/MO		28 MA/MO (56%)	35 MA/MO (70%)
Arzabal et al. (81)	37 MA/MO	3 mo	MA (75%)	No data provided
			MO (31%)	No data provided
			MA/MO (60%)	MA/MO (76%)

Abbreviations: MA, migraine with aura; MO, migraine without aura.

MA only, having at least five attacks per month, refractory to at least two different accepted prophylactic drugs. Eligible patients underwent a transthoracic echocardiograph (TTE) with bubble study (see p. 142) to detect right-to-left shunts [including PFOs, atrial septal defects (ASDs), and pulmonary shunts] and to provide semiquantitative assessment of shunt size, because a meta-analysis had shown a significant association between shunt size and prevalence of migraine with aura (80). Patients with "large" PFO shunts (defined by the bubble number on the freeze frame of the ultrasound) were randomized to either shunt closure using a patented "umbrella-like" device placed by a simple transvenous procedure under local anesthetic ("transcatheter closure"), or to sham operation. The frequency of migraine attacks in the two groups was then monitored for a three-month period, following an initial three-month postprocedure "healing period."

The study found that:

- almost 60% of the eligible patients had shunts, 40% having large PFOs,
- another 17% had smaller shunts,
- 5% had large pulmonary shunts,
- 1% had ASDs.

These results were similar to those of an earlier study that found that almost half the migraine patients examined had a PFO, some 40% being moderate to large, significantly more than nonmigraineur normal controls (about 10%) (81).

In the MIST I study, 147 patients were found to have a "large" PFO. Seventy-four were randomized to PFO closure and 73 underwent sham operation. On review at six months, the primary end point of a 40% elimination of migraine attacks had not been achieved, but 42% of the PFO closure patients reported a 50% reduction in headache days, compared to only 23% of the sham-operated patients; and the "migraine burden" (number of headaches multiplied by headache duration in hours) had been reduced by 37% in the PFO closure patients compared to 17% in the placebo group. The observed benefit of PFO closure in this randomized controlled trial was thus more modest than reported in the uncontrolled studies (as might be expected), but it clearly showed that selected patients, having migraine with aura refractory to prophylactic medication and with a substantial right-to-left shunt on bubble TTE may well benefit from this low-risk intervention. At the time of publication of this book, it is unclear whether this procedure will have more general application and the exact mechanism of the beneficial effect remains to be defined.

CONCLUSIONS

In this book, we have proposed that the migraine mechanism is the basis for all primary headache. We would argue that the prime target for treatment is that unifying mechanism—the upstream target. The closer our treatment is to that target, the more effective the treatment should be. Downstream treatments may help symptoms, often very effectively, but probably only if given early in the attack when pain mechanism activation and neural windup is minimal. As the attack develops, and the migraine mechanism becomes fully engaged, simple downstream treatments tend to be progressively less effective and problems such as headache rebound are likely to develop. The problem of medication-misuse headache is already immense and might develop further when triptans go "OTC." We need a better understanding of this and many other areas in headache.

In the last few years, there have been enormous strides in headache research and drug development. The interest among physicians has grown proportionately. Nevertheless, there is still plenty of room in headache for opinions, ideas, and controversies. We hope this book adds to the discussion.

REFERENCES

1. Von Klein CH. The medical features of the Papyrus Ebers. J Am Med Assoc 1905; 45:1928–1935.
2. Critchley M. Migraine from Cappadocia to Queen Square. Background to Migraine. Vol. 1. London: Heinemann, 1967:28–38.
3. Edmeads J. The treatment of headache: a historical perspective. In: Gallagher RM, ed. Drug Therapy for Headache. New York: Marcel Dekker Inc., 1991:1–8.
4. Diener HC, Pfaffenrath V, Schnitker J, et al. Efficacy and safety of 62.5 mg t.i.d. feverfew CO_2-extract (MIG-99) in migraine prevention—a randomised, double-blind, multicentre, placebo-controlled study. Cephalalgia 2005; 25:1031–1041.
5. Gowers WR. A Manual of Diseases of the Nervous System, Vol. 2. Churchill: London, 1888:793.
6. Flatau E. Die Migräne. Berlin: Springer, 1912.
7. Horton BT, Peters GA, Blumenthal LS. A new product in the treatment of migraine: a preliminary report. Mayo Clin Proc 1945; 20:241–248.
8. Sicuteri F. Prophylactic and therapeutic properties of 1-methyllysergic acid butanolamide in migraine. Int Arch Allerg 1959; 15:300–307.
9. Hargreaves R, Beer M. 5-HT receptors in brain and vasculature. In: Humphrey P, Ferrari M, Olesen J, eds. The Triptans: Novel Drugs for Migraine. Frontiers in Headache Research. Vol. 10. Oxford University Press, 2001:11–22.
10. Terrón JA. Is the 5-HT$_7$ receptor involved in the pathogenesis and prophylactic treatment of migraine? Eur J Pharmacol 2002; 439:1–11.
11. Humphrey P. The discovery of sumatriptan and a new class of drug for the acute treatment of migraine. In: Humphrey P, Ferrari M, Olesen J, eds. The Triptans: Novel Drugs for Migraine. Frontiers in Headache Research. Vol. 10. Oxford University Press, 2001:3–10.
12. Peatfield RC, Fozard JR, Clifford Rose F. Drug treatment of migraine. In: Clifford Rose F, ed. Handbook of Clinical Neurology. Headache. Vol. 4. Amsterdam: Elsevier, 1986:173–216.

13. Brandes JL, Saper JR, Diamond M, et al. Topiramate for migraine prevention. A randomized controlled trial. JAMA 2004; 291:965–973.

14. Silberstein SD, Neto W, Schmitt J, et al. Topiramate in migraine prevention. Results of a large controlled trial. Arch Neurol 2004; 61:490–495.

15. Lampl C, Katsavara Z, Diener H-C, Limmroth V. Lamotrigine reduces migraine aura and migraine attacks in patients with migraine with aura. J Neurol Neurosurg Psychiatr 2005; 76:1730–1732.

16. Reidenberg M, Lowenthal D. Adverse non-drug reactions. N Engl J Med 1968; 279:678–679.

17. Rasmussen BK, Jensen R, Schroll M, et al. Epidemiology of headache in a general population—prevalence study. J Clin Epidemiol 1991; 44:1147–1157.

18. Evans RE, Lipton RB, Silberstein S. The prevalence of migraine in neurologists. Neurology 2003; 61:1271–1272.

19. Sacks O, Evans RW, Lipton RB, et al. The prevalence of migraine in neurologists. Neurology 2004; 62(2):342.

20. Lipton RB, Goadsby PJ, Sawyer JPC, et al. Migraine: diagnosis and assessment of disability. Rev Contemp Pharmacother 2000; 11:63–73.

21. Steiner TJ, Scher AI, Stewart WF, et al. The prevalence and disability of adult migraine in England and their relationships to age, gender and ethnicity. Cephalalgia 2003; 23(7):519–527.

22. Zwart JA, Dyb G, Hagen K, et al. Analgesic use: a predictor of chronic pain and medication overuse headache: the Head-HUNT Study. Neurology 2003; 61(2):160–164.

23. Hopkins A, Ziegler DK. Headache—the size of the problem. In: Hopkins A, ed. Headache: Problems in Diagnosis and Management. W.B. Saunders Company, 1988:3–7.

24. Wells NE, Steiner TJ. Effectiveness of eletriptan in reducing time lost caused by migraine attacks. Pharmacoeconomics 2001; 18:557–566.

25. Packard RC. What does the headache patient want? Headache 1979; 19:370–374.

26. Davies PTG, Glynn CJ, Kadry MA. Expectations of patients attending a combined headache clinic. J Headache Pain 2003; 4:79–82.

27. Lipton RB, Stewart WF. Acute migraine therapy: do doctors understand what patients with migraine want from therapy? Headache 1999; 39:S20–S26.

28. Linn FHH, Wijdicks EFM, van der Graaf Y, et al. Prospective study of sentinel headache in aneurismal subarachnoid haemorrhage. Lancet 1994; 344:590–593.

29. Hughes PJ, Davies PTG. Exertional Headaches. Clin Sports Med 1990; 2: 37–40.

30. Mokri B. Low-cerebrospinal fluid volume headaches. In: Goadsby PJ, Silberstein SD, Dodick DW, eds. Chronic Daily Headache for Clinicians. London: BC Decker, 2005:155–166.

31. Shinohara Y, Takahashi W, Takagi S, et al. Present status of brain check-up system for apparently healthy people in Japan. J Neurol Sci 2001; 187(suppl 1):S208.

32. Pickering T. Headache and hypertension—something old, something new. J Clin Hypertens 2000; 2:345–347.

33. Reveiz-Herault L, Cardona AF, Ospina EG, et al. Effectiveness of flunarizine in the prophylaxis of migraine: a meta-analytical review of the literature. Rev Neurol 2003; 36(10):907–912.

34. Evers S, Mylecharane EJ. Non-steroidal anti-inflammatory and miscellaneous drugs in migraine prophylaxis. In: Olesen J, Goadsby PJ, Ramadan NM, et al., eds. The Headaches. 3rd ed. Philadelphia: Lippincott Williams and Wilkins, 553–566.

35. Tfelt-Hansen P, Henry P, Mulder LJ, et al. The effectiveness of combined oral lysine acetylsalicylate and metoclopramide compared with oral sumatriptan for migraine. Lancet 1995; 346:923–926.

36. Geraud G, Compagnon A, Rossi A, COZAM study group. Zolmatriptan versus a combination of acetylsalicylic acid and metoclopramide in the acute oral treatment of migraine: a double blind, randomised, three-attack study. Eur Neurol 2002; 47:88–98.

37. Dowson A, Ball K, Haworth D. Comparison of a fixed combination of domperidone and paracetamol (Domperamol) with sumatriptan 50 mg in moderate to severe migraine: a randomised UK primary case study. Curr Med Res Opin 2000; 16:190–197.

38. Ellis GL, Delaney J, DeHart DA, et al. The efficacy of metoclopramide in the treatment of migraine headache. Ann Emerg Med 1993; 22:191–195.

39. Waelkens J. Dopamine blockade with domperidone: bridge between prophylactic and abortive treatment of migraine? A dose-finding study. Cephalalgia 1984; 4:85–90.

40. Dahlof CG, Hargreaves RJ. Pathophysiology and pharmacology of migraine. Is there a place for antiemetics in future treatment strategies? Cephalalgia 1998; 18:593–604.

41. Heinrichs L. Linking olfaction with nausea and vomiting in pregnancy, recurrent abortion, hyperemeisis gravidarum, and migraine headache. Am J Obstet Gynaecol 2002; 186(5 suppl):S215–S219.

42. De Lignieres B, Vincens M, Mauvais-Jarvis P, et al. Prevention of menstrual migraine by percutaneous oestradiol. BMJ 1986; 293:1540–1543.

43. Sances G, Granella F, Nappi RE, et al. Course of migraine during pregnancy and the postpartum: a prospective study. Cephalalgia 2003; 23(3):197–205.

44. Loder E. Safety of sumatriptan in pregnancy: a review of the data so far. CNS Drugs 2003; 17:1–7.

45. Hopkinson HE. Treatment of cardiovascular diseases. In: Rubin P, ed. Prescribing in Pregnancy. London: BMJ Publishing Group, 1995:98.

46. Editorial. The placebo effect. Clin Med 2003; 3:397–398.

47. Editorial. Using placebo in headache management. Cephalalgia 2005; 25:321–322.

48. Ernst EP. The Desktop Guide to Complementary and Alternative Medicine. An Evidence-Based Approach. Amsterdam: Elsevier, 2001.

49. Whitmarsh TE, Coleston-Shields DM, Steiner TJ. Double-blind randomised placebo-controlled study of homeopathic prophylaxis of migraine. Cephalalgia 1997; 17:600–604.

50. Alecrim-Andrade J, Maciel-Junior JA, Cladellas XC, et al. Efficacy of acupuncture in migraine prophylaxis: results from a placebo-controlled pilot trial. Cephalalgia 2004; 24:775–814.

51. Goadsby PJ. Pathophysiology of cluster headache: a trigeminal autonomic cephalgia. Lancet Neurol 2002; 1:251–257.

52. Hardibo JE, Suzuki N. Anatomy and pathology of cluster headaches. In: Olesen J, Goadsby PJ, Ramadan NM, et al., eds. The Headaches. 3rd ed. Philadelphia: Lippincott Williams and Wilkins, 751–753.

53. Robbins L. Intranasal lidocaine for cluster headache. Headache 1995; 35:83–84.

54. Kudrow L. Response of cluster headache attacks to oxygen inhalation. Headache 1981; 21:1–4.

55. Goadsby PJ. Cluster headache and the clinical profile of sumatriptan. Eur Neurol 1994; 34(suppl):35–39.

56. Prusinski A, Kozubski W, Szulc-Kuberska J. Steroid treatment in the interruption of clusters in cluster headache patients. Cephalalgia 1987; 7(suppl 6):332–333.

57. Tfelt-Hansen P. Prophylactic pharmacotherapy of cluster headache. In: Olesen J, Goadsby PJ, eds. Cluster Headache and Related Conditions. Oxford: Oxford University Press, 1999:257–263.

58. Ekbom K, Sakai F. Management. In: Olesen J, Tfelt-Hansen P, Welch KMA, eds. The Headaches. New York: Ravens Press, 1993:591–599.

59. Matharu MS, Boes CJ, Goadsby PJ. Management of trigeminal autonomic cephalalgias and hemicrania continua. Drugs 2003; 63:1637–1677.

60. Cohen A, Matharu MS, Goadsby PJ. Suggested guidelines for treating SUNCT and SUNA. Cephalalgia 2005; 25:1200.

61. Evers S, Goadsby PJ. Hypnic headache. Clinical features, pathophysiology, and treatment. Neurology 2003; 60:905–910.

62. Diener H-C, Limmroth V. Medication-overuse headache: a world-wide problem. Lancet Neurol 2004; 3:475–483.

63. Green Al, Owen SLF, Davies P, Molr L, Aziz TZ. Deep brain stimulation for neuropathic cephalalgia. Cephalalgia 2005; 26:561–567.

64. Leone M, Franzini A, Broggi G, et al. Hypothalamic deep brain stimulation for intractable chronic cluster headache: a 3 year follow-up. Neurol Sci 2003; 24:143–145.

65. Bogduk N, Bartsch T. Headaches of cervical origin: focus on anatomy and physiology. In: Goadsby PJ, Silberstein SD, Dodick DW, eds. Chronic Daily Headache for Clinicians. London: BC Decker, 2005:129–143.

66. Matharu MS, Bartsch T, Ward N, et al. Central neuromodulation in chronic migraine patients with suboccipital stimulators: a PET study. Brain 2004; 127:220–230.

67. Bahra A, Goadsby PJ. Cough headache responsive to methysergide. Cephalalgia 1998; 18:495–496.

68. Dodick DW. Indomethacin-responsive headache syndromes. Curr Pain Headache Rep 2004; 8:19–26.

69. Diener HC. Almotriptan in migraine patients who respond poorly to oral sumatriptan: a double-blind, randomized trial. Headache 2005; 45(7):874–882.

70. Pietrobon D, Striessnig J. Neurobiology of migraine. Nat Rev Neurosci 2003; 4:386–439.

71. Goadsby PJ. New targets in the acute treatment of migraine. Curr Opin Neurol 2005; 18:283–288.

72. Akerman S, Goadsby PJ. Topiramate inhibits cortical spreading depression in rat and cat: impact in migraine aura. Neuroreport 2005; 16(12):1383–1387.

73. Kaube H, Herzog J, Kaufer T, Dichgans M, Diener HC. Aura in some patients with familial hemiplegic migraine can be stopped by intranasal ketamine. Neurology 2000; 55(1):139–141.

74. Wilmshurst P, Nightingale S. Relationship between migraine and cardiac and pulmonary right-to-left shunts. Clini Sci (Lond) 2001; 100:215–220.

75. Sztajzel R, Genoud D, Roth S, et al. Patent foramen ovale: a possible cause of symptomatic migraine. A study of 74 patients with acute ischaemic stroke. Cerebrovasc Dis 2002; 13:102–106.

76. Morandi E, Anzola GP, Angeli S, et al. Transcatheter closure of patent foramen ovale: a new migraine treatment? J Interv Cardiol 2003; 16:39–42.

77. Post MC, Thijs V, Herroelen L, et al. Closure of patent foramen ovale is associated with a decrease in prevalence of migraine. Neurology 2004; 62: 1439–1440.

78. Reisman M, Christofferson TD, Jesurum J, et al. Migraine headache relief after transcatheter closure of patent foramen ovale. J Am Coll Cardiol 2005; 45: 493–495.

79. Arzabal B, Tobis J, Suh W, et al. Association of interatrial shunts and migraine headaches: impact of transcatheter closure. J Am Coll Cardiol 2005; 45: 489–492.

80. Wilmshurst P, Pearson M, Nightingale S. Re-evaluation of the relationship between migraine and persistent foramen ovale and other right-to-left shunts. Clin Sci (Lond) 2005; 108:365–367.

81. Schwerzmann M, Nedeltchev K, Lagger F, et al. Prevalence and size of directly detected patent foramen ovale in migraine with aura. Neurology 2005; 65: 1415–1418.

Appendix 1

**INTERNATIONAL HEADACHE SOCIETY (IHS)
CLASSIFICATION (IHC-2)**

1. Migraine
   1.1 Migraine without aura
   1.2 Migraine with aura
      1.2.1 Typical aura with migraine headache
      1.2.2 Typical aura with nonmigraine headache
      1.2.3 Typical aura without headache
      1.2.4 Familial hemiplegic migraine
      1.2.5 Sporadic hemiplegic migraine
      1.2.6 Basilar-type migraine
   1.3 Childhood periodic syndromes that are commonly precursors of migraine
      1.3.1 Cyclical vomiting
      1.3.2 Abdominal migraine
      1.3.3 Benign paroxysmal vertigo of childhood
   1.4 Retinal migraine
   1.5 Complications of migraine
      1.5.1 Chronic migraine
      1.5.2 Status migrainosus
      1.5.3 Persistent aura without infarction
      1.5.4 Migrainous infarction
      1.5.5 Migraine-triggered seizures
   1.6 Probable migraine
      1.6.1 Probable migraine without aura
      1.6.2 Probable migraine with aura
2. Tension-type headache and new daily persistent headache
   2.1 Infrequent episodic tension-type headache
      2.1.1 Associated with pericranial tenderness
      2.1.2 Not associated with pericranial tenderness

(*Continued*)

(Continued)

6.1 Ischemic stroke and transient ischemic attacks
    6.1.1 Ischemic stroke (cerebral infarction)
    6.1.2 Transient ischemic attacks (TIAs)
6.2 Nontraumatic intracranial hemorrhage
    6.2.1 Intracerebral hemorrhage
    6.2.2 Subarachnoid hemorrhage (SAH)
6.3 Unruptured vascular malformations
    6.3.1 Saccular aneurysm
    6.3.2 Arteriovenous malformation
    6.3.3 Dural arteriovenous fistula
    6.3.4 Cavernous angiomas
    6.3.5 Encephalotrigeminal or leptomeningeal angiomatosis (Sturge Weber Syndrome)
6.4 Arteritis
    6.4.1 Giant cell arteritis (GCA)
    6.4.2 Primary central nervous system (CNS) angiitis (isolated CNS angiitis, granulomatous CNS angiitis)
    6.4.3 Secondary central nervous system angitis
6.5 Carotid or vertebral artery pain
    6.5.1 Arterial dissection
    6.5.2 Postendarterectomy headache
    6.5.3 Carotid angioplasty headache
    6.5.4 Headache associated with intracranial endovascular procedures
    6.5.5 Angiography headache
6.6 Cerebral venous thrombosis (CVT)
6.7 Other intracranial vascular disorders
    6.7.1 CADASIL (Cerebral Autosomal-Dominant Arteriopathy with Subcortical Infarcts and Leukoencephalopathy)
    6.7.2 MELAS (Mitochondrial Encephalopathy, Lactic Acidosis and Stroke-like episodes)
    6.7.3 Benign angiopathy of the central nervous system
    6.7.4 Pituitary apoplexy
7. Headache attributed to nonvascular intracranial disorder
  7.1 High cerebrospinal fluid pressure
    7.1.1 Idiopathic intracranial hypertension
    7.1.2 ICH secondary to metabolic, toxic, or hormonal causes
    7.1.3 ICH secondary to hydrocephalus
  7.2 Low cerebrospinal fluid pressure
    7.2.1 Postdural puncture headache
    7.2.2 CSF fistula headache
    7.2.3 Spontaneous (or idiopathic) low CSF pressure
  7.3 Noninfectious inflammatory diseases
    7.3.1 Neurosarcoidosis
    7.3.2 Aseptic (noninfectious) meningitis
    7.3.3 Other noninfectious inflammatory disease
    7.3.4 Lymphocytic hypophysitis

(*Continued*)

(Continued)

9. Headache attributed to infection
    9.1 Intracranial infection
        9.1.1 Bacterial meningitis
        9.1.2 Lymphocytic meningitis
        9.1.3 Encephalitis
        9.1.4 Brain abscess
        9.1.5 Subdural empyema
        9.1.6 AIDS
    9.2 Extracranial infection
        9.2.1 Bacterial infection
        9.2.2 Viral infection
        9.2.3 Other infection
    9.3 HIV/AIDS
    9.4 Chronic postinfectious headache
10. Headache attributed to disorder of homeostasis
    10.1 Headache attributed to hypoxia and/or hypercapnia
        10.1.1 High-altitude headache
        10.1.2 Diving headache
        10.1.3 Sleep Apnea
    10.2 Dialysis
    10.3 Arterial Hypertension
        10.3.1 Headache attributed to pheochromocytoma
        10.3.2 Headache attributed to hypertensive crisis without hypertensive encephalopathy
        10.3.3 Headache attributed to hypertensive encephalopathy
        10.3.4 Headache attributed to pre-eclampsia
        10.3.5 Headache attributed to eclampsia
        10.3.6 Headache attributed to acute pressor response to exogenous agents
    10.4 Headache attributed hypothyroidism
    10.5 Headache attributed to fasting
    10.6 Cardiac cephalgia
    10.7 Headache attributed to other disturbance of homeostasis
11. Headache or facial pain attributed to disorder of cranium, neck, eyes, ears, nose, sinuses, teeth, mouth, or other facial or cranial structures
    11.1 Cranial bone
    11.2 Neck
        11.2.1 Cervicogenic headache
        11.2.2 Retropharyngeal tendinitis
        11.2.3 Craniocervical dystonia
    11.3 Eyes
        11.3.1 Acute glaucoma
        11.3.2 Refractive errors
        11.3.3 Heterophoria or heterotropia (latent or manifest squint)
        11.3.4 Ocular inflammatory disorders

(Continued)

11.4 Ears
    11.4.1 Primary otalgia
    11.4.2 Referred otalgia
11.5 Rhinosinusitis
11.6 Teeth, jaws and related structures
11.7 Temporomandibular joint disease
11.8 Headache attributed to other disorder of cranium, neck, eyes, ears, nose, sinuses,teeth, mouth, or other cranial facial or cervical structures
12. Headache attributed to psychiatric disorder
    12.1 Headache Attributed to Somatization Disorder
    12.2 Headache Attributed to a Psychotic Disorder
13. Cranial neuralgias and central causes of facial pain
    13.1 Trigeminal neuralgia
        13.1.1 Classical trigeminal neuralgia
        13.1.2 Symptomatic trigeminal neuralgia
    13.2 Glossopharyngeal neuralgia
        13.2.1 Classical glossopharyngeal neuralgia
        13.2.2 Symptomatic glossopharyngeal neuralgia
    13.3 Nervous intermedius neuralgia
    13.4 Superior laryngeal neuralgia
    13.5 Nasociliary neuralgia (Charlin)
    13.6 Supraorbital neuralgia
    13.7 Other terminal branch neuralgias
    13.8 Occipital neuralgia
    13.9 Neck–tongue syndrome
    13.10 External compression headache
    13.11 Cold stimulus headache
        13.11.1 External application of a cold stimulus
        13.11.2 Ingestion of a cold stimulus
    13.12 Constant pain caused by compression, irritation, or distortion of cranial nerves or upper cervical roots by structural lesions
    13.13 Optic neuritis
    13.14 Ocular diabetic neuropathy
    13.15 Herpes zoster
        13.15.1 Acute herpes zoster
        13.15.2 Postherpetic neuralgia
    13.16 Tolosa–Hunt syndrome
    13.17 Ophthalmoplegic migraine
    13.18 Central causes of facial pain
        13.18.1 Anaesthesia dolorosa
        13.18.2 Central poststroke pain
        13.18.3 Multiple sclerosis
        13.18.4 Persistent idiopathic facial pain
        13.18.5 Burning mouth syndrome
        13.18.6 Other cranial neuralgia or other centrally mediated facial pain
14. Other headache, cranial neuralgia, central or primary facial pain
    14.1 Headache not elsewhere classified
    14.2 Headache unspecified

Appendix 2

International Headache Society, IHS, www.i-h-s.org
The World Federation of Neurology, WFN, www.wfneurolgy.org
The World Health Organisation, WHO, www.who.int
The World Headache Alliance, WHA, www.w-h-a.org
The European Headache Federation, EHF, www.ehf-org.org
The American Headache Society, www.ahsnet.org
The British Association for the Study of Headache, BASH, www.bash.org
Migraine in Primary Care Advisors, MIPCA, www.mipca.org
The Migraine Trust, www.migrainetrust.org
Migraine Action Association, MAA, www.migraine.org.uk
The Organisation for the Understanding of Cluster Headache, OUCH,
  www.ouchuk.org
Headache UK, HUK, www.headacheuk.org
MIDAS, www.midas-migraine.net
HIT6, www.headachetest.com

Index

333